VITAL CONNECTIONS
IN LONG-TERM CARE

VITAL CONNECTIONS IN LONG-TERM CARE

Spiritual Resources for Staff and Residents

by

Julie Barton, M.A.
Marita Grudzen, M.H.S.

and

Ron Zielske, M.Div.

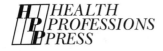
HEALTH
PROFESSIONS
PRESS

Baltimore • London • Winnipeg • Sydney

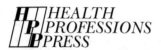

Health Professions Press, Inc.
Post Office Box 10624
Baltimore, Maryland 21285-0624

www.healthpropress.com

Typeset by Auburn Associates, Inc., Baltimore, Maryland.
Manufactured in the United States of America by
Versa Press, Inc., East Peoria, Illinois.

Most cases described in this book are composites based on the authors' actual experiences. In these instances, individuals' names have been changed and identifying details have been altered to protect confidentiality. Real names and stories are used by permission.

The excerpt in Chapter 6 on page 84 is from **I Can't Remember: Family Stories of Alzheimer's Disease**, by Esther Strauss Smoller. Reprinted by permission of Temple University Press. © 1997 by Temple University. All Rights Reserved.

Library of Congress Cataloging-in-Publication Data

Barton, Julie.
    Vital connections in long-term care : spiritual resources for staff and residents / by Julie Barton, Marita Grudzen, and Ron Zielske.
       p.   cm.
    Includes bibliographical references and index.
    ISBN 1-878812-79-3
    1. Church work with the sick.   2. Sick—Religious life.   3. Long-term care of the sick.   I. Grudzen, Marita.   II. Zielske, Ron.   III. Title.
    [DNLM: 1. Religion and Medicine.]
    BV4335.B32   2003
    261.8'321—dc21

                                    2003041749

British Library Cataloguing in Publication data are available from the British Library.

Contents

About the Authors

Julie Barton, M.A., ELC Associates, Post Office Box 2699, Cupertino, California 95015 E-mail: jgelc@earthlink.net

Julie is a consultant in the field of gerontology and is an adjunct faculty member in the Religious Studies Department at Santa Clara University, California.

Julie has been active in the field of gerontology for more than 25 years. At Santa Clara University, she developed a Religious Studies course titled "The Spiritual Journey of Aging." She has also taught "Aging and Mental Health" at San José State University and "The Psychology of Multigenerational Families" at Santa Clara University.

As a result of her work with the growing number of grandparents who are raising their grandchildren and her increasing concern about elder abuse in any setting, Julie designed classes for the California State Board of Corrections on juveniles living in grandparent-headed households and on elder abuse.

Julie has been an adult education teacher in retirement and long-term care facilities, specializing in drama and poetry therapy. As supervising case manager and program director for two aging services at Catholic Charities in San José, California, she designed and implemented a volunteer respite care program for family caregivers and went on to offer elder care planning services to a number of corporations.

Julie is also a board member of the Center for Gerontology, Spirituality and Faith, which sponsors numerous seminars on spirituality and aging, and she has frequently been a presenter at the annual meetings of the American Society on Aging.

Marita Grudzen, M.H.S., Stanford Geriatric Education Center, 1215 Welsh Road, Stanford, California 94305 E-mail: mgrudzen@leland.stanford.edu

Marita is the Associate Director of the Stanford Geriatric Education Center and Lecturer and Research Training Program Officer in the Division of Family and Community Medicine, Stanford University School of Medicine, California.

A founding member of Stanford Geriatric Education Center, Marita now plans and implements multidisciplinary trainings in ethnogeriatrics and is a frequent presenter for national and regional professional organizations and conferences.

Marita is co-author of a chapter in *Aging and the Meaning of Time: A Multidisciplinary Exploration* by Susan H. McFadden and Robert C. Atchley (Springer, 2001) and is a frequent contributor to publications in the field of gerontology.

Marita has co-chaired several regional conferences at Stanford University including "Cultural Diversity and End-of-Life Issues" and "Spirituality and Aging." She is chair of the Advisory Council for the Center for Gerontology, Spirituality and Faith and is an adjunct faculty member at Pacific Lutheran Theological Seminary.

As Lecturer and Academic and Research Training Program Officer for the Center for Education in Family and Community Medicine, Stanford University School of Medicine, Marita develops curricula and coordinates pre-clinical courses and clerkships in family practice for Stanford medical students. She and her collaborator, Bruce Feldstein, M.D., were awarded the Templeton Award in 2001 for the medical school curriculum they developed titled "Spirituality and Meaning in Medicine."

Marita's work and writing are also influenced by her former roles as a Maryknoll Sister (1959–1967), the co-president of national leadership in the Federation of Christian Ministries (1974–1978), and a respiratory therapist and manager in acute and long-term care settings (1974–1979).

Ron Zielske, M.Div., Sunny View Manor/Sunny View West, 22445 Cupertino Road, Cupertino, California 95014 E-mail: ron@sunny4care.com

Ron is the President and Chief Executive Officer of Sunny View Lutheran Home and an adjunct faculty member at Pacific Lutheran Theological Seminary, Berkeley, California.

Ron has been in leadership positions at Sunny View Lutheran Home for more than 25 years. Prior to being at Sunny View Lutheran Home, he served as a parish pastor for 10 years.

Ron is a licensed nursing facility administrator and a licensed administrator for residential care facilities for older adults in California. He is also a founding member of the Center for Gerontology, Spirituality and Faith and has served on several other boards relating to aging and spirituality issues.

Ron is currently a member of the advisory board for the Center for Aging, Religion and Spirituality. He has presented workshops for various organizations including the American Society on Aging and the California Association of Homes and Services for the Aging.

Foreword

The stated purpose of this book is "to assist the staff in understanding the spiritual nature of all human beings, especially in caring for older adults, and to assist the staff in exploring the spiritual dimensions of their work" (see page xi). Rarely do authors carry out their stated purpose as well as Julie Barton and co-authors Marita Grudzen and Ron Zielske. The 14 chapters of this workbook cover a full gamut of topics relevant to wholistic care of residents in a long-term care setting.

This is indeed a timely book, considering the regulations of such agencies as the Joint Commission of Accreditation of Healthcare Organizations (JCAHO) that require long-term care settings to provide a continuum of care that flows from the belief that attention to the human spirit, including mind, heart, and soul, contributes to the goals of health. There is a growing recognition that one's spirituality and values are part of being a healthy human. In the 1980s, only a handful of the nations' 126 medical schools taught anything about the spiritual dimension of health. It is significant that at the start of the 21st century more than 50 medical schools currently offer courses in spirituality and health.

In other words, the biomedical paradigm, which has long been the lens through which aging and growing old have been viewed, is being challenged. The biomedical model has resulted in the "medicalization" of aging. A new model has emerged that enlarges and enriches the understanding of the aging process. This wholistic (holistic) model is a dynamic blend of the spiritual, physical, mental, emotional, and social dimensions of human personhood. The spiritual dimension is increasingly being recognized as the most important dimension in health care today. It is gaining recognition as a critical component of "successful aging."

The new paradigm includes images and understandings, symbols and rituals, and ministry and caring that emphasize the transcendent meaning of life conveyed by an Ultimate Being. We are challenged to respect the image of God in people through what is sacred in sickness and suffering, and, yes, even what is sacred in aging and dying. The human body is God's most perfect icon, created in His image.

In the midst of writing this foreword, I received a telephone call from a long-term care setting on whose board I serve. I was informed that a special meeting was scheduled to discuss the drastic cuts that would have to be made because of the governor's proposed reduced budget for older adult services. Among the many programs and departments affected by these reductions is the Pastoral Care Department, which must reduce the hours of the part-time chaplain and alter the projected plans to enlarge pastoral care services.

These days of tight budgets make this volume all the more relevant and valuable. This volume is *truly a workbook* to be used in developing and assisting long-term care staff in exploring the varied and often overlooked spiritual dimensions of their respective roles. It is brimming with insights and suggestions for programs of wholistic pastoral care to assist staff in understanding the multifaceted potential of their jobs and roles to incorporate spirituality into daily tasks of service delivery.

This volume clearly recognizes that spiritual care in long-term care settings cannot be limited to chaplains or visiting clergy. It is a primary responsibility for every health care provider. It should not be viewed as separate from the other health care needs of residents. In keeping with the JCAHO's espoused mandate for wholistic care, this volume offers a very complete overview and outline for introducing and training staff to understand and implement wholistic spiritual care in their daily roles and functions.

During these early years of this new century, the recognition that spirituality is a very important ingredient to the total well-being of older adults will continue to be developed by scholars, researchers, and practitioners. This workbook will be an important exhibit of how spiritual well-being can be wholistically introduced into a long-term care setting and become a shared responsibility of each person working in such a setting. It is innovative and insightful in setting forth ways to enhance spiritual well-being through various service roles. I know of no other volume that comprises such helpful and creative ways of introducing spiritual well-being into a long-term care setting.

Melvin A. Kimble, Ph.D.
Professor Emeritus of Pastoral Theology
Director, The Center for Aging, Religion and Spirituality
Luther Seminary, St. Paul, Minnesota

Introduction

This book is intended to assist staff in understanding the spiritual nature of all human beings, especially in caring for older adults, and to assist staff in exploring the spiritual dimensions of their work, thus enhancing the total well-being of nursing facility residents. Although a wholistic (holistic) approach to care has become popular since the late 1990s, the spiritual dimensions of life are not always included. The whole person is not only mind and body, but mind, body, and spirit. Some would argue that a person's spirituality is the very foundation of the physical, mental, and emotional components of the self.

Everyone is spiritual; however, not everyone has a religious belief. Spirituality can include a specific religious practice of a specific group or denomination (e.g., Presbyterian) in that group, but spirituality includes all that creates meaning in one's life.

Consider the following story: A speaker once began a seminar by holding up a $20 bill and asking who wanted it. Every hand in the audience went up. Next, he took the $20 bill and crumpled it in his hand and then asked who wanted it. Again, everyone's hand went up. Then, he took the $20 bill and threw it on the floor and stepped on it and asked who wanted it. Of course, everyone's hand went up. The $20 bill does not lose its value despite its condition. Likewise, human beings, though dropped, crumpled, and stepped on during the course of their lives, never lose value. Their worth is determined by who they are more than by what they have done. This intrinsic value and worth is a large part of how we define spirituality.

Kathleen R. Fischer, author of *Winter Grace: Spirituality and Aging* (1998), said that spirituality is how we live out the relationship we have with a higher being or what we claim to be meaningful in life. Rabbi Samuel Seicol (1996), Director of Religious Services at the Hebrew Rehabilitation Center for Aged in Boston, offered this definition: "Spirituality is the internal sense of wellness, the sense of commonality among all people. In religious terms, it is that aspect of a person that is created in God's image. Spirituality is the process of connecting to our sense of meaning, value, and purpose to create a sense of identity." The National Interfaith Coalition on Aging (1975) defined spiritual well-being as the "affirmation of life, . . . a relationship with God, self, community, and environment . . . that nurtures and celebrates wholeness."

The value of lifelong learning is included in the concept of spirituality and holds true for residents, staff, and families. Life is about growth, and all learning is mutual. We are sometimes the teachers, sometimes the students, and sometimes both at once! Good teachers often say, "I learn more from my students than I could ever teach them." This mission can be extended to our care facilities: We learn from each other, simply through the art of listening, by learning to express an emotion through poetry or painting, or by coming to know the history of a person or place. All of this is a vital part of spiritual growth and well-being, a "vital connection" because it honors both teacher and student. This concept is central to the chapters in this book.

Sometimes, we have difficulty realizing that residents in a long-term care facility can and should go on learning. Perhaps this true story will illustrate our point: In a California facility, a female resident who was considered particularly difficult was invited to participate in a poetry writing class in which each resident contributed a line or two to an original group poem. Not only did this woman, who was severely impaired, rise to the challenge, but she shared what she had written on a videotape that the teacher made. When the aide who was assigned to this resident happened to walk through the room in which the tape was playing, she stopped in her tracks and her mouth literally fell open. She had previously not been able to see past the resident's difficult behavior to see her possibilities. Now, she, too, was able to participate in a learning process: She learned to look at a fellow human being in a completely new way, and the resident learned to express herself in a beautiful and constructive manner. The staff and residents no longer thought of the resident as "the difficult patient in Bed A!" In addition, the teacher learned never to write off anyone as unsuited to a particular learning experience.

Our hope is that long-term care facilities will avail themselves of community teachers, volunteers, and professionals. Adult education and community college programs are usually offered at no cost to many long-term care facilities. Art docents and music teachers may also be willing to share their expertise, and high school or college interns may be of great intergenerational value. In addition, many residents may have experiences that they are willing to share with others. The idea of lifelong learning invites us to participate in the creation of something beautiful and useful, which is truly a spiritual necessity for us all.

This book presents an opportunity to explore and address spiritual well-being in relationship to the physical, mental, and emotional needs of individuals receiving long-term care services; their families; and the staff. The spiritual well-being of all three is the goal of this book. The spirituality and ethical and multicultural issues of older adults with Alzheimer's disease and dementia are also addressed.

This very practical book is for caregivers who perform the hands-on work of caring for elders. The chapters in this book contain Objectives, Discussion questions, Exercises, illustrative stories, Action Steps (for implementing new knowledge and skills), Recommended Reading, and Resources. The Discussion questions and Exercises bring to light the sacredness of spiritual growth and suggest new ways of developing meaning and value in life. As staff members go through the Discussion questions and Exercises, we would like them to envision that they are caring for their own parents. The chapters illustrate the importance of incorporating spiritual concerns into models of wholistic care for elders. The contents of these chapters will also assist the director of staff development in meeting the regulatory requirements for the education of nursing assistants about the issues involving spirituality.

You are undoubtedly already familiar with and practicing some of the suggestions in this book. We hope that these chapters will increase your knowledge and enhance your practices. Significant spiritual interconnections and growth occur each day among residents, staff, and families, and as such, long-term care facilities become sacred spaces.

REFERENCES

Fischer, K.R. (1998). *Winter grace: Spirituality and aging.* Nashville: Upper Room Books.

National Interfaith Coalition on Aging. (1975). *Definition of spiritual well-being.* Retrieved January 31, 2003, from http://www.ncoa.org (click on "Constituent Units," then click on "NICA," then click on "News & Resources").

Seicol, Rabbi S. (1996). *Spirituality, health, and aging: The health of the human spirit.* Paper presented at the American Society on Aging annual conference, Anaheim, California.

For the Reader

The following suggestions may make using this book easier and more efficient for the staff developer in providing training for facilities that offer care to older adults and comfort to their families.

- Read the entire text before beginning trainings to have a clearer picture of the format and goals. You may also wish to review the topics that seem especially important to the staff in your facility and to pay particular attention to the objectives at the beginning of each chapter.

- The book does not need to be followed sequentially. Some facilities may find that selecting topics of specific concern or moving through chapters in a different order better meets the needs of the staff.

- Conversation and participation among those attending the training in which this book is used is very important, but no one should be urged to share beyond his or her comfort level.

- A smaller group of participants usually works better (10 or fewer), especially in discussing controversial or emotionally laden subjects. Work toward a relaxed, informal atmosphere.

- People usually love to share their stories. It may be helpful to suggest time limits for some of the book's exercises and to discourage domination of group discussion.

- Some of the exercises may result in the surfacing of strong or suppressed emotions. Having a referral list for counseling is always wise.

- Consider the development of an evaluation instrument for the trainings, as well as a mechanism to see how well new or revised practices are working. For example, if you decide to set aside a room or space for prayer or meditation, how are residents and/or their families using this space?

We hope you will enjoy the opportunity to share the richness and importance of spiritual care and its often beneficial effects on staff, residents, and families. It is comforting to know that our work and our lives have meaning and purpose and that there is another dimension to all that we do.

Vital Connections in Long-Term Care: Spiritual Resources for Staff and Residents was inspired by presentations made at the American Society on Aging and the

California Association of Homes and Services for the Aging. The authors of this book are members of the Advisory Board for the Center for Gerontology, Spirituality and Faith (CGSF) in Cupertino, California. The CGSF exists to provide training in the areas of spirituality to those who work with elders. These training events include workshops, retreats, and seminary courses.

Vital Connections in Long-Term Care: Spiritual Resources for Staff and Residents is a complementary education tool for the course titled "Aging and Spirituality." This mini-course is a certificate program designed for professionals (e.g., social workers, nurses, administrators, clergy) working with elders. Additional information can be obtained by writing to Gerry Roy, Center for Gerontology, Spirituality and Faith, 22445 Cupertino Road, Cupertino, California 95014.

Acknowledgments

I would like to acknowledge my friend and co-teacher, Virginia Daugherty, for her tireless support, honesty, and humor, especially during the writing of this book. She has been an equal partner in all of our endeavors and has brought a sense of fun and truth to our teaching. She is always ready, with her artistic sense of detail, to make any work that comes out of our office look not only professional, but beautiful as well. I look forward to many more days of working together.

I also have very much enjoyed working on this book with my friends and colleagues Marita Grudzen and Ron Zielske. Their critiques, commiseration, and above all, their sense of humor, have been both valuable and joyful. Our colleagues on the board of the Center for Gerontology, Spirituality and Faith have also been an ongoing source of inspiration to me.

I am very grateful for the patience and support of my husband and family during this last year and a half. I know that just as they supported me through the preparation of this book, they are rejoicing with me at its publication.

—J.B.

While I cannot identify and thank all of the people who have made the vision and publication of this book possible, there are those who have been *terribly* significant.

Mary Magnus, Director of Publications for Health Professions Press, invited us to submit the manuscript and has supported and shepherded the lengthy process. Amy Kopperude has been a skilled and gracious editor, ensuring that our intentions were clear in the editing process.

Ron Zielske and Julie Barton have been marvelous collaborators. Without their vision and commitment, this book would not exist. Gwen Yeo, Director of the Stanford Geriatric Education Center (SGEC), understood well over a decade ago how essential spirituality, in all of its forms, is to the lives of older adults, most especially elders of ethnic minority. She encouraged SGEC collaboration with the Center for Gerontology, Spirituality and Faith. This book is one of the fruits of that collaboration.

I am especially grateful to my husband, Gerry Grudzen, who, more than any other individual, supported my work in so many small and large ways *every day*. He also embodied, in his familial relationships, the work described in these pages.

I can't go without thanking the other individuals in my life who so beautifully model these practices of spiritually informed care and healing, often at great personal cost. They include, but are not limited to, Bob Andersen, Alan Cole, Judy Clarence, Bruce Feldstein, Carolyn Grassi, Charlea Massion, Sandi Peters, Joan Randall, Marge Reilley, Mary Lee Reilley, Patricia Reilley, Shanti Rubenstone, Susan Slack, Phyllis Soto, Sharon Waller, Judy Walter, and Manuel Yaniz. Our daughters, Corita and Simone, provide me with a constant source of joy, energy, and hope.

—M.G.

I am grateful to my wife, Marian, for her support, patience, and encouragement, not only during the formation of this book but during my entire ministry. She helps me create balance and reminds me of the need for self-care. She shares the vision and passion for elders' well-being.

I want to give many thanks to Marita and Julie, who are most excellent friends. They know how to support others with hugs and words. Marita has been a co-presenter at many workshops and classes, and I am grateful for her expertise in developing programs. I also want to thank all of the members on the board for the Center for Gerontology, Spirituality and Faith for their hard work in implementing the Center's mission and vision.

—R.Z.

For Anita Frank, of blessed memory. A dear friend and a role model of humor and dignity, she possessed a sparkling wit, conversed elegantly, and was generous with her hugs well into her nineties. She was often in my thoughts as I wrote, and I miss her dearly.
—J.B.

For my mother, Mary Alice (O'Brien) Reilley, who stepped through her dementia to bless me as only a mother can bless her daughter. My mother and father have given me the template for all that I have gone on to learn.
—M.G.

For Mel Kimble, Professor Emeritus of Pastoral Theology and head of the aging concentration at Luther Seminary, St. Paul, Minnesota. I consider Mel to be the grandfather of aging and spirituality work and my mentor as well as a mentor to many others who share the passion of guiding elders into abundant living.
—R.Z.

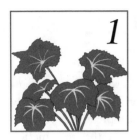

Spiritual Transformations

*Insights, Support, and
Healing for Spiritual Well-Being*

Ron Zielske

OBJECTIVES

As a result of reading this chapter and working through the exercises, participants will be able to

1. Define spiritual well-being

2. Recognize core values that are universal to residents and necessary for supporting their spiritual health

3. Understand the possibilities for wellness and healing within the context of aging, illness, and even death

4. Discover new insights for their own spiritual transformation

5. Understand their role in supporting the well-being of residents

DEFINING SPIRITUALITY

Perhaps spirituality, in its broadest definition, is that which brings meaning to life and that which forms values for an individual. There certainly are as many definitions of spirituality as there are people and perhaps as many different ways to define spiritual well-being. (See the introduction for more definitions of spirituality.)

A particular religion, together with its beliefs and rituals, may be the expression of spirituality for some people. Others may not belong to a particular religion, but they still have spirit inside that directs their values. That which helps people become connected in meaningful ways to other people is in itself spiritual. Spirituality is also that which defines people's belief systems and what is valuable and meaningful for daily living. In relating to others, being able to identify and understand the history of one's own spirituality is important.

DISCUSSION

1. What do you think about your spiritual journey thus far?

2. Do you practice a particular religion or a specific form of that religion?

3. How did you come to that faith and that expression of the faith?

4. Do you define all of your spirituality in terms of that practice?

5. What are the three most important values in your life?

6. What do you think is the reason for you to be alive on earth at this time?

7. What brings meaning to your life?

8. What do you take pride in?

9. Who are the people who have influenced you the most? Why?

10. Are you aware of the spiritual practices of the residents, families of residents, and other staff?

EXERCISE

List or draw the major events that have formed your spirituality (e.g., a personal revelation, a religious ceremony such as a baptism or confirmation, special insight given by a family member or friend). Share your answers with others in your group. At the end of the discussion, think about what you have learned from others in the group that applies to your life.

In addition to understanding their own spiritual journey and spiritual expressions, people need to be aware of the overt and subtle biases they may have about certain other religions, about expressions of other religions, or about certain types of spiritual expression. One must recognize that prejudices about particular ethnic and cultural groups may factor into attitudes about certain faiths. It is also important to refrain from thinking that if a person is of a particular ethnic or cultural group, he or she also belongs to a particular religion or expression of that religion. In order to relate well to others, it is important for staff to understand and respect residents' different religious views and beliefs in order to be attuned to their spiritual needs.

KATIE AND ZHELA

Katie works as a nursing assistant and considers her role of helping residents as her calling from God. She is a fervent evangelical Christian and often has discussions with residents about their need to accept Jesus as their Savior in order to go to heaven. On the other hand, Zhela, another nursing assistant, was raised in the Islam faith and feels strongly that Christianity is wrong. She believes that the only religious truth is the Muslim truth. She often speaks to other staff about her beliefs. Zhela and Katie often discuss and sometimes argue during breaks about their religious convictions.

DISCUSSION

1. As the head of the unit, what would you say to Katie and Zhela to help them see what they are doing and

honor the residents' and staff's own religious or spiritual perspectives?

2. What prejudices were you exposed to about religion and race during your childhood?

3. What negative feelings have you collected during your life as a result of how you saw others treated based on their behavior, personality, ethnic group, or religious faith? Think about how those negative attitudes may have prevented you from relating to others or from understanding other people's spiritual and religious needs.

DEFINING WELL-BEING

What does it mean to have well-being? Many people associate this with not having any illness or disease. Many people have the attitude that elders with multiple disabilities and diseases cannot have well-being. Some independent adults in their late eighties and early nineties who go to nursing facilities to visit residents, as well as many others in this society, equate *old* with diseases and disabilities common among older adults that lead to dependency on other people. They associate being old and dependent with a lack of well-being. That very attitude can prevent older adults from having well-being. Everyone ages. Old age and death come to all in one form or another. People were not made to live forever; each person does wear out and eventually die. That is natural to all life. Having physical infirmities does not preclude a person from experiencing well-being.

DISCUSSION

1. Discuss the biases of old age and illness that you grew up with. What attitudes have changed over the years? Which ones changed as a result of your own aging and which ones as a result of others' aging?

2. Describe elders you know who are very healthy and active even in their eighties and nineties. What would they tell you have been the keys to their healthy and active lives?

3. Give an example of someone who has multiple disabilities and still possesses well-being.

CORE VALUES OF SPIRITUALITY

In 1975, the National Interfaith Coalition on Aging started defining spirituality with two key words: 1) *affirmation,* in that spirituality is an affirmation of life that would lead to wholeness, and 2) *relationship* with other people, the self, the community, the environment, and perhaps God or a supreme being.

At the very center of spiritual well-being is the word *hope.* This core value is more than optimism; it is the expectation of things getting better (e.g., *I hope I win the lottery, I hope my telephone gets fixed today*). We have all heard hopefulness expressed over a very sick person, "There is nothing to do but hope." Although these are popular examples of hope, the way in which hope relates to spirituality is different. In this case, hope implies that there is a meaning to what the future holds and that the future may hold more possibilities than one can imagine or understand. It is also the confidence that a higher being or a higher level of existence will be present in our future. Hope is linked to *trust* and *meaning* and is often associated with *patience.* Hope is linked to *trust* as in trust and belief in God or a higher power who is ultimately compassionate. Hope is linked to *meaning* in that if a person has discovered meaning and purpose in life, he or she is hopeful even in difficult times. Hope is also associated with patience in that hope produces patience in hard times and confidence that a higher being will be present. Hope is further connected with yearning and longing and eager expectation. Hope is often found when everything else is stripped away and when there seems no logical reason to hope.

The former Czechoslovakian leader Vaclav Havel believed that people cannot necessarily change things with hope but that they can make a difference. When human beings are in close proximity to each other, a "soul-to-soul" connection takes place even when words are not spoken. When one person supports another person, hope grows in their lives.

DISCUSSION

1. What keeps you going? How do/did you survive difficult times?

2. Who do you know who has been hopeful even when the world around them was collapsing?

3. In the movie *The Shawshank Redemption,* when Andy DuFresne is asked, after 60 days in solitary confinement, how he survived, he answers, "Hope." What stories can you tell from real life or fiction that are examples of hope?

4. Talk about a time when you were able to make a difference in someone's life.

5. Can you describe a time when you felt a "soul-to-soul" spiritual connection with someone and knew that your presence made a difference? Describe the last time someone made a difference in your life and brought you hope?

Another core value is the concept of *integration*. Integration means to recall, celebrate, or grieve over the past events of one's life, plan the future but live in the present, and be open to what the future may bring. It does not mean to constantly dwell on the past either with longing or regret or with a desire to relive it. Nor does it mean to plan obsessively for or live constantly in dreams of the future. This definition of integration can be compared with visiting treasures from the past in the attic or visiting the planning table and workbench in the basement: A person does not live in either place but sojourns to these locations to reminisce or complete certain tasks.

DISCUSSION

1. Where do the residents for whom you care currently spend most of their time? Where did they spend most of their time before they lived in a nursing facility?

2. What do you spend most of your time thinking about?

3. If you spend a great deal of time regretting the past or planning the future, what or who will help you stay more focused in the present and help you be present to those around you?

Another core value is found in the word *relationships*. A person experiences wholeness by having healthy relationships with a higher being, other people, and him- or herself. An important understanding of relationships is to recognize that people are interdependent, not independent or dependent. Throughout life, people take turns being care givers and care receivers. To be well, all human beings need the abilities and personhood of others with whom they come in contact.

Perhaps one of the most difficult realities for long-term care residents is having to accept the help of others in the basic activities of daily living such as bathing, grooming, and toileting. Allowing others to provide care often seems contrary to western society's emphasis on rugged independence. Allowing others to provide care, however, lets them experience meaning, satisfaction, and well-being. In a sense, this creates a sacred "spiritual" space for those involved. The Christian scriptures record Jesus washing the feet of the disciples despite their protests. Allowing others to serve themselves enables them to fulfill a personal mission and contributes to their well-being.

A person is valuable because he or she exists and not for what he or she produces. People are called human beings and not human doings. People are spiritual beings on a human journey. It is not uncommon for people to have negative or self-degrading opinions of themselves, especially when they do not feel that they are productive members of society any longer. Acting superior is not the antidote to low self-esteem. A healthy appreciation of one's intrinsic worth and special abilities and an understanding that one is equal to others in the community is the antidote. One of the many ways to appreciate the self is to make a list of a person's gifts and abilities and to recall times when those were used to help others. This approach works as well for residents as it does for staff.

EXERCISE

Wash each other's feet, or perform some other caregiving task that is typically performed for residents. Discuss how it feels to be the one who serves and how it feels to be served.

DISCUSSION

1. Recall times when you have been a care giver and times when you have been a care receiver. Share

these experiences with the group, as well as your feelings and self-image at the time.

2. Can you let others serve you without feeling depressed, violated, or angry; without refusing help; or without refusing to ask for assistance when you need it?

3. Is there any kind of help you could use right now?

4. Explore how you feel about being both the server and the one served based on your spiritual beliefs. Share these explorations with the group.

The fourth core value is compassion. The word *compassion* means to be passionate with or suffer with another and thus is cause for more involvement than pity, just as empathy is cause for more involvement than sympathy. The empathy experienced with compassion involves trying to understand the suffering of another person, whereas pity involves feeling sorry for someone in a judgmental way that involves little or no emotion or urge to help.

A main task that promotes healthy spiritual well-being is that of caring. The word *care* does not mean "to save," be responsible for another's life, or dictate that certain beliefs and values become theirs. Compassion occurs when a person is present with others in their need, listening to them and touching them in a caring way. Love, at its most profound level, demonstrates compassion. Those who are wounded by trials and problems are best able to heal the wounds of others who are suffering. Author Henri J.M. Nouwen (1972) called these people "wounded healers." Regardless of a person's level of compassion, however, he or she can never really understand how another person feels. The commonly used phrase, "I understand how you feel," simply is not true, even if two people experience the same event. Each person has his or her own physical, emotional, and spiritual experience of an event. Nevertheless, caring can be expressed in many compassionate ways.

DISCUSSION

1. Discuss times when you felt pity from someone when you really wanted compassion. Share with the group the difference between these two in your example.

2. What are the ways in which you show compassion now?

3. When is it difficult for you to show compassion?

4. How do you practice loving acts without making decisions for other people or running their lives?

5. The last time someone told you that they knew how you felt, what were your thoughts and feelings?

HEALING AND CURING

The word *healing* is often used as a synonym for curing. There is a difference between the two. People cannot be cured of some things; however, acts of healing can take place that may create a sense of well-being. When the staff brings food and water to residents or dresses, bathes, grooms, talks with, hugs, or caringly touches residents, the staff brings a form of health and well-being to each resident, in spite of any incurable disease or disability that a resident may have. Even a loving attitude and kind personality can create spiritual well-being. These are all spiritual gifts that one person can share with another. This kind of spiritual well-being may change the atmosphere of the entire facility, and visitors can sense this as they walk in the front door.

DISCUSSION

1. What are some of the small ways that you bring healing and well-being into the lives of residents each day?

2. What are the ways that you bring well-being to other staff members?

Even when curing does take place, there may or may not be healing of the mind and spirit, and, thus, the person will still not experience wholeness. Being present with a person, listening, and giving a caring touch are healing acts. Spiritual or religious comfort in the form of prayer, Scripture reading, poetry, and inspirational messages bring healing. Healing also occurs if one finds meaning in suffering. Life review can bring healing as well as recognition of what has been done for others in the past. The arts, music, poetry, and inspirational literature bring healing. Some religions and faiths have rituals of healing that promote healing even if curing does not take place.

One cannot expect a cure for all ills, but that does not preclude healing of various kinds taking place. Acts of caring bring healing, and healing brings spiritual well-being. Harold Koenig (2000), a physician at Duke University, has said that physicians are to cure sometimes, relieve often, and comfort always. In some Christian traditions, the sick and dying are anointed with oil while prayers and Scripture are read, and special worship services are held in which people are invited to be anointed with oil for healing the mind, body, and spirit.

EMILY AND MATILDA

Emily Yang, a resident in a dementia unit, is in need of a healing experience. She rarely speaks and needs to be fed and toileted. If you look carefully into her eyes, you can sometimes glimpse a sparkle when she is excited or a frown when she is experiencing pain from her cancer.

Matilda, a staff member who often communicates with Emily, walks with her to the bathroom. Matilda holds Emily's hand and talks to her with simple words and a mild tone without being condescending. She handles her gently as she puts her on and off the toilet. She reminds Emily when her son will be visiting to take her out for ice cream. Matilda turns on Emily's favorite kind of music as she puts her in bed for a nap. By doing these things, Matilda has brought healing to Emily.

DISCUSSION

1. Can you describe ways in which you and residents have experienced healing without being cured?
2. Can you describe ways that a person was healed in spirit or mind after his or her body was cured?
3. How do residents live with their disabilities? What helps them? Who helps them?

SPIRITUAL TRANSFORMATION

It is important for staff to recognize how residents might be feeling about entering a facility and about how their views of aging may be changing.

SPIRITUAL SELF-ASSESSMENT FORM

1.   List 10 people or events that have most influenced your life in a good or bad way, and briefly discuss how they have done so.

2.   What have been your experiences of physical, spiritual, or mental distress or suffering, and how have these affected your attitude or values? Identify your experiences of powerlessness, forgiveness, or weakness.

3.   Identify what means you use to find comfort or support. If this has changed over the years, discuss how and why.

4.   What have been your experiences of loving others and being loved?

5.   How have your beliefs changed over the years about God, about your relationship with God, about your relationship with others, and about your place in the world?

6.   Identify what positive traits you most appreciate about yourself and how they have developed.

7.   Identify your greatest source of joy. Who or what is responsible for it, and how do you protect it?

8.   Are you at peace with your relationship with God? If yes, how did you achieve it? If no, what factors contribute to it?

9.   What part does religion play in your life now? If your religious expressions changed, how or why?

10. Is anything especially frightening or meaningful to you now?

11. Identify for yourself
     • Something to hope for
     • Something to work for
     • Something to love
     • Your purpose in being

Figure 1.   Spiritual self-assessment form. (From Kathryn Scott, Director of San Mateo Secure Seniors Project, Sunny View Lutheran Home, Cupertino, California; reprinted by permission.)

When a resident enters a facility, his or her spiritual values and practices can be discovered during the intake process as part of his or her social history. A comprehensive spiritual assessment can be made using various questions (see Figure 1). This will allow the needs of the resident to be met in a complete way and open the door for continued spiritual growth. With the permission of the resident, this information is ideally shared with the entire staff, not just visiting clergy.

Residents' spiritual well-being also grows through the environment in which they live. The meaning of their lives comes from a profound spiritual search. The need to have pictures and other personal objects from their past and present is vital. The need to review the past and make sense out of their lives is also a significant task toward the end of life (see Figure 2). A qualified person made available by the facility can lead residents through reminiscence and life review to greatly enhance their spiritual growth.

QUESTIONS TO ASSIST RESIDENTS IN REFLECTING ON THEIR SPIRITUALITY

1. How have you found meaning and purpose in your life?

2. What are your most important values, and how have you tried to apply them to your life?

3. From where and whom do you derive your spiritual strength?

4. How have you managed to come through difficult times? What have you learned from these times? Have these times brought you closer to your spirituality or separated you from your beliefs and practices?

5. Do you belong to a particular religion? If so, what practices, rituals, and/or prayers are important to you? Do you have a close relationship with a higher being?

6. What stories from the scriptures of your religion are your favorite and why?

7. Does a spiritual guide (e.g., pastor, priest, rabbi) visit with you? If not, would you like one to visit?

8. Has your faith had a positive or negative effect on your life?

9. How does the practice of your faith or spiritual beliefs support any close personal relationships that you have with others?

10. What do you do when you feel angry or hurt by others?

11. How do you practice forgiveness with others? How do you experience forgiveness?

12. Do you feel hopeful about the future? What or who has been helpful when you have felt hopeless?

13. What would you like to do to increase your spiritual health and well-being?

14. What are the most important things about you as a person and your life that you would want others to remember after your death?

Figure 2.   Questions to assist residents in reflecting on their spirituality.

Innovators in the long-term care field have introduced alternative management styles for nursing facilities, such as The Eden Alternative, that stress a more home-like environment and help the facility move away from the traditional medical model of a hospital-like environment where medical procedures seem to be the most important part of a resident's life. The Eden Alternative is designed to eliminate the three plagues of long-term care institutions: helplessness, loneliness, and boredom. Its mission statement includes "We must teach ourselves to see the environments as habitats for human beings rather than facilities for the frail and elderly. We must learn what Mother Nature has to teach us about the creation of vibrant, vigorous habitats" (from The Eden Alternative web site at http://www.edenalt.com/home/index.htm). The presence of plants and animals and resident involvement in caring for plants makes facilities feel more like home. One of the other transforming ingredients of The Eden Alternative model is empowerment of residents and staff in joint decision making, which enhances relationships between the two.

DISCUSSION

1. Does your facility gather religious and spiritual information?

2. Does the social worker or clergy use a comprehensive survey?

3. Do you know about your residents' religious beliefs? If so, how does knowing help you address the needs of the residents? How do you support the spirituality of the residents?

4. How does the family support the religious or spiritual life of the resident?

5. What spiritual resources come into your facility for the resident?

6. Is your facility engaged in implementing The Eden Alternative or a similar program? If not, how can such programs be explored?

The resident will experience spiritual growth and well-being depending on how his or her particular spiritual and religious needs are directly met and how well the caregiver provides for the resident's needs. Nursing facility staff and others who work in a facility can experience their own spiritual growth and well-being through the everyday care of residents. Successful caregiving is the result of the spiritual values of the staff and is modeled by simple rewards such as a smile, words of thanks, or touch from residents. Even for those residents who will not or cannot respond positively, the staff need to know that the acts of caring enhance the quality of life of the residents. The staff members invest their own life's meaning into the care of residents. In every instance in which residents, families, management, or other staff express gratitude, the caregiver is spiritually affirmed and experiences well-being.

The most frequent and significant personal contact and communication for residents comes from the staff and especially from the nursing assistants who spend the majority of their time with residents. The spiritual life of both the resident and the staff are enhanced by the communication—words, body language, and touch when appropriate—that takes place when staff members help change residents' clothes, get them ready for bed, take them to meals, and bathe them. Some residents will experience spiritual growth when they are actively engaged by staff members who ask them about their life and express concern and care for them.

SAMMY

Sammy has been a nursing assistant in his facility for more than 10 years and is a prized staff member because of his sensitivity, kind words, friendly manner, and caring skills. Sammy finds deep fulfillment and meaning in life in his relationships with residents and other staff who rely on him for knowledge and a steady positive attitude even in times of crisis. Sammy will say that he learns a lot about life from the residents, and some of them respond to his kindness with their own kindness. Several of the residents pray for him and his family on a regular basis and ask him about his two boys.

DISCUSSION

1. Why do you do work in long-term care, and what meaning does it have for you? Why do you stay in this line of work?

2. How do you contribute to resident well-being through daily tasks? Does that contribute to your own well-being in some way?

3. Tell others in the group about when you have received positive feedback from residents or other staff members and how that made you feel.

4. Reflect on the words *care* and to *care fully*. Describe how you carefully relate and serve the needs of the residents. List all of the things you would do to be fully caring.

The other ingredient to residents' spiritual growth is their positive experiences with family and friends. Since relationships are vital to spiritual well-being, the staff members need to welcome visitors with open arms and smiles and thank them for coming rather than see visitors as an intrusion on the daily routine. In addition to having a format for resident involvement in the care, there needs to be a way in which families and friends can be involved in doing things with the residents (e.g., caring for plants and birds in residents' rooms). Families also need to be invited for occasional social gatherings and celebrations, as residents would have done in their own homes. For a short period of time, the sign on one nursing facility door read: Love is Ageless, Come and Visit.

DISCUSSION

1. How have you greeted family and friends today? How can you be more welcoming even if your language skills are limited?

2. Contribute to the group ways in which the family and friends of residents can be more involved with their loved one.

Up to this point, this chapter has focused on examples of positive relationships; however, relationships are not always positive. Residents sometimes are critical, staff members sometimes are grumpy, and some family relationships are destructive. There may be little that staff can do about some residents' dysfunctional family relationships except to give comfort and a listening ear to the resident, which supports well-being. If the staff has a good relationship with residents and their families, someone can suggest a meeting with the clergy or a family counselor. Staff members can also enhance the spiritual well-being of a resident who is hostile. Treating the person as a whole human being with a spirit regardless of harsh words or physical abuse by the resident is a key to resident and staff well-being. This does not mean that staff should be doormats for residents, but boundaries that are enforced with love and care will create spiritual growth. Caring continues even with difficult residents, but the spiritual growth and well-being of the staff involved need the support of other staff and of other, more positive residents. When people care, beauty is all around.

DISCUSSION

1. How do you handle hostile residents and how do you feel about them?

2. Have residents or family members complimented you for your caring? How does that make you feel? How does that give you encouragement for continuing your work?

3. Can you give yourself a pat on the back during times when no one else does and, if so, how?

THE ROLE OF CHAPLAINS

Because spirituality is pervasive and extends into all aspects of daily life, simply holding a few religious services for residents will not necessarily meet their spiritual needs. Professionally trained chaplains trained in clinical pastoral education who are on the premises full time can be a great asset and the primary moving force in promoting spiritual transformation and growth. The nursing staff has precious few minutes each day to dedicate to the spiritual growth of residents, whereas the chaplain's major responsibility is to attend to the residents' spiritual needs. Chaplains for retirement and nursing facilities, such as pastors, priests, shamans, and rabbis, function the same way that hospital chaplains do in that they are there for people of a variety of religions, and for those of no religion, to serve as midwives for the spiritual process.

DISCUSSION

1. Have you worked in places where there have been professionally trained chaplains? If so, what difference did it make in the lives of the residents and staff?

2. In what ways could a chaplain at your facility make a difference in the lives of residents and staff? Choose several residents as examples and suggest ways in which a chaplain would enhance the spiritual growth of those individuals.

3. In what ways could this chaplain assist the staff in care planning and care conferences?

4. How would your facility go about finding and funding a chaplain?

Even when a qualified chaplain or other spiritual leader is not available, there are many things that can be done by staff, family, and friends to bring spiritual care to residents. See Table 1.

Table 1. Ways to provide spiritual care when there is no chaplain

1. Have volunteer groups from local churches provide worship experiences.
2. Have volunteers provide one-to-one room visits.
3. Have volunteer clergy provide regular Bible study.
4. Have a community hymn sing.
5. Display paintings from a local senior center.
6. Provide mini-concerts from a local school of music.
7. Have a religious heritage day during which residents share their personal heritage.
8. Have celebrations of religious holidays relating to all residents in the nursing facility.
9. Promote life review that evokes reflection and meaning-making that is more than reminiscence.
10. Lead finger-painting (or collage) activities displaying abstractions such as forgiveness, death, and/or life beyond death.
11. Host meditation prayer groups.
12. Encourage resident-led devotions.
13. Publish an "I Met God When..." booklet of residents' experiences.
14. Foster the development of ethical wills.
15. Hold a "Celebration of Aging Festival" with local speakers.
16. Teach a tai chi class.
17. Develop a ritual for celebrating the life of a resident who has died.
18. Develop a ritual for welcoming residents to their new home.

(continued)

Table 1.   *(continued)*

19. Provide prayer cards at meal tables appropriate for different religious traditions.
20. Give staff the overt freedom to talk about religion and faith (without proselytizing).
21. Provide a dedicated space for worship and/or prayer.
22. Ensure that residents are not only asked but are provided the means of attending religious activities and ceremonies held on campus.
23. Make one's spirituality a part of the intake assessment.
24. Have at least one television in the facility tuned to religious programming when appropriate.
25. Mail a letter to local faith groups inviting them to partner with the facility.
26. Take residents for a walk in the park.
27. Provide a variety of devotional literature (often available free through faith groups).
28. Present videotapes of stories that promote meaning-making. Don't forget to discuss their meaning afterward.
29. Provide audio- and videotapes of sermons from local faith groups.
30. Hold a workshop for residents and families on end-of-life choices, including advance directives.
31. Sponsor a grief support group.
32. Hold a "Caring and Sharing Group" for resident discussion of the meaning of life events.
33. Ask a local synagogue to sponsor a Passover Seder.
34. Encourage local faith group choirs to sing at the facility. They often have "concerts" at their place of worship during special times of the year and are looking for a place for a "dress rehearsal."
35. Hold a "Religious Expression Festival" and invite local clergy from differing faith groups to participate.
36. Secure from residents the names of the clergy of their faith groups and invite them to extend their ministry to your facility.
37. Provide in-service training for staff on spirituality, and make spiritual care one of the expectations of a staff's work.
38. Ask residents to write a "This I Believe" article for your facility's newsletter.
39. Have a Chinese New Year celebration.
40. Develop a policy on Spiritual Formation and Pastoral Care that gives guidelines for participation of clergy and faith groups from the community.
41. Have a concert using local talent (e.g., high schools, elementary schools, churches, individuals).
42. Identify and use existing staff who have been trained within their own faith traditions to provide spiritual care and development.
43. Encourage guided imagery through a painting exercise.
44. Discuss the meaning found in favorite TV programs.
45. Develop a "Meditation Walk" (mental journey) with pictures, thoughtful sayings, poetry, and verses from religious texts.
46. Have volunteer residents become telephone friends to home-centered people.
47. Have residents volunteer to fold and stuff bulletins for a local religious organization.
48. Make and use memory prayer beads that represent an important event.
49. Have residents write, as a group, a poem describing something common to resident life and give it a title such as "Ode to a Walker."

From: Reverend Donald Koepke, Director of the Center for Spirituality and Ethics in Aging, A Program of California Lutheran Homes and Community Services, Burbank, California; adapted by permission.

SPIRITUAL ETHICS

Ethical considerations, whether they are centered on clinical care, end-of-life issues, or the ethics of the organization, are about meaning for and the values of individuals, groups, and organizations. As such, they are spiritual in nature. Remembering that ethical considerations are important for the meaning and values of those involved is an important mindset in approaching the subject of ethics and also in staffing ethics committees. The ethics committee membership should include the clergy and social worker or others who can bring spiritual issues into discussions. Ethics committees deal with the difficult and conflicting issues surrounding care and the policies of the facility, especially the options of treatment toward the end of life.

In considering ethical issues, it is necessary to remember to give up the use of power. Ethics has everything to do with justice and equal access and treatment of residents to care and services in the facility as well as in the community or nation. Ethics deals with cultural and ethnic issues and concerns as part of valuing the individual and the family or clan. Ethical considerations move past prejudices and look at the body, mind, and spirit of the individual as a whole.

Organizational ethics help the facility look at its own mission and especially its values. What are the underlying principles that guide the organization in decision-making about policies that govern the residents' lives, and what are the principles that gird up the personnel policies?

DISCUSSION

1. Does your facility have an ethics committee?

2. Who is on this committee? Who needs to be on the committee but is not?

3. Does the committee deal with organizational ethics as well as bio-ethics?

4. Does the facility have published value statements, and, if not, can they be inferred from the personnel policies and from the everyday actions of the management staff?

TRANSFORMATION OF THE COMMUNITY

When staff, residents, and families recognize that the work in the facility is sacred and has much to do with spirituality, not only are they transformed, but also the community in which the facility resides begins a transformation.

In very practical ways, transformation comes about from the words spoken by staff, families, and residents to neighbors about the spiritual aspects of their work and the value of the people whom they serve. This is the beginning of neighbors seeing the facility as a sacred place. Further transformation can take place as the facility focuses its attention on the whole person—mind, body, and spirit—and makes known its participation in either The Eden Alternative or other philosophies that change a facility's focus from a medical model of care to a social model.

Another part of the transformation comes about when volunteers from the community can, for example, visit, assist with programs, and take residents for walks. These volunteers will themselves be transformed by their relationships with residents and will begin to see the facility as a sacred place.

Volunteers from a variety of cultural, ethnic, and language backgrounds can make a profound difference in the lives of residents by giving them someone with whom they can identify and relate on a personal and shared cultural basis. Remember, relationships are at the very heart of spiritual growth.

Volunteers can be valuable assistants to the activity directors or can even lead some of the activities after training. Volunteers are very valuable in one-to-one activities such as writing letters and sending cards, playing games such as checkers and cards, reading books, and listening to the residents' stories. In addition, volunteers can use their own special talents such as playing musical instruments for residents and can supplement the regular activity programs at a time when scheduled activities are not taking place and when the activity staff is absent.

All human beings are spiritual even if they do not participate in an organized religion. The spirituality of each person has to do with the meaning and purpose he or she finds in life and his or her sense of contributing to other people and the world in general. Rather than thinking of a person as comprising three parts—mind, body, and spirit—it may be helpful to think of the spirit as that which underlies the physical, emotional, mental, and social aspects of a human being.

ACTION STEPS

1. Look for opportunities to talk to others about how working in your facility brings meaning to your life. Discuss ways to improve the quality of care that takes place.

2.   Discuss what efforts are being made by the facility for positive public relations. Propose additional strategies.

3.   How can volunteers be used? How will they be invited, trained, and honored?

REFERENCES

Koenig, H. (October 4, 2002). Religion, spirituality, and medicine: Applications to clinical practice. *Journal of the American Medical Association, 284*(13), 1708.

Koepke, D. (2001). *49 ways to provide spiritual care when there is no chaplain.* Handout presented at California Homes and Services for the Aging annual conference, Incline Village, Nevada.

Nouwen, H.J.M. (1972). *The wounded healer, ministry in contemporary society.* Garden City, NJ: Doubleday.

Scott, K. (1999). *Spiritual self-assessment format.* Director of Secure Seniors Project, Sunny View Lutheran Home, Cupertino, California.

Thomas, B., & Thomas, J. *What is Eden? Our mission statement.* Available on The Eden Alternative web site at http://www.edenalt.com/about.htm.

RECOMMENDED READING

Aging as a spiritual journey by Eugene C. Bianchi (The Crossroad Publishing Company)

The aging experience: Diversity and commonality across cultures by Jennie Keith et al. (Sage Publications)

Aging, spirituality, and religion: A handbook edited by Melvin A. Kimble et al. (Augsburg Fortress Press)

Another country: Navigating the emotional terrain of our elders by Mary Bray Pipher (Riverhead Books)

Articles from the Spring 1997 issue of *Spirituality and Aging, IX*(I):

   Aging and spirituality: A response by David O. Moberg, p. 8

   Designed to be imprecise by Martin Marty, p. 3

   Limited by theological language by Rabbi Sam Seicol, p. 4

   Spiritual well-being: A psychological perspective by Reymond F. Paloutzian, p. 7, 8

   Spiritual well-being: An experience of lived story by Anne Streaty Wimberly, p. 5

   Spiritual well-being defined by Reverend James W. Ellor, pp. 1–2

   What spiritual well-being means to me by Reverend Donald F. Clingan, p. 6

Assessing spiritual needs: A guide for caregivers by George Fitchett (Augsburg Fortress Press)

The development of spiritual awareness programs in long-term care settings, A White Paper for the Forum on Religion, Spirituality and Aging by Reverend James W. Ellor, Reverend Margaret Munci, and Rabbi Samuel Seicol (1993). Available from American Society on Aging, 833 Market Street, Suite 511, San Francisco, California 94103.

Elder wisdom: Crafting your own elderhood by Eugene C. Bianchi (The Crossroad Publishing Company)

The five stages of the soul: Charting the spiritual passages that shape our lives by Harry R. Moody (Anchor Books)

In the ever after: Fairy tales and the second half of life by Allan B. Chinen (Chiron Publications)

The Oxford book of aging edited by Thomas R. Cole & Mary G. Winkler (Oxford University Press)

Spiritual dimension of ageing by Elizabeth MacKinlay (Jessica Kingsley Publishers)

Spiritual passages: Embracing life's sacred journey by Drew Leder (Putnam Publishers)

A work of heart: Understanding how god shapes spiritual leaders by Reggie McNeal (Jossey-Bass)

RESOURCES

The Eden Alternative
742 Turnpike Road
Sherburne, New York 13460
Telephone: 607-674-5232
E-mail: contact@edenalt.com
Web site: http://www.edenalt.com

Pioneer Network
Post Office Box 18648
Rochester, New York 14618
Telephone: 585-271-7570
E-mail: RoseMarie.Fagan@PioneerNetwork.net
Web site: http://www.pioneernetwork.net

Wellspring Innovative Solutions
607 Bronson Road
Seymour, Wisconsin 54165
Telephone: 920-833-1833
E-mail: wellspring@goodshepherdservices.org
Web site: http://www.wellspringis.org

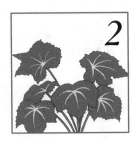

The Face of Dignity

Honoring the Individuality of Residents and Staff

Marita Grudzen

OBJECTIVES

As a result of reading this chapter and working through the exercises, participants will be able to

1. Appreciate the opportunities that providing personal care allows for engaging, listening to, showing respect for, and honoring the resident

2. Understand the value of touching with permission, awareness, and support

3. Recognize and respond to cultural differences in giving and receiving care

4. Appreciate and enhance the aesthetics of care and the environment of the older adult

5. Understand different models of resident care and the benefits of each

6. Recognize and work toward reconciling inevitable conflicts between institutional versus resident needs and rhythms

7. Recognize the need for caregivers to "pause and refresh" and understand the strategies for doing so in the work environment

8. Enhance resident awareness of nature and a sense of place

9. Develop a personal "toolkit for healing" specific to the staff caregivers' knowledge and talents

DIGNITY

What is dignity, and how can it be affirmed in residents? Simply put, dignity is a sense of personal worth and value. Many pathways exist to affirming and mirroring the dignity of residents. Affirming dignity starts with acknowledging the person on admission to a facility. When the admission can be planned, one or more welcoming initiatives can be incorporated. Examples of these are

- Inviting family members to stay for the next meal

- Blessing the new resident's space by a chaplain, rabbi, minister, or another member of the person's faith community

- Placing flowers, a plant, or other signs of welcome in the room

- Assigning a resident to be a guide or "big sister/big brother" for the new resident

- Surrounding the new resident with personal items (e.g., framed family photos or favorite artwork, religious objects, cosmetics, pillows)

Even for the most ill elder, some expression of welcoming the person into a safe and healing environment, a new home, is necessary. Recognizing someone's dignity, however, should not end upon entry into the facility. Every time a resident is awakened, greeted, touched, lifted, or engaged is an opportunity to show respect. How often are residents asked how they would like to be addressed, or, if they are unable to respond, is the family member consulted? If a resident is non–English-speaking, efforts must be made to provide for his or her language needs. And at all times it is appropriate to ask permission to enter residents' rooms or to search their closets and drawers for needed items.

DISCUSSION

Ask for a volunteer recorder or assign one to record staff members' responses to the following questions on a large board.

1. For whom is English a second language in your facility? How are elders viewed in their culture? Is there a word for dignity in their mother tongue, and does this change as elders become more frail?

2. How does your religion view elders?

3. Discuss your family's attitudes about elders or ancestors.

Summarize the rich, diverse perspectives that staff have expressed (referring to the board or list). Define *dignity* based on any one definition. Remember the expressions that others have shared.

EXERCISE

Have participants change places in the room. Then, say: *Let's relate the topic of dignity to our practices here at [name of facility] and to the everyday interactions with one another and with residents. To provide the opportunity for everyone to participate, we will break up in pairs. Pick someone whom you don't know very well, and spread out in the room. Each person will have 5 minutes to respond to the questions. Remember, this isn't a test; rather, it is an opportunity to express your point of view and for all of us to learn from one another. You don't need to write down anything. Listen deeply to one another. I will announce when the first 5 minutes are up so that both individuals in a pair have 5 minutes to generate answers.*

Have participants answer the following questions in pairs.

1. How do you experience your self-respect or dignity?

2. When do you feel disrespected? What offends or threatens your dignity?

3. How do you experience the dignity of our residents? How do residents reflect its presence to us? What seems to threaten their dignity?

4. How do you show respect for residents and protect their sense of dignity? Do you have suggestions for other ways staff can show respect for residents?

5. How are we doing as a facility? Are there other things we could do to reflect the dignity of the residents and the contributions of the staff?

6. How is your facility and the work you do viewed in the community? How can we strengthen our relationship to the community?

After 10 minutes, bring the group back together and ask how the sharing in pairs went. If participants do not respond, ask, "What was the most difficult question?" Draw out the mood of the group with similar questions. If staff members were confused by the questions, clarify the questions and the process. Encourage staff to rewrite the questions to better suit their situation. It is important to validate staff members' ways of knowing and to develop ways of building a safe learning circle.

Encourage staff members to implement one of the new approaches they learned from this discussion and report back at the next training on their experience of implementation.

DISCERNING RHYTHMS

In the course of aging, ordinary daily events of life typically acquire greater significance. People's lives become more circumscribed and their energy more limited. They also become vulnerable to pain and to loss of privacy. The person who has little independence and is unable to perform the activities of daily living (e.g., eating, toileting, bathing, grooming, transporting to and from a chair) experiences a profound loss of control. It is difficult for younger, more able people to imagine the personal adjustment these changes require. The adjustment or maladjustment to losses can take considerable time and may take many forms, for instance, lack of initiative, withdrawal, outbursts of anger, or depression. The institutional character of a long-term care setting may exacerbate a person's feelings of loss, which can extend to losses of independence, a former living environment, and control over a new environment, as well as a diminishing sense of personhood and individuality.

One of the secrets of good care—because it reestablishes a sense of control and comfort to the individual receiving care—is identifying and strengthening the natural and preferred rhythms of the older adult. Consider the universal physical activities of breathing and circulation to understand how integral rhythm is to human existence and well-being. The biopsychosocial and spiritual rhythms of each person vary, for example, in which part of the day a person is typically most alert and energetic or how easily he or she establishes rapport and engages with others. Spiritually, rhythms can take different forms during daily practices, but on a larger scale people frequently cycle from times of spiritual connection to experiences of alienation and disconnection. Individuals differ in many of their everyday rhythms due to both biology and preference. These differences contribute to each individual's character. Usually, the more a person is in touch with and honors these rhythms, the better he or she deals with life's demands and opportunities.

Institutions also have observable rhythms. Specific circumstances of the day's events or the institution's functioning sometimes supersede personal rhythms. The necessity of shift changes, mealtimes, bath times, medication rounds, activity times, and so forth drive the rhythms of nursing facility routines. Staff and residents alike are affected. But residents' rhythms frequently are masked by the institutional time clock. Moreover, caregivers must be aware of the tendency to impose their own schedules on residents. The benefits of discerning and strengthening the resident's rhythms include enhancing resident well-being as well as caregiver satisfaction.

The first instance in which to begin attuning oneself to residents' rhythms is while administering personal care. Through observation, inquiry, and listening to what residents say about these daily rituals, and by examining a resident's lifestyle prior to admission, staff can become more aware, not only of the residents' pace but also of the associations, practices, and pleasures that have accompanied their rituals of daily living.

Social rhythms pertain to the patterns of how and when a person chooses to interact with others. Some people need the constant reassurance of others. Others, although having a social side, may prefer to have time alone in the first part of the day or may need periods of quiet throughout the day. Providing for these personal preferences encourages a sense of individuality, pleasure, capability, and control.

Although not as directly observable as social or personal preferences, determining the spiritual rhythms of residents is also desirable. The FICA (Faith, Influence, Community, Address) model of documenting a spiritual history (Puchalski & Romer, 2000) is a good way to collect this information (see Resources on p. 44). It can be part of the social history taken during admission. This spiritual history tool helps identify a resident's values and beliefs, the person's support community, and his or her spiritual practices and needs, as well as how the facility might meet those needs.

Doubters may ask, "All well and good, but how can we ever consider residents' personal rhythms in the context of institutional life?" Rather than an "either/or" perspective, the goal is to envision a "both/and" world. Before considering what this would look like, it may be helpful to examine one's personal experiences more closely.

DISCUSSION

Provide pens and paper to participants and ask for a volunteer recorder or assign one. Encourage participants to jot down a few answers to questions 1 and 2 before sharing with the group.

1. What daily activities are important to you (e.g., morning walk, cup of hot coffee on rising, daily call to a friend or relative, evening bath, favorite television program)?

2. Now ask yourself, if you became disabled, which of these routines would be most important to maintain? Share your responses to this and question 1 with the person sitting next to you (allow 1 minute for each person).

3. What daily, weekly, and yearly rhythms are you aware of (e.g., how many meals you have and when you eat them, keeping the Sabbath, annual family gatherings, ethnic and religious holidays)? Include the different rhythms of your life: the physical and biological, emotional, mental, social, and spiritual. These rhythms touch on your personal needs, such as whether you like to read the newspaper, how often and what time of day you bathe, your need for hugs, your need to see family and friends, and so forth. The answer here is not important; rather, it is important to see that everyone develops personal rhythms and, for the most part, has control over maintaining them.

EXERCISE

Write the following categories on a board or newsprint pad: 1) physical/biological, 2) emotional and/or psychological, 3) mental, 4) social, and 5) spiritual and/or religious. Encourage staff members to generate a list of manifestations of these rhythms in their lives (e.g., rest or sleep under physical/biological).

Assignment before next in-service: Ask staff members to identify three to four rhythms of one of the residents in their care and to be ready to discuss how they were able to identify the rhythm. Ask at the next in-service whether they have been able to integrate the resident's rhythms into the care plan. Provide an example of what is expected and ask if there are any questions.

TOUCH

Touch is one of the most powerful healing modalities. It must not be forced on others without their assent, however. Asking for permission to touch or move a resident shows respect, as does informing and engaging the person in what is about to be done. Such measures respect a person's cultural and personal boundaries and the sacredness of his or her body. Being intentional in one's movements has the added advantage of providing better support in assisting an elder with movement. It gives residents a sense of security.

Staff members have probably observed in their own experience how the emotional state of the one touching is communicated to the person being touched. The resident receiving care can sense if the caregiver is angry, stressed, or emotionally drained. Checking one's emotional state is necessary before administering personal care to someone else. One way of doing this is for the staff member to take a few deep breaths and scan for inner feelings while washing his or her hands *before* giving personal care. The practice of focused breathing helps to release stress and tension.

At a professional meeting, a former nursing assistant in a long-term care facility shared the following anecdote, which spoke volumes to those present: A female resident who hadn't spoken during her 6-month stay was presumed to be unable to speak. To everyone's amazement, this resident began to speak in response to the respectful and tender care she was given by one of the nursing assistants. Families also need to be encouraged to provide caring touch. They are often at a loss for ways to offer comfort or to engage with the older adults whom they are visiting. Many of the older residents, especially women, have given and received touch all of their lives. Now, even their visiting children sometimes sit at a distance, out of touch. Encourage visitors, when appropriate, to engage in "hands-on" activities. This will remedy the touch deprivation that so many of the elders in care facilities experience. Examples of "hands-on" activities include simply holding the hand of the person or applying lotion and gently massaging his or her hands. This can also be done with the feet and back, unless there are contraindications. Combing (and even setting) hair, shaving, or providing a manicure or pedicure offer other possibilities for touch. For patients with cognitive impairment, a comforting hand can be very reassuring and can facilitate a significant connection. When a resident is in a comatose state, holding hands or touching can be particularly helpful to the grieving process of family members and to their need to express their love.

It is important to be aware that many cultures and religions have specific guidelines or expectations about who can touch a man or a woman, where on their bodies either can be touched, and under which circumstances. In one long-term facility, when a male attendant was helping a Chinese American woman put on her shoes, the woman blushed. After cultural consultation it was discovered that in Chinese culture it is not appropriate for a man to touch a woman's feet. In traditional Mexican families, it is not appropriate for a daughter to provide personal care for her father, so in a long-term care environment, it may not be appropriate for a young Latina to offer care to an older Latino male. Sometimes it is difficult to elicit these cultural mores. Another example is that of a pregnant Japanese nursing assistant who declined repeatedly to care for a dying elder. Upon inquiry, she expressed that it is considered bad luck in her culture for a pregnant woman to be in the presence of a dying person. It is easy to unknowingly overstep cultural and religious boundaries.

AESTHETICS AND PERSONAL SPACE

Jaber Gubrium (1995), an anthropologist, made a significant breakthrough in understanding quality-of-care issues in long-term care through extensive interviews with nursing facility residents, specifically about their life experience. He found that aspects of their past informed their attitudes. Gubrium identified relationships between residents' personal histories and their perception of the quality of care in their nursing facility. In residents relating their personal histories, he heard "narrative links" that tended to manifest "horizons of meaning," which served as personal lenses for evaluating quality of care. His work provides a rationale for listening to the individual resident's life stories for clues to his or her perception of what quality care is and discussing how it relates to the resident's present living situation. Making corresponding adjustments in care could produce a high return in satisfaction.

An important dimension of resident care is honoring residents' space. It can be helpful to reflect on how, during the life cycle, people move from a small crib to larger worlds of home, school, work, community, and worldly influence. Then, as people age and, particularly, become more frail, their space and influence on the world begins to shrink. For some, the realm of influence becomes restricted first to the home, then to a few rooms, and then to a bed. For most residents in long-term care facilities, their sense of space has become limited to one half of a room with a few drawers that hold their few personal belongings. In appreciating the losses that these changes represent and respecting residents' space and belongings, staff should acknowledge this space and ask residents if they would allow staff to get a particular item from a drawer or cupboard. Sometimes, a resident will make what seems like unreasonable demands (e.g., keeping a particular wheelchair for their use, coveting a particular chair in the activity room). In negotiating these requests, it helps to acknowledge the losses of personal space and control that this individual has experienced. The resident may not be conscious of this need motivating his or her demands. Nonetheless, staff members can bring a more informed perspective to the situation.

One way for residents to experience a sense of belonging is to be allowed to create their own sense of order and beauty in their living space. Staff may enhance this experience by bringing residents' attention to the presence of nature outside their window or to patterns of daylight. Many residents have one or more framed pictures of family, a religious object, or some other treasured object that they may want in view. Many residents take great pleasure in flowers as sources of beauty and important pathways of connection—a single blossom in a small vase when staff can manage it can be enough. Music is another important avenue for many elders.

Finally, the opportunity to enhance the personal appearance of residents in ways that respect their individuality and give them pleasure is also key. Family members can be involved in providing personal care items: moisturizers, lipstick, nail polish, or a preferred shaving cream. Certain gifts are also appropriate: clothing, a cassette tape or CD player, plants, pillows, prints for the wall, and so forth. When the resident is involved in selections, it fosters his or her sense of self.

EXERCISE

Write the following three headings across the top of the board or newsprint:

Issues of Aesthetics, Personal Space, and Belonging	Approaches	Results

Ask staff members to identify examples of each. Provide some of the following examples to help prompt suggestions.

Resident requests a manicure.	Suggestion is made to the activity director to involve families and volunteers to make this available to residents.	Manicures become a new activity for residents and families.
Buddhist resident wants to burn incense during her daily prayer.	Arrangements are made for resident to be able to use a patio for an altar, for prayer, and for burning incense.	Resident is satisfied with the outcome.
Resident complains that her favorite nightgown is missing.	Resident's attachment to her nightgown is acknowledged and validated. A nursing aide takes responsibility for contacting the laundry unit and discovers that the nightgown has been	Resident and family are appreciative of facility's concern and communication.

| | damaged and discarded. The aide contacts the family, who purchases a similar gown. | |
| Vietnamese male resident refuses to be bathed indoors; he prefers a bath outside in a private garden. | A family meeting is called. After much discussion, a family elder convinces the man that in the United States, this is shameful to a family and that deceased elders would not be happy. | The resident reluctantly accepts showering indoors. |

DISCUSSION

Identify situations similar to those described above that occur in the context of personal care or present themselves in a social activity in which a wish, conflict, or need is expressed. These would be listed in the column *Issues of Aesthetics, Personal Space, and Belonging*. Ask the participants to generate possible *Approaches* and describe *Results*. After describing five or six situations, starting with the issue, and then possible approaches and expected or actual outcomes, ask participants about the level of satisfaction for both the resident and the caregiver when the resident's issues were addressed. Discuss how much extra effort was required to meet these needs and wishes and if the caregiver's addressing of the need was reasonable. Was the family or a friend involved in solving the issue? Did any issues need to be referred to administration? Beginning the next in-service training with a review of this content and discussion is recommended to both reinforce the material and to identify new perspectives resulting from implementation.

RELATIONSHIP-CENTERED CARE

A close examination of the framework for the delivery of resident nursing services reveals a very task-oriented structure. Within this task-oriented model, success is measured by the number of baths given, beds made, meals fed, medications delivered, and so forth. This is understandable given what needs to be accomplished in any one day, but the approach can be mechanical and not conducive to recognizing the personal, social, environmental, and spiritual needs of residents as discussed in this chapter. One remedy to this task orientation is a person-centered approach, which emphasizes holistic care and more effective ways of communicating with and engaging residents and their families. When implemented in facilities, the person-centered model has improved the care given and has made staff members much more aware of the whole person in their care.

Beginning in the 1990s, a new model was developed that highlights the *relationship* of the caregiver and the care receiver as the *container* for quality care. This model fosters healthy relationships and honors preference and choice, self-awareness and nonjudgmental presence, trust and interest in learning, cooperation and negotiation, special needs and special talents, appreciation and satisfaction, and a sense of beauty and joy. The well-being of the facility's staff, as well as its residents, needs to be a priority for this model to be effective. Staff and resident councils, therefore, need to be involved in accommodating this model to a specific facility. The goals for a facility adopting this model include empowering residents and staff, welcoming responsibility, elevating the status of residents and staff, improving coordination among staff and services, and increasing the potential for healing and personal satisfaction.

PAUSE TO REFRESH

Relationship-centered care is only possible when the staff is committed to self-care. It may seem impossible to pay attention to staff needs in the midst of so many other demands in the facility. David Kundtz (1998), however, in his work with health and social service professionals, stresses how critical the practice of "stopping" is. Stopping is doing nothing as much as possible for a definite period of time (e.g., from one second to one month) for the purpose of becoming more fully awake and remembering who one is (Kundtz, 1998). He invites people to practice stopping often throughout each day as well as to schedule time apart from the work setting and the demands of others. According to Kundtz, the benefits of stopping include enriching one's sense of purpose and the capacity for renewal and relaxation.

Many people prefer to take their breaks with others and find that the socializing helps them relax. Time spent alone, however, is an option that should not be forgotten. A simple headset with CDs of nature music can turn break time into a time of deep relaxation and peace. A staff break room can include this type of equipment at a very low cost to encourage staff meditation and stress reduction.

Chapter 11 provides in-depth information about self-care. It explores self-care from many perspectives and suggests not only personal remedies but educational and administrative strategies as well.

SENSE OF PLACE

The isolation that residents may experience often has to do with living within the confines of an institution, having little, if any, sense of place. Connecting with the particularities of a place offers many potential healing dimensions and ways of enriching spirituality.

Different people define place in different ways. For many, a connection to the natural world supports their own life or natural cycles. Another definition of place focuses on the part of the country and state where a care facility is located, along with characteristics of this unique physical location including the seasons of the year, natural inhabitants, weather patterns, bird migrations, soil composition, terrain, flowers and plants, and insects.

A social and cultural definition of *place* is the particular city, town, or neighborhood with its distinct population, history, community leaders, parks, community gardens, colleges, temples and churches, libraries, orchestras and bands, and museums. This also includes community sports teams, popular and cultural folkways, local heroes, newspapers, celebrations, ethnic foods, parades, schools, corner markets and other small businesses, and local restaurants. Each small or large city and neighborhood has its distinct characteristics: the way the streets are laid out, the number and type of schools, the types of trees that line the streets, and even its animals and birds.

One way to help residents feel more comfortable in their "place" is by helping them connect to life outside of the nursing facility. Each staff member can encourage this connection through his or her interaction with the residents (e.g., pointing to a newly blooming plant outside a resident's window, purchasing items at a local farmer's market, reading news from the local paper about a political election, identifying birds in the area). The possibilities are limitless and very rewarding.

One of the most tangible connections of people to a place can be created through a horticulture or gardening circle. Residents can become part of an annual seasonal planting cycle in at least some small area of the grounds or in an enclosed atrium located on the premises. They can see how the seasonal changes affect plants and can have some involvement in planting or designating certain areas for planting. In some cases, local school children can become involved in these projects and earn credit for their participation. Park rangers from the County Park Commission can be invited to discuss the natural environment of the local area. In some cases, residents can be taken on a field trip to see the beauty of nature in a local preserve with a guide from a local environmental organization or a park ranger. Residents can also be given responsibility for the care of plants in their own room. This will help to define their sense of place in their personal environment.

The sense of place has a lot to do with feeling at home in the place where a person lives. This feeling of belonging to a specific community can be encouraged and developed by the staff in many ways. Each person has particular needs, desires, and expectations that help him or her to feel comfortable, and these needs, wants, and expectations help to define a person's identity and relationship with others (see Chapter 3). It can be something as simple as helping a resident to mount a family picture on his or her wall or prepare a collage of pictures for display in his or her room. Pictures can be a wonderful way to help residents connect with one another as well as to connect with family. Staff can arrange times for residents to share their pictures of family members, particularly during holiday seasons when there is so much emphasis on family coming together to celebrate.

A sense of place can also be fostered during holiday celebrations. (e.g., Chinese New Year, Juneteenth, Day of the Dead; see Chapter 8). At Christmastime each year, residents can add their own particular decoration to the Christmas tree. Chinese New Year is a time for decorating and sharing food, song, and family rituals. For residents who are alert but frail, staff can help them make a very simple decoration that has their name on it. Local churches, schools, and choral groups are often willing and eager to have their choirs come to a nursing facility to sing with residents for different holidays and holy days. For each holiday celebration, staff and residents create traditions that become part of a long-term care community. Residents and staff look forward to these times of year, and they can always add or modify certain elements of a celebration as new residents enter the facility.

Other resources in the surrounding community can be tapped to enrich the sense of place for residents. The immediate neighborhood of a nursing facility can be a fertile ground for development of outreach programs that connect the home to the surrounding community. As staff members visit nearby businesses, schools, and churches, they can explore what new roles these groups might play in the lives of the facility residents. For example, businesses could be encouraged to donate simple gifts for use as prizes in the recreational programs of the residents. Representatives from churches, synagogues, or temples can become part of a visiting program that supports those residents who have very few family members in the immediate area. Schools can arrange visits by children, who greatly influence the morale in a nursing facility. Be aware, however, that volunteers and children need some orientation to the facility and guidance in appropriate activities with residents.

DISCUSSION

1. What sights, sounds, smells, and memories do you associate with places where you have lived? Be as specific as possible.

2. What vivid memories do you have of the locale in which you grew up? What were the social and cultural interactions that took place in that environment?

3. What kinds of involvement did you and your family have with nature and with the activities and festivities of those areas?

Write the following two headings on the board:

Natural surroundings   **Social connections**

Ask participants to generate a collective list of experiences under each category based on their answers to the discussion questions about place. Encourage specificity.

EXERCISE

Ask for a volunteer recorder or assign one. Ask the recorder to write staff members' responses to the following questions on the board:

1. How important might the connections be with nature and the local neighborhood, with all of its particular activities, small businesses, and local events?

2. Write the following headings on the left side of the board, making room for additional headings on the right side of the board (use the examples under *Natural surroundings* and *Social and cultural connections* to help prompt suggestions from staff):

Present Connections for Residents

Natural surroundings	**Social and cultural connections**
After their morning bath, residents are encouraged to sit in the sun room or outside	A gospel choir sings for the residents every third Friday

How connected are the residents in your nursing facility to their natural setting and to the local community and its activities and folklore? List on the board the present ways that residents are connected and how those ways might be emphasized in the nursing facility.

3. What new connections to this particular place can be envisioned and implemented in the course of providing care for residents? Write the following headings on the right side of the board (use the examples under *Natural surroundings* and *Social and cultural connections* to help prompt suggestions from staff):

Potential Connections for Residents

Natural surroundings	**Social and cultural connections**
Someone from a local environmental group, who has knowledge of birds, is invited to share pictures of and information about local birds	A representative from a local community garden serves as a guide for residents to start a small vegetable garden on the nursing facility property

Note: For questions 2 and 3, generate a list of at least five suggestions in each column. Then, have the group evaluate the lists and prioritize suggestions for implementation. Select one specific intervention from each of the two subjects, *Present Connections for Residents* and *Potential Connections for Residents*.

Identify the steps for implementation, resources for implementation, and an appropriate estimate of time for follow-through. Identify someone in the group who would like to participate in the implementation. This individual will explore the resources for implementation with the director of nursing or director of in-service education.

TOOLKIT FOR HEALING

Caregiving is a healing art and, like any other art, requires self-knowledge. Each staff member brings particular gifts to the caregiving relationship. Some of these talents flow from personal attributes; others have been learned. Many people are unaware of their healing talents until a situation or relationship evokes or demands them. The idea of a *toolkit for healing* can help individuals be more aware of these personal talents for healing and encourage the appropriate use of them. Following are just a few examples to get staff members thinking about their own talents:

- Words: Using a resident's mother tongue, addressing a resident in a respectful way, a gentle awakening, expressing compassion through appropriate tone of voice and body language, using humor appropriately, providing mediation, and being reassuring

- Smiling: A way of greeting, an expression of warmth that evokes a presence of joy

- Celebration: A festive atmosphere with decorations, involving residents and families in activities such as music, singing, storytelling, and other expressive arts

- Breathing: Releasing pain and anxiety through focused use of breath

- Nature: Gardening, bird watching, animal visits, and floral arrangements

- Religious connections: Inviting a gospel choir to sing at the facility; rides to worship such as a Shabbat service, rosary circle, Bible study, or Buddhist chanting; and planning memorials for deceased residents

- Wellness: Gentle movement, relaxation, imagery, tai chi, yoga, and physical strength building that has an impact on a person's physical, emotional, and mental wellness

The idea of the toolkit is for each staff member to identify specific qualities, talents, and skills that characterize and create a healing experience. Any experience that may be described as comforting, pleasurable, and uplifting or that restores dignity and provides joy, peace, encouragement, hope, and connection could be considered healing. Staff can be encouraged to create physical "kits" that contain reminders about healing practices. Such a kit can be individualized for the unique abilities of each staff member or can be a collection of helpful ideas.

EXERCISE

Guide participants through a relaxation exercise for about 8–10 minutes. This exercise focuses on understanding how to use focused breathing to care for the self and for residents. The facilitator can say: *Let's begin by putting down anything that we are holding and placing our feet flat on the floor. Assume a comfortable position with your back as straight as possible. This exercise is meant to support and refresh you, so don't worry about whether you are doing it correctly.*

Gently close your eyes and bring your attention to your breathing. Simply focus on your breathing without trying to change it.

(Pause)

Now that your attention is on your breath, think about your process of inhaling, or taking a breath in and then exhaling, or letting go of a breath. Focus on inhaling and exhaling for a few breaths. Again, you are not trying to change your breathing; you are just focusing your attention on your breathing cycle.

(Pause)

As you exhale your next breath, think of letting go of any stress, worry, or discomfort that you may be experiencing. If it helps, you can exaggerate exhaling by slightly bending over as you exhale and making your exhalation audible (demonstrated by the facilitator). *As you do this, imagine that, as you let go of your breath, you are letting go of any negative experiences that are being held in your body. Let's just do that for a minute.*

(Pause)

Now, I want you to focus on some quality that you want or need at this time and imagine that you can inhale that quality (e.g., peace, energy, joy) as you take in a breath. Now, we are just going to focus on inhaling that quality with a few in-breaths. Realize that you can use your breath as a way of opening and receiving this quality, this peace or strength, that you need at this time.

(Pause)

Now, as we focus our attention on our breath, we want to think about what we have learned together. Starting with exhalation, we want to let go of worry, pain, fatigue, or distress as we breathe out. Immediately after that, inhale whatever it is that you feel you need. We will just continue that together for a minute.

(Pause)

Let's gently bring ourselves back together now, opening our eyes and slowly returning our attention to the room. You have just been introduced to a healing tool.

DISCUSSION

1. How was the relaxation exercise for you? Does anyone want to share their experience?

2. Was focusing on your breathing a helpful way to relax?

3. Can you think of any times that relaxation or breathing techniques such as this could be helpful to residents? In what specific ways? Would you like more training in relaxation through breathing?

EXERCISE

Provide participants with the following materials:
plastic pocket liners (one per participant; these can be purchased at uniform shops)
a variety of stickers
file cards (3" x 5")
colored pens and markers
a large work table

Encourage participants to close their eyes and recall positive experiences that they have had as nursing assistants with their residents. Ask them to think about how they would describe that experience (e.g., Did they feel a connection? A sense of gratitude on the part of the resident for something they had done? Some sensitivity they brought to the interaction?) and what contributed to the positive, and possibly healing, quality of the experience. Perhaps it was something they did or brought to the interaction or something they were able to foster in the relationship. Encourage participants to identify what they did or what talent or personal quality they brought to the care that seemed to have this desired effect. (See list of personal talents for healing on p. 39.)

Distribute the plastic pocket liners. Put the other materials in the center of the table, available to all. Reintroduce the concept of the "toolkit for healing"—a way of making explicit the healing ways that each staff member cares for residents. Encourage staff members to mirror each other's gifts in a noncompetitive way. Allow sufficient time for everyone to decorate their pocket liner and decorate and write out some cards to represent their talents and tools for healing. Ask everyone to share some new understanding or image of healing that has come to them from working on their own toolkit for healing. Encourage participants to share one of their tools (e.g., "My smile puts others at ease").

Everyone has daily rituals that guide many of their personal activities (e.g., a morning walk or run, a cup of tea before going to bed) from the time they first awaken in the morning until they go to sleep at the end of the day. The vast majority of people have the physical ability and the personal resources to enact these rituals in routine ways. Nursing facility residents typically have neither the ability nor the resources to control their daily rhythms, which can deprive them of a sense of identity.

It is important to recognize the profound loss and disorientation that institutionalization represents. One of the most basic ways to include spirituality in long-term care is through respect and support for personal preferences, individual differences (e.g., getting out of bed early each day), and autonomy as often as possible. Through honoring such specific requests, care providers restore the face of dignity to residents.

ACTION STEPS

1. Which of the learning objectives from this chapter do you believe are most valued by your facility? By the instructor? By the participants?

2. Which exercises were most useful? Think of ways to use what you have learned in your daily care practices.

3. Discuss methods for identifying cultural and ethnic viewpoints among residents and staff and how this knowledge can be communicated effectively throughout the facility.

4. Describe other forms that the "toolkit for healing" could take in your facility. How can the healing gifts of nursing assistants, especially, be recognized?

5. How will positive changes that result from this training be identified, rewarded, and maintained?

REFERENCES

Gubrium, J.C. (1995). Perspective and story in nursing home ethnography. In J.N. Henderson & M.D. Vesperi (Eds.), *The culture of long term care: Nursing home ethnography* (pp. 23–26). Westport, CT: Bergin and Garvey.

Kundtz, D. (1998). *Stopping: How to be still when you have to keep going.* Berkeley, CA: Conari Press.

Puchalski, C., & Romer, A.L. (2000). Taking a spiritual history allows clinicians to understand patients more fully. *Journal of Palliative Medicine, 3*(1), 129–137.

RECOMMENDED READING

Culture & Nursing Care: A Pocket Guide edited by Juliene G. Lipson, Suzanne L. Dibble, and Pamela A. Minarik (Available from UCSF Nursing Press, School of Nursing, University of California–San Francisco, 521 Parnassus Avenue, San Francisco, California 94143; Telephone: 415-476-4992; http://nurseweb.ucsf.edu/www/book.)

Healing Words: The Power of Prayer and the Practice of Medicine by Larry Dossey (HarperSanFrancisco)

Irresistible Communication: Creative Skills for the Health Professional by Mark King, Larry Novik, and Charles Citrenbaum (W.B. Saunders)

Kitchen Table Wisdom: Stories that Heal by Rachel Naomi Remen (Riverhead
   Books)

RESOURCES

Diversity, Healing and Health Care
Web site: http://www.gasi.org/diversity.htm

Diversity, Healing and Health Care is a resource for clinicians who work
with patients whose cultures and religions are different from their own.

The George Washington Institute for Spirituality and Health (GWISH)
The George Washington University Medical Center
Warwick Building, Room 336
2300 K Street, NW
Washington, DC 20037
Telephone: 202-994-0971
Web site: http://www.gwish.org

This web site addresses the FICA model of taking a spiritual history (spiritual assessment).

Pioneer Network
Post Office Box 18648
Rochester, New York 14618
Telephone: 585-271-7570
Web site: http://www.pioneernetwork.net
E-mail: rosemarie.fagan@pioneernetwork.net

The Pioneer Network seeks to change the culture of aging for the 21st
century to one that is "life-affirming, satisfying, human and meaningful."

Eldergivers
1755 Clay Street
San Francisco, California 94109
Telephone: 415-441-2650
Web site: http://www.eldergivers.org
E-mail: info@eldergivers.org

Eldergivers is a reciprocal model of giving and receiving in interactions
with older adults living in nursing facilities, assisted living facilities, and
residential care facilities.

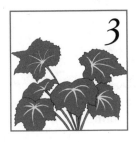

Circle of Support

Creating a Caring Community for Residents, Staff, and Families

Julie Barton

OBJECTIVES

As a result of reading this chapter and working through the exercises, participants will be able to

1. Broaden conventional definitions of *family*

2. Describe the advantages of creating a caring community for residents, families, and staff

3. Develop a greater understanding of spiritual concerns in long-term care settings

4. Identify the issues that entering long-term care may present to the resident, family, and staff

CONCEPTS OF FAMILY

How in the world can the word *family* be defined? Does family refer only to blood relatives? Who else might be included in the definition? The answer may depend on a particular culture, family upbringing, or expectations of how society in general defines family.

EXERCISE

Write on paper your personal definition of *family,* and compile a list of the people whom you would consider family. This exercise shows us that we tend to evaluate others' notion of family by what we each deem important to us. It also shows us that we can expand our horizons if we remain open-minded.

DISCUSSION

1. Are you surprised by others' definitions of family or by the people on others' lists?

2. How has hearing other people's opinions affected yours?

3. What changes, if any, might you make to your definition(s) as a result?

4. What do you think are your reasons for your original definitions?

In working with the families of residents, staff may need to expand some of their personal notions of family. Many long-time friends, especially in some cultures, are considered family, and certainly gay or lesbian partners need to be included as family. Members of volunteer groups, churches, or religious and fraternal organizations may be considered family over time. Neighbors and former co-workers may also assume this status, especially if blood relatives live at a distance or are uninvolved or deceased. If a family member is defined as someone who has had a long and perhaps loving relationship with a resident, then a more inclusive definition of family emerges.

The word *loving* does not necessarily mean free from tension or anger, but it does imply a certain staying power that is usually part of the concept of family. Indeed, staff in long-term care facilities often assume the role of surrogate family after a time, and this can be both a desirable and beautiful thing. This relationship is not in competition with relationships among actual family members but can often be a way for the resident to continue feeling valued and loved when family cannot be present.

THE CONCEPT OF MUTUALITY

The interface for residents, families, and staff, no matter how it is defined, provides a unique opportunity to focus on the spiritual well-being of everyone concerned, rather than on the issues that can bring misunderstandings and tension. Everyone has a role in this system of interaction, and everyone can give as well as take. The customary perception within various roles of caregiving that one is "caring for" instead of "caring with" other individuals may require a radical shift in thinking and possibly in training before it gives way to the concept of mutuality in long-term care. Perhaps even more difficult for members of helping professions may be relinquishing caregiving roles and accepting care for oneself. Family members often have the same reluctance to accept care and help, even when they are worn out by the caregiving role.

It is understandable to fear that a policy of mutual care and inclusion will not be cost or time effective and will create more work for staff. However, it is possible that just the opposite may happen: Including residents and families in the loop of effective communication around care and well-being may actually free staff time and lighten task loads.

DISCUSSION

1. What are some ways of including residents and family members in certain tasks or decision-making processes as well as in activities?

2. In what ways are you already practicing this?

3. If this is not yet a policy, what would it take to include family members as a part of the care system in your facility?

Consider the following more specific discussion questions:

1. At home, Mr. R always provided special treats for his wife around mealtime: a flower, a funny story,

favorite candy. How could the facility consult with Mr. R to continue giving Mr. R's wife some form of treat?

2. Mrs. Z is used to having certain things done at particular times: fresh sheets and towels in the morning, a clean nightgown at bedtime. If this does not fit the facility's schedule, how could the facility bring in a family member to plan a way to accommodate Mrs. Z?

3. Ms. H eats a hearty breakfast and a good lunch. At dinner, however, she picks at her food and seems depressed but claims to be fine. How can you find out what might be causing this, and how might family members contribute to a solution?

MEETING THE NEEDS OF FAMILY

Families are usually intimately involved in the decision to place a relative in a long-term care setting and are naturally concerned with their family member's well-being during this time. We know that these decisions and responsibilities often come with emotional baggage: grief, guilt, reluctance, and sometimes relief. Including family members, whenever possible, in the system of day-to-day long-term care can be of enormous benefit. It is often a family member who can share a story, provide an explanation of certain behavior, and shed a little light on the personality of a particular resident. By so doing, family members can ease the task load of a staff member who is concerned about the spiritual and physical well-being of a resident and, at the same time, can be present as an advocate for the resident. Many family members will also find that being included in their relative's care plan will meet their own spiritual and emotional needs, as well as the needs of the resident. They will feel included again in the caregiving that they may have once provided themselves.

Family members do have needs of their own. Their long history with a loved one, whether a difficult relative or a treasured spouse or partner, gives rise to emotional and spiritual needs that can easily go unrecognized and unmet in the pressure of tasks at hand. We often hear the phrase "unfinished business"; for family members, this can be the need to forgive or be forgiven, to talk out old grievances, to deal with their guilt about placing their loved one in a nursing facility, to remember and celebrate the good times, and to say their thank-yous and good-byes.

EXERCISE

Complete the first two questions as a private writing exercise. Then, share your answers for the third and fourth questions with the group.

1. Think of your own family situation, if you are willing. What are some areas of unfinished business for you or other family members?

2. How do you deal with these issues?

3. How might your experience guide you in talking with families of the resident?

4. Try to see this in the light of spiritual needs. What might some of those needs be?

In order to better understand this type of situation, consider the following practical case example.

MRS. SANCHEZ

Mrs. Sanchez has had several strokes, the most recent one quite severe. She is no longer able to walk by herself, her speech is significantly impaired, and she is incontinent. Her daughter, Rafaela, has been providing care but, as a recent widow, needs to return to work in order to support herself and two teenage children. The present level of care that is needed is also beyond what Rafaela can safely provide, and she has reluctantly talked with her mother about nursing facility care. Her mother is devastated at the prospect and fears that Rafaela will abandon her if she enters the nursing facility. Rafaela and Mrs. Sanchez visit a facility to discuss the options.

DISCUSSION

1. What sort of emotions do you think Rafaela is feeling at this time? Why? What would be some ways for staff to work with Rafaela and these emotions?

2. What about Mrs. Sanchez's emotions?

3. What might staff need to know about the ongoing relationship between Mrs. Sanchez, her daughter, and the grandchildren in order to honor both the individuals and their particular family system?

4. What cultural considerations might there be in this situation?

5. What spiritual needs might arise for Mrs. Sanchez, Rafaela, and their family?

6. What are some respectful ways in which these needs could be met or at least acknowledged?

7. Can you think of any advantages for staff in trying to meet these needs?

Some additional thoughts about what to look for in this discussion:

1. Rafaela's emotions may include various types of grief. She is a recent widow with many responsibilities. She may also feel that she is failing in her duty to both her mother and her children.

2. Loss is evident in Mrs. Sanchez's life. She has lost mobility and health and now must part from home and family. She may feel abandoned by God as well as by her family.

3. We might wonder about lifelong relationships here, especially the one between Mrs. Sanchez and her daughter. Has it been one of duty or exceptional loving? Have the grandchildren's needs been displaced by Mrs. Sanchez's needs in the home? The stress of being pulled in different directions may be taking a toll on each member of the family.

4. Does Rafaela feel that she is unworthy because of needing to place her mother in others' care? Have the grandchildren been able to maintain traditional respect throughout this time?

5. Spiritual and emotional needs intertwine here and are almost indistinguishable. Dealing with pain, loss,

guilt, and feelings of abandonment are issues in both areas.

6. The most respectful thing we can do is listen and honor these legitimate feelings and, eventually, stress that the family is still a part of the care process. Known and respected clergy might also be consulted if staff can be sure of clergy's willingness to be non-judgmental.

7. By honoring the needs of the Sanchez family, steps will be taken to ward off problems in the future. *After truly being heard,* it is doubtful that family members would displace guilt or anger on the facility.

MEETING THE NEEDS OF STAFF

We also need to consider the spiritual needs of the staff person. He or she may be expected to meet everyone else's needs, to always be cheerful and courteous. Staff members have their own set of concerns and losses: Providing care on a daily basis is not only physically and emotionally challenging but spiritually challenging as well. It is sad to lose a resident, to watch an inevitable decline, or to be aware of rifts in family relationships that are difficult to mend. It is also sometimes hard to put personal problems aside when attending to others' needs. What are some ways that staff in a facility can be attentive to each other's needs, with due respect for privacy? Staff members can learn to see this as a spiritual task.

EXERCISE

1. Try to list at least three ways that you find satisfaction or joy in your work.

2. Now list three areas that are difficult for you or that make you sad in your daily work.

3. How do you take care of yourself or care for others when they are sad?

4. How do you share joyous moments?

5. Would you say that these areas are spiritual in nature? Why?

6. What are some ways that administration can support
    staff members in their daily work?

See Chapters 1 and 11 for more information on spiritual well-being
and self-care.

THE RESIDENT IS CENTRAL

The resident is in the middle of the care system. The greatest impact of
placement in a long-term care facility naturally falls on the resident. It is
she who has had to give up her home; it is he who has had to confront and
adapt to growing infirmity or to live apart from a spouse. The emotional
and spiritual needs may, in fact, be greater than the physical needs and yet
may go unexpressed or unacknowledged. (See Chapter 7 for information
about the effects of change and transitions.)

What does all of this say? It seems to illustrate the need for a kind of
"mutual presence," an opportunity for a care system to create something
that is more than just the sum of its three parts: residents, families, and
staff. It is a chance for residents, families, and staff to join together in creating a sacred space; a place of safety, well-being, and hope; in short, a
community of *healing* even when *cure* is not possible.

CONSIDERING OPTIONS

Table 1 illustrates some options for each group—residents, staff, and families—as well as the importance of creative choices that can be made in trying to meet the day-to-day needs of all concerned.

EXERCISE

How creative can *you* be in bridging the gap between the
two columns in Table 1 and in bringing about positive
change that will further the well-being, especially the spiritual well-being, of members of the care community?
Notice that the words in the opposing columns are not
always really opposite to each other in meaning. Some may
be simply a different way of looking at the situation. For
example, is there really any reason that someone cannot be

Table 1.   Effecting transformation

How can staff help residents transform feelings of	to a sense of
isolation	inclusion
illness	well-being, wholeness
limitations	possibilities
depression	hope
finality	fulfillment
resignation	acceptance
disruption	completion

How can staff help themselves effect transformation from feeling	to feeling
busy	engaged
distracted	prioritized
pleased	enjoyment
weary	self-caring
efficient	flexible
task oriented	person centered

How can staff help families effect transformation from feeling	to feeling
like strangers	like a community
interfering	consulting, supporting
exhausted	creative
guilty	grief
needy	fulfilled

both "efficient" and "flexible"? Perhaps flexibility can even improve our efficiency! Read the words in the left-hand column and briefly jot down any feelings that come up. Now read the words in the right-hand column. What feelings do you have? Can you begin to come up with a plan for building a "bridge" from the left column to the right? How can you help to create such a plan? Think about Mrs. Sanchez and her family or an actual resident in your facility as you come up with answers to these questions.

As a result of thinking through some of the points in this chapter and doing some of the suggested exercises, staff should now have a truly broad definition of *family*, one that recognizes the possibility that all three components of a care setting—residents, families, and staff—can become a community, a family in the truest sense of the word. And this is just the type of setting that becomes transformed into a sacred space, where spiritual and emotional needs, as well as physical needs, can be met.

ACTION STEPS

1. Discuss ways your facility can promote a "circle of support" as part of good spiritual care.

2. Look at ways an expanded notion of "family" could alter the way care is provided for each resident.

3. Think of ways that your facility can broaden the idea of family by inviting members of the community into the "circle of support."

RECOMMENDED READING

Multigenerational family therapy by David S. Freeman (Haworth Press)

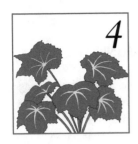

Messages of Truth and Hope

Promoting Effective Communication

Julie Barton

OBJECTIVES

As a result of reading this chapter and working through the exercises, participants will be able to

1. Increase their knowledge and use of good communication skills

2. Understand both the aids and barriers to good communication

3. Apply new skills in working with staff, residents, and families

4. Gain greater insight into cultural patterns of communication

5. Understand how good communication promotes spiritual care

TRUTHS, UNTRUTHS, AND MISCOMMUNICATION

Someone once said that communication takes place when the message received is the same as the message sent. Remember that old game, Telephone, in which everyone sits in a circle and a message is whispered from one person to another? Anyone who has ever played that game knows that when the last person in the circle gets the message and says it aloud, it is nothing like what the first person whispered. Everyone has a good laugh and wonders how in the world that message got so garbled. How, indeed, do messages get so garbled?

How often do people say or hear, "Oh, I didn't mean it that way!" Family quarrels, political calamities, and even wars have been started by miscommunication or misunderstandings of one kind or another. And perhaps not enough attention is paid to acceptable forms of communication from one culture to another, either. There is another, more subtle, point to be made here: Communication really depends on truth telling. Shading the truth, or telling outright lies, even to protect another's feelings, means people have not truly communicated. When an untruth has been discovered, trust can be lost; even if an untruth has not been discovered, the teller still knows that an untruth has been spoken.

It is a commonly held belief that communication presupposes a person's right to know certain things: the accuracy of a bank statement, when a child will be home after a date, and certainly, the accuracy of information from caregivers and health care providers about the state of one's health. In some cultures, such as some Asian cultures, however, it is not considered respectful to inform an older person of a serious or life-threatening diagnosis. It is important, therefore, to be sensitive to individual and cultural preferences. In doing this, effective communication becomes a delicate and spiritual issue.

EXERCISE

1. Examine your own feelings about being misinformed or uninformed about something that was important to you. What would your immediate reactions be if you knew that you had not been told the truth?

2. Think about the culture in which you were raised. How does your upbringing affect your thoughts and feelings about being told the truth?

3. Now write down an opinion you may have in this area regarding a person of a different culture. Would he or she want to know the truth? What would be his or her family's role in this situation? What is your role as a staff member?

4. Share your perceptions about the way that other cultures might deal with these questions.

Situations such as being told or not being told the truth may serve as real or perceived barriers to good communication. Other situations or problems might also inhibit communication. What if a resident has a hearing or visual impairment? What are some ways to ensure that the message received is the same as the message sent? There can be language difficulties, either because of cultural and ethnic differences or, possibly, damage caused by a stroke. Sometimes, the best policy is for staff members to acknowledge their inability to understand a resident. Simply saying, "I'm so sorry. I can't seem to understand" is honest and avoids blaming the resident for the difficulty. It also communicates a desire to care and to understand—both of which carry spiritual overtones.

EXERCISE

How can staff, in institutional settings, practice good communication? How can you make sure that the message received is indeed the message sent and that it is sent with compassion and care?

To begin, let's compare these two sentences:

1. You did a good job.

2. I know how busy you are this morning, and you still took the time to do this well.

Both sentences are examples of positive communication. Which one would you rather hear? Why? Now, compare these sentences:

1. You should have given Mrs. Jones a bath this morning.

2. I see that Mrs. Jones has not been bathed this morning. Can you tell me what happened?

If you had been the person who did not follow the schedule, which communication would you prefer hearing? Why? In the latter communication, the speaker will probably be able to get the information that he or she wants without the assistant becoming defensive. Why?

Much has been said about "I" messages and what powerful communication tools they can be. They are powerful because the speaker takes responsibility for his or her own thoughts and feelings, rather than putting the burden on the listener. In this way, a compliment gains momentum, a correction or disagreement loses its sting, and the listener feels validated. Consider the effect of "I'm so sorry that happened to you" rather than "Too bad that happened." Or, "Excuse me, I believe you dropped this" rather than "You dropped this." A subtle difference, perhaps, but one that can enhance how messages are received.

EXERCISE

Try to convert the following statements to "I" messages:

1.   You should fold the blanket this way.

2.   You need to pay more attention to details.

3.   That tray is not attractively arranged.

4.   Mr. Jones' room needs cleaning.

The following example is good for practice in communicating with "I" messages.

MRS. ARNOLD

Mrs. Arnold is a resident who has lived in a long-term care facility for 2 years and has recently been complaining to everyone, including family, staff, and residents, about the quality of the food. The staff knows that the quality of the food has not changed and that Mrs. Arnold has always been pleased in the past. Her discontent is puzzling.

EXERCISE

Break into dyads, with one person acting as Mrs. Arnold and one as a concerned staff member. The staff member will use "I" messages to get the following information:

1.   What are Mrs. Arnold's concerns about the food?

2.   Is the food her real concern, or is there a deeper problem or problems? What might those problems be?

Depending on the answers, how can you best communicate your care and concern to Mrs. Arnold if the food is not the real issue and you know Mrs. Arnold has enjoyed the food in the past?

HEARING METAMESSAGES

The previous exercise may also reveal another aspect of communication: the *metamessage*, or the underlying meaning of what a person actually says. The metamessage is often the real message unconsciously cloaked in a cover story. Consider how the staff addresses a spiritual need by looking for Mrs. Arnold's metamessage. A common complaint adults hear from children is "I have a tummy ache!" when what they might really mean is that they don't want to go to school or participate in an event. It doesn't take long for a clever parent to decipher what a child really means! Another classic: "You never bring me flowers!" Metamessage: "You don't love me!" Similarly, Mrs. Arnold may be using the food complaint to communicate distress of a different kind: Perhaps she is depressed or feeling neglected or ignored. She may also be trying to tell staff that she is lonely or not feeling well and that eating seems like a chore or is unappetizing. If staff members take the time to "hear" Mrs. Arnold's metamessage and to communicate to Mrs. Arnold that they have heard her concerns, they will surely have contributed to her physical and spiritual health and well-being and perhaps even have averted a greater health or morale problem.

EXERCISE

In what ways do we communicate? (Some answers might include body language [e.g., crossing our arms on our chests], silence, handshakes, eye contact or lack of it, and touch.) Record these answers on a piece of paper. Now break into dyads. Each person in turn picks an emotion and tries to communicate it to his or her partner using only nonverbal messages. Discuss this method of communication. Was it easy? Difficult? Was the message received just as it was sent?

Return to the idea that communication is about truth. Most people can recall from personal experience a time when someone in authority or in a position of trust failed to tell the truth or glossed it over. Chances are they felt upset and possibly even betrayed upon learning the truth. How does this play out with an older adult or resident as staff members, in their desire to "protect" the person, fail to honor the person's need for truth? Much of the staff may be too uncomfortable with the issues that confront older or chronically ill residents and their families and thus avoid any mention of them. It becomes a challenge to honor the resident's right to truth and overcome personal discomfort with the realities. It is helpful to keep in mind the goal of patient-centered care while practicing effective communication techniques.

OVERCOMING BARRIERS TO EFFECTIVE COMMUNICATION

In their article on good patient care and communication around difficult issues, Dale Larson and Daniel R. Tobin spoke to this issue and recognized that "no single health care professional can successfully undertake all aspects of this challenge" (2000, p. 1577). They further suggested that it is helpful to focus on the patient's experience of his or her situation, asking what his or her fears and worries might be, and to talk about practical issues.

The staff is trying to navigate the two-way stream of communication, and that is not always easy, especially if there are cultural considerations with which staff may not be familiar. In these cases, the staff needs to respect areas of privacy. Perhaps a simple statement might suffice: "Mr. Jones, I'm not sure whether you want to talk about this now. Could you tell me if you do?" or "Mr. Jones, I wonder if I could help to explain some of the information you've been given. Is that something you'd like?" If such a approach is not feasible, there are other ways to obtain needed information. Residents' charts are available, but staff can also obtain information respectfully by keeping eyes and ears—and hearts!—open. For example, what do a resident's keepsakes, such as plants or pictures, say about his or her preferences and history? A gentle inquiry can be a useful gateway: "I see you have a picture of a little dog. I'd love to know something about him. Would you be willing to tell me?" That being said, staff members need to take their cue from the resident's willingness or reticence and be willing to drop the subject if that is the signal they receive.

In the area of spiritual care, staff members can also note whether the resident has pictures, religious articles, books, or perhaps a small altar to respectfully inquire about. Again, staff must be willing to take a cue from the resident. If the resident is unwilling to reveal the meaning of his or her belongings, that is communication enough.

The staff also needs to consider altering communication styles to fit a resident's culture, needs, and capabilities, while simultaneously avoiding the temptation to exclude or infantilize the resident. It is inappropriate to talk with a third party in the presence of a resident as if he or she were not there. It is unkind to speak in a different language so that a resident is shut out entirely. A resident's visual or hearing impairments must be taken into consideration. Determining a resident's dominant "sensory modality" may be useful. In other words, does the resident rely more on hearing, seeing, or perhaps his or her sense of touch? Even if a person is now visually impaired who previously was not, he or she will still use and respond to visual words such as "I see!"

EXERCISE

The five modalities are visual, auditory, kinesthetic (tactile), olfactory (smell), and gustatory (taste). Do you know what your own dominant sensory modality is? Take this test: Write the word *lemon* on the board, and say the word. Then, ask each participant to cite the first thing that comes into his or her mind. If the participant's dominant sensory modality is visual, his or her response might be "yellow" or "round." If auditory, the response might be "the sound of a squirt" or "a knife slicing through it." If kinesthetic, the response might be "bumpy" or "cool." If olfactory, the response might be "fresh" or "pungent." If gustatory, the answer might be "sour."

DISCUSSION

1. What words can you use to reflect your own and possibly a resident's dominant sensory modality?

2. How does sensitivity in this area reflect good spiritual care?

Using words that reflect the senses most important to a resident honors and augments that resident's understanding of what has been said. Doing this offers and reflects good spiritual care: Residents will very likely feel heard and understood, and there may even be a spark of friendship between a staff member and a resident.

THE VALUE OF LISTENING

This chapter on communication cannot be concluded without acknowledging that there is such a thing as too much communication and perhaps even too much truth telling. It is not up to staff to shatter a resident's illusions about him- or herself, especially without consultation with other professionals or family members. This is especially important when a resident's capacity to understand is impaired or when a resident is coping with a difficult situation by using a healthy form of denial.

EVELYN

Evelyn had been placed in a skilled nursing facility by her son. She was in the early stages of dementia, and her son never came to visit her. In the course of his visits to Evelyn's nursing facility, the chaplain learned from the staff that the son did not come to visit, but Evelyn informed the chaplain that her son was very attentive and visited often. This was *her* truth, and the chaplain realized that it would be cruel indeed to impose the objective truth on her. Instead, he just listened.

"He just listened." It is impossible to overestimate the value of "just listening," especially in a chapter on communication. Too often, and understandably, people tend to think of communication as doing something, rather than just being with someone. But consider how a smile can brighten a day; think about the person who sits down next to another upon learning he is sad and takes his hand, about the friend who opens her arms wide and gives a huge hug of congratulations, and about the person who really pays attention and doesn't try to "fix" anything when a friend pours out troubles. So much can be communicated by just listening, just being with someone.

In the early 1990s, David Freeman, a social worker and therapist who has worked with Holocaust survivors and their families, coined the phrase *safe witness,* a truly spiritual concept. By being a safe witness, a person becomes truly present to another's pain or joy, allowing that person to be secure in the knowledge that someone is listening with his or her heart. This is perhaps the best and purest form of communication that people can ever practice.

Good communication is truly a spiritual issue in care facilities. When people care enough to make sure that the message received is the same as the message sent, whether between staff members or between staff and residents or families, they are honoring those other people. When people truly listen to another's joy or pain without intruding with their own agenda, and when they honor and remember that people in cultures other than their own might choose to communicate in different ways, then people develop the sensitivity that is part of good spiritual care and that contributes to the well-being of everyone involved.

ACTION STEPS

1. Think of a time in your life when someone was a safe witness for you. Discuss your remembered feelings. How was it helpful to you at the time?

2. How have you been a safe witness to a friend or a resident? What was the result?

3. Using some of the ideas in this chapter—or your own ideas—discuss ways that communication might continue to improve in your facility.

REFERENCE

Larson, D.G., & Tobin, D.R. (2000). End-of-life conversations: Evolving practice and theory. *Journal of the American Medical Association, 284*(12), 1577.

RESOURCES

Contact a local adult education district or community college for classes on effective communication. Most of these institutions publish and mail detailed brochures and have web sites that are easily accessible. Many adult education and community college personnel actually conduct classes on numerous subjects for residents and staff in long-term care facilities, often without charge to the facility.

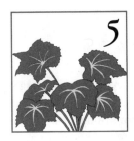

The Need for Connection

Examining Attitudes and Values About Intimacy and Sexuality

Julie Barton

OBJECTIVES

As a result of reading this chapter and working through the exercises, participants will be able to

1. Expand their insights into their own personal attitudes and values in the areas of sexuality and intimacy

2. Continue to develop understanding and tolerance for others' values in these areas

3. Differentiate between sexuality and intimacy

4. Explore ways to include sexual and intimacy needs in assessment and interview settings

5. Clarify spiritual and ethical implications when dealing with sexuality and intimacy in the facility

6. Review and discuss current facility policies regarding sexuality and intimacy

SEXUALITY AND INTIMACY

People's sexual identities help to define who people are as human beings, and sexual expression is one of the pathways to meaning and joy in life. Similarly, the need for intimacy—with oneself, a loved one, or a higher being—is basic to human nature. Each person needs to feel known, understood, touched.

Both intimacy and sexuality are about connection. Yet, when working with older people, staff members sometimes, possibly because of their own discomfort, ignore, label as "inappropriate" or fail to honor these very human needs. To relieve such discomfort and to acknowledge that these areas touch both residents' physical and spiritual beings, facility staff need to become educated. The desire for closeness, belonging, and intimacy does not diminish with age and should not be ignored. Good spiritual care will allow for understanding, compassion, and openness toward these often misunderstood and under-valued areas of a person's very self-hood. Informing staff attitudes and setting policies regarding sexuality and intimacy in long-term care settings is admittedly not easy but well worth the effort.

Simply put, sexuality and intimacy are basic human needs—needs of the spirit and psyche, as well as the physical body. Human beings are not seen with their spirits sitting on one chair, their bodies on another, and their thoughts and emotions on still another. The physical body is home to the spirit and the psyche, and these three elements cannot be separated.

MRS. D.

Mrs. D. never smiled or reached out to anyone until a volunteer in her nursing facility brought a young boy along to do magic tricks. Mrs. D. looked at the boy, and her face lit up in a huge smile as she reached out to grasp his hand.

What can be learned from this? Perhaps Mrs. D. had no way of expressing her need to touch and be touched until she saw the boy, when her need for human contact took over. She may have perceived the child as a safe person, and if that is so, the adults in this setting have somehow failed in whatever attempts they have made to meet her needs. Mrs. D.'s story happens over and over again, and because the need for connection, for intimacy, is so fundamental to the human spirit, this topic is included in this book.

A beautiful example of intimacy was provided by a woman who came every evening to visit her husband, who had Alzheimer's disease, in a nursing facility. She would prepare him for sleep and then gently lie down beside him, holding him and snuggling until he fell asleep. This closeness undoubtedly meant a great deal to both husband and wife and grew out of a long and loving life together.

JIM AND ALICE

Jim and Alice met one another in their nursing facility. They each have some dementia involving short-term memory loss and occasional confusion. They are not married to each other but have formed a trusting friendship and often hold hands as they sit together. Jim's wife, Grace, who does not reside in the nursing facility, and other members of Jim's family became very upset when they discovered this and demanded that the two be separated.

DISCUSSION

1. What are the issues here?

2. Who will be most affected by allowing the situation to continue?

3. Who will be most affected by separating Jim and Alice?

4. Perhaps a similar situation has happened in your facility. What did you do?

5. What should staff do when confronted with this situation?

Sexuality and intimacy can be closely related, but they are not necessarily the same. The need for intimacy, for connection with not only the inner self but with others and with a transcendent being, encompasses physical needs and enriches life in other ways. It may seem strange to speak of intimacy with oneself when the focus of interactions is usually on relating to others. However, self-knowledge and self-acceptance precede meaningful relationships with others and are part of late life development, what Erik Erikson (1986) referred to as the stage involving *integrity versus despair,* the search for integrity, or wholeness. People can work toward this integrity, or wholeness, by developing an acceptance of who they are and who they have been: not perfect, by any means, but at some sort of peace with their mistakes as well as their achievements. Through this acceptance, people can gradually become intimate and comfortable with themselves and able to relate to others in a deeper way. This task may be difficult indeed for elders who see themselves as burdens or as no longer needed, and it is for this reason that good spiritual care is essential—not to talk anyone out of their feelings but to acknowledge that this time of life can be difficult and to offer safe witness to emotional or spiritual pain. Becoming a companion to a family member or a resident in this developmental stage can be a richly rewarding experience and may, in the long run, work toward a more harmonious atmosphere in a care setting. It may also prepare staff for making a similar journey.

EXAMINING PERSONAL ATTITUDES

It may be helpful for each person to reflect on the attitudes and beliefs that he or she has picked up from present society and to understand, as well, that family, ethnicity, culture, and religion help to shape these attitudes and beliefs. It has been said that American society is preoccupied with sexual issues and, at the same time, woefully ignorant in the areas of both sexuality and intimacy. Fashion magazines seem to exploit sexuality, and the number of self-help books on the subject of sexuality and intimacy seem to indicate that Americans are seeking ever more information.

The lack of awareness or understanding is especially apparent in how these needs in older people are viewed. This ignorance becomes hurtful when the needs of older people are expressed in catch phrases such as "dirty old man," "foxy lady," and "act your age." No one stops to think about their implications. They suggest that sexual expression is inappropriate after a certain age. They label as *cute* an older man and woman holding hands. The attitude that intimate behavior is *inappropriate* spills over into care settings, especially if a man and woman are not married to each other.

Must all expressions of affection after a certain age and in certain communities be frowned upon? It is essential to reflect compassionately—and accurately—on these important matters.

EXERCISE

One or more of the following questions are to be answered in a private writing exercise. Staff can be asked to share their responses if they feel comfortable doing so.

1. What are my beliefs concerning sexual expression at any age? What informs these beliefs (e.g., culture, family, gender, religion, society)?

2. How do I feel about same-sex relationships? Again, what informs my beliefs?

3. How do I feel about sexual expression among older people? Among those who are not married to each other? Among those who may have cognitive impairments?

4. If I have noticed sexual activity among residents in my facility, what were my thoughts and feelings at the time?

5. What is the difference between sexuality and intimacy? Why is it important to reflect on the differences?

INFORMING FACILITY POLICIES

Sexuality, intimacy, and spirituality are not separate and distinct. It is only recently, however, that these issues have begun to be included in assessment forms and strategies. It is high time for it, but how to do it appropriately, kindly, and respectfully in an institution, especially in an era in which everyone is especially concerned about "inappropriate" behavior, is a challenge.

Granted, there will always be residents who cannot exercise a sexual form of intimacy or who do not, for whatever reason, wish to. These very same residents, however, may still have the need for some form of intimacy (e.g., a welcome touch; a gentle hug; time spent together in conversation, silence, or prayer), whether spiritual or physical, with another human being. Residents who are able to be sexual, however, may need to have this at least acknowledged by a conversation with a trusted staff member or in some type of support group or perhaps by a tactful assessment question.

It is not the purpose of this book to suggest how each and every facility should shape or change policy regarding sexual activity. It is, however, a resident's right and an ethical issue: Some residents may have a justifiable need for sexual expression, and others may need protection from unwanted overtures.

DISCUSSION

1. Think about your feelings when the word *intimacy* is spoken. What are they? What does the word mean to you?

2. What are some ways we connect with others? Have you observed residents trying to make connections to others in the facility? How?

3. What might be some ways that staff could facilitate these connections?

4. When you feel the need for some form of spiritual refreshment or connection, what do you do?

5. What are some ways the facility might offer spiritual refreshment to residents?

6. What practices do you use to accept and forgive yourself when you make a mistake?

7. Make a list of some of your achievements and some of your mistakes. Think about and/or talk about how you felt during this exercise.

THE NEED FOR THE DIVINE

Perhaps the most difficult area of intimacy to address is the need for connection with the divine, however that concept is understood by each individual. As seen in previous chapters, spirituality and religion are not necessarily the same, although they may be closely related for many people. Facilities that offer various religious opportunities, such as church services or chaplains' or Eucharistic ministers' visits, are indeed performing a real service. The chance to "sit shiva" with those who mourn, the provision of quiet space for meditation, or the opportunity to face toward Mecca during prayer will undoubtedly be appreciated. But for some, this may not be enough or appropriate. Many forms of spiritual needs and practices may be present in a care community. Such spiritual needs may include meditation, different ways of praying, being at one with nature, or listening to or seeing something of beauty (e.g., music, art, poetry). Residents and families may also experience other pressing spiritual needs at this time of life: the need to forgive and be forgiven; the need to understand where God is in the midst of suffering and loneliness; and opportunities to say good-bye to a loved one in a meaningful way. All of these areas speak of a striving for connection and intimacy, even if they are not connected to a specific religion.

It is a basic human need to feel connected to people, places, and traditions that have played significant roles in one's life. For the most part, each person lives in a community and experiences some form of interdependence. People who have had to leave their family or their community and traditions may feel disoriented and adrift (see Chapter 3). The care facility becomes a new, and perhaps frightening, milieu, and the resident may feel cut off from everything and everyone familiar to him or her. In order to reestablish a feeling of connection, intimacy, and community, staff members need to be good listeners and safe witnesses to memories, joy, and pain.

Sexuality and intimacy are not easy topics for care facilities to address. Not all residents will have a need to express their sexual feelings, and in some other cases, it will be necessary to carefully monitor sexual expression. But all residents will have intimacy needs. No one, not even the most saintly hermit, lives in a vacuum. According to the late therapist Virginia Satir in her book, *The New Peoplemaking,* "We need to love and be loved, to be noticed, recognized, and respected, to be literally and figuratively touched.... We need to have satisfying and intimate relationships.... We need to belong.... We need to be in touch with our life force, our religion, our divinity" (1988, p. 355).

ACTION STEPS

1. Are there assessment or interview procedures in place that acknowledge the legitimacy of sexual feelings and needs? If not, how could they be implemented?

2. Does current policy allow open staff discussion on this subject? Discuss ways to enhance openness.

3. Does the facility have a plan to discourage unwanted sexual advances, to respect staff boundaries, and to protect frail residents?

4. What staff discussions are needed regarding sexuality and people with dementia?

5. If there is a well spouse or life partner still at home, what policies could be developed to meet the couple's needs?

6. What is the staff attitude regarding same-sex relationships? Is a policy statement or enforcement needed?

7. Discuss whether a staff member or consultant should be designated with whom residents or family members can discuss these matters.

8. Make sure a referral policy to an ethics committee exists for difficult situations.

9. What training is available and/or required regarding the issue of sexuality?

REFERENCES

Erikson, E. (1986). *Vital involvement in old age.* New York: W.W. Norton & Company.
Satir, V. (1988). *The new peoplemaking.* Mountain View, CA: Science and Behavior Books.

RECOMMENDED READING

From age-ing to sage-ing: A profound new vision of growing older by Zalman Schachter-Shalomi and Ronald S. Miller (Warner Books)

Love and sex after 60, Revised edition by Robert N. Butler and Myrna I. Lewis (Ballantine Books)

Sister age by M.F.K. Fisher (Vintage Books)

RESOURCE

AARP/Modern Maturity Sexuality Survey
Web site: http://research.aarp.org/health/mmsexsurvey_1.html

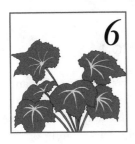

6

The Long Good-Bye

Enhancing Relationships with People with Alzheimer's Disease and Dementia

Ron Zielske

OBJECTIVES

As a result of reading and working through the material in this chapter, participants will be able to

1. Develop relationships with residents in a nonverbal way

2. Understand the individuality of each resident with dementia

3. Understand the benefit of living in the moment

4. Relate to residents with dementia so that their spiritual well-being is enhanced

METHODS OF COMMUNICATION

Marty Richards, in a lecture at the 2001 American Society on Aging and National Council on Aging Conference, said that when he asked a nursing assistant if it was depressing working with people who had dementia, she responded, "No, it is not. I just connect soul to soul." This thought opens a doorway for a new understanding about a caring connection between staff and residents. Another way to describe this kind of caring is "listening with your heart."

There are many ways to communicate. Most people first think of words when they think of communication. However, there are many nonverbal ways to communicate. Body motions and gestures, also referred to as body language, can convey a message to others. Nonverbal motions and facial expressions, sometimes more than words, convey the real message and feelings of a person. People sometimes say "yes" or "okay" only to have their body language communicate their real, deeper feeling of "no."

Staff members can maintain a soul-to-soul connection even with residents who have advanced dementia or visual impairment. Residents will always sense if another person is genuine in his or her communication, whether it is verbal or nonverbal. When two human beings are close to each other in friendship, something takes place that contributes to the well-being of both of them.

The nursing assistant who spoke of having a soul-to-soul connection with her residents sees a sacred spiritual connection taking place, and even though it cannot be measured, she is very positive about her contribution to residents' lives. She knows that the ground supporting both of them is holy ground and that their connection is a sacred one.

A variety of practical steps can aid good communication. Here are many appropriate and sensitive examples:

- Stand where a resident can see you and introduce yourself

- Make sure residents' hearing aids are functioning properly

- Obtain and maintain eye contact that is culturally acceptable

- Touch the resident, if culturally appropriate, to make him or her aware of your presence and to assure the resident of your friendship

- Demonstrate or act out what you want the resident to do. For example, you may have to drink from a glass to help a resident who has severe dementia understand that she should drink from a glass as well.

- Learn to talk in a tone of voice that is appropriate (e.g., a calm and soothing tone)

- Speak clearly and use simpler speech, but do not address residents as if they are children. Avoid referring to residents as "sweetie" or "honey"; call them by their names. In addition, don't use baby words such as "going bye-bye" instead of going for a ride or "going nighty night" instead of going to bed.

- Find the resident's level of verbal skills and use words that fit that level for good, effective communication.

- Allow adequate time for a resident to respond; it may take a while for him or her to process a question or comment.

- Be sure to speak in a positive way by asking a resident for what you want rather than telling him or her what you don't want. Rather than saying, "Do not go to the bathroom outside," say, "I'll take you to your bathroom." Instead of saying, "Don't make such a mess when you eat," say, "Use your spoon; it will make it easier for you to eat."

- Avoid arguing with residents. Instead of telling a resident that he or she cannot go out for a walk, walk with him or her or find someone who can.

- Don't grab, push, or yell at a resident who wanders away. Walk with the resident for a while and gently lead him or her to the original path.

- Guide a resident to another activity or another place if he or she is being disruptive in a group or activity. Don't insist that he or she stay and behave, which will lead to further disruptions.

GEORGE

George is frequently agitated. He tries hard to say what he means, but his speech comes out all mixed up with words that are not sentences and it is difficult for staff to understand what he wants to convey. Once in a while, staff can guess what he means by the time of day (e.g., mealtime), by his body posture (e.g., if he needs to use the bathroom), or by some other means. Sam, a nursing assistant, makes sure that George can see him and talks calmly to George, making guesses at what George might be trying to say. When Sam is right, George nods his head. When Sam cannot understand, George's face muscles tighten and he stomps his foot and becomes very loud. In a case such as this, Sam continues to talk in a calm tone of voice and puts his hand on George's arm as an expression of friendship. He leads George back to his room and puts on classical music, George's favorite. In a short while, George calms down and is back out in the activity room again.

DISCUSSION

1. Describe to the group times when you knew or could feel that communication was taking place even when no words were spoken.

2. Describe one or more of the methods of communication you have used that have been successful and those that have not been successful.

3. If you can sing or play an instrument and have done so with a resident, describe to the group how you think that assists communication and how it is a method of communication.

EXERCISE

Sit in silence with your eyes closed and experience the presence of other group members. Then, describe to others what being in their presence means to you.

THE VALUE OF HUMANITY

All residents have gifts and abilities. They have used these gifts throughout their lives to earn a living, relate to others, and contribute to society (e.g., being an elected city official, feeding the homeless, volunteering at a local senior center) and to organizations (e.g., religious, charitable). A resident may have Alzheimer's disease or another dementia, but that does not totally define who he or she is any more than a resident is defined by a broken hip. Although Alzheimer's disease and other dementias are not a normal part of aging, a person doesn't stop being a human because of them, even though he or she is very different from who he or she was before. People with dementia, like all others, are people of great value. They still have gifts to bring to the community in which they live and to the staff and other residents in their nursing facility community. They have a name, a spirit, feelings, a unique personality, and a life story. They give and receive love and attention, can be compassionate and concerned, may respond to new information, may possess old skills and learn new ones, may be able to remember and tell stories, and may have humor and possess social graces.

TINA

Tina is in the middle stage of dementia and can still follow simple directions about the basics of everyday living such as eating, grooming, and following a simple activity when she is reminded. Her great gift to the residents and staff is humor. You can "kid around" with her, and her laughter comes from deep within her soul. Her laugh is infectious and all other residents laugh with her, even though they don't understand why they are laughing. Her other gift is music. She can no longer play the violin as she once did, but she can sing. She enjoys singing in and listening to the facility's musical groups. Her voice is strong and she helps others sing by being a song leader.

DISCUSSION

1. What makes a person a human being?

2. Do you have a loved one with dementia? If so, describe that person and how you relate to that person.

3. What do you like best about working with residents with dementia?

4. What do you find difficult about working with these residents?

5. What would you like to know about working with residents with dementia?

6. Can you describe the coping skills that a particular resident uses? What are your coping skills in working with residents with dementia?

7. Can you identify a gift that each resident has to give?

8. What gifts have been given to you from the residents?

There is a saying, "When you have seen one person with dementia, you have seen only one person with dementia." A person with dementia still has his or her unique personality even if much of it seems to have gone away. A person's facial expressions, particular laugh, and many other characteristics still identify him or her as distinct or unique from any other human being. People with dementia will still sense who a person fundamentally is, which requires being genuine in their presence. The most important thing to a person with dementia is having a caregiver with a caring, loving, and accepting attitude. The words spoken and the tone of voice are important, regardless of whether the person with dementia can participate in the conversation. All these things—physical presence, a caring voice, and participation in a resident's daily life and activities—bring health, life, and meaning to a person with dementia.

A person with dementia will progress through various stages of the disease (see Table 1). The person will move from thinking of the society around him or her to focusing on his or her immediate, physical needs; from self-reliance and productivity toward dependence on others; from altruistic love toward self-protection and attachment to caregivers; from finding meaning in the disease toward letting go; from looking for a hopeful future toward coping with the current stage; and from having access to a religious tradition toward discovering simpler spiritual expression.

As a resident's dementia increases, others can nourish the person by affirming his or her unique history; respecting his or her preferences and expressed values; assuming responsibility when a resident's judgment is incapacitated; remembering that errant behavior is caused by the disease and has nothing to do with the person's intentions; supporting the resident's social connections; and adapting religious and spiritual practices to nurture her or his spirit.

Table 1. Stages of symptom progression in Alzheimer's disease

Stage	Symptom	Example
Early	Recent memory loss begins to affect job performance	Cannot remember what he or she was just told to do; forgets telephone numbers
	Confusion about places	Gets lost on the way to work; arrives at wrong place or time or constantly rechecks calendar
	Loses spontaneity—the spark or zest for life; loses initiative	Family and friends notice person's withdrawal and disinterest; person shows less interest in hobbies and volunteer activities
	Experiences mood/personality changes	Becomes anxious about symptoms; avoids people
	Has poor judgment; makes bad decisions; misinterprets a situation	Makes odd purchases; does unsafe things
	Takes longer with routine chores	Spends all day making dinner; labors over fixing a pot of coffee
	Has difficulty handling money, paying bills	Forgets which bills have been paid, overpays bills, or forgets to pay bills for several months
	Loses things	Misplaces valuables
Middle	Has increased memory loss and confusion; has shorter attention span	Can't remember visits immediately after visitors leave; has lapses recognizing family and friends
	Repeats statements and/or movements; cannot follow a sequence of steps	Asks the same question repeatedly; may continue to put on unnecessary layers of clothing
	Is restless, especially in late afternoon and at night	Paces; may get up to wander at night
	Experiences perceptual motor problems	Has difficulty getting into a chair or setting the table for a meal; experiences occasional muscle twitches or jerking
	Has difficulty organizing thoughts, thinking logically	Cannot find the right words to say something, so may substitute words; uses a circumlocution to describe a word that he or she cannot think of
	Has problems with reading, writing, and numbers	Cannot follow written signs, write name, or add or subtract numbers

(continued)

Table 1. *(continued)*

Stage	Symptom	Example
	May be suspicious, irritable, fidgety, tearful, or silly	May accuse spouse of hiding things or of infidelity; may act childish
	Experiences loss of impulse control	Has sloppier table manners; unzips pants in public
	Gains and then loses weight	May have a huge appetite for other people's food, forget when last meal was eaten, then gradually lose interest in food
	May experience delusions	May see or hear things that are not there
	Needs full-time supervision	May not recognize surroundings and continually attempt to "escape"
Late	Has almost complete memory loss and confusion	Doesn't recognize family, friends, or own self in the mirror
	Experiences increased weight loss	Loses weight even with a good diet; may experience difficulty with swallowing
	Has little capacity for self-care	Cannot control bowels or bladder; needs help with bathing, dressing, eating, and toileting
	Cannot communicate with words	May groan, scream, or make grunting sounds
	Processes only very basic sensory input	May put everything in his or her mouth or touch everything
	May experience a variety of physical problems	May have seizures, contract skin infections; sleeps often

Source: Gwyther (1985).

DISCUSSION

1. Share an example of a resident you have cared for who was in each of the three stages of Alzheimer's disease—early, middle, and late—and how you related to him or her.

2. Identify what you have learned from each other in this process and what you have discovered that you can do differently that promotes well-being.

3. Share a time when working with a person with dementia was particularly distressing, and relate your feelings to the group. Ask others in the group to offer suggestions for dealing with such a situation when it arises again.

THE MEANING OF WORSHIP

Tim Brennan said of his own descent into Alzheimer's disease,

> I am less Catholic now. I still take comfort from the touch of a rosary, but don't know how to make it work. I no longer remember prayer I once recited automatically. The prayers frequently get mixed up with each other. However, God is in your heart. There is a sixth sense at work that "feels" his presence. I don't understand how one could become less religious and possibly more spiritual. Yet, this appears to be happening. (1999, p. 1)

Even though a person with Alzheimer's disease loses his or her memory, God remembers that person's history and life, and that person is instantly blessed. God does not forget even when people forget. God remembering is a frequent theme in the Judeo-Christian Scriptures. God is even expressed as suffering with a person with problems or a disease and shedding tears for him or her. Family and friends of a person with dementia tend to think that their loved one is lost. However, those who believe that a person's soul still exists realize that there is no such thing as being totally lost. The absence of trouble and grief is not the basis of hope or the fulfillment of life, as some might think. The basis for hope is in God's remembrance and God's presence and the comforting presence of others.

The law of karma is one of the central beliefs of Buddhism, and this law determines what happens to people in a future life based on their behavior in their current life. Some people believe that a person has dementia because he or she was bad in a former life. But, another explanation for the existence of dementia is that we are susceptible to disease through genes, the environment, or illness. Realism is also a hallmark of Buddhism, so if change is inevitable, we must accept the condition and move on with life. As in other religious traditions, the Amida Buddha is compassionate and his love is unconditional and offers help to those in need. One of the comforts for many Buddhists is that birth in the Pure Land (known as enlightenment) is already assured. The concept of heaven is also a theme in many other religions, and although a person with severe dementia probably will not remember this as a source of comfort, those in the early stage of dementia can be strengthened by thinking about the time when all disease, war, and hurtful things will be replaced by health, perfect well-being, and peace. This doesn't mean, however, that we are to be complacent or fatalistic about dementia.

TRAN

Tran has been a devout Catholic all of his life, attending mass at every possible opportunity. He actively served in various committees and was especially active in evangelism efforts for the local parish. He is now in the late stage of Alzheimer's disease and seems to recognize very little of the worship services and does not participate at all. However, when the priest greets him after the service, Tran grasps the cross and kisses it. At the same time, his face relaxes and there is a special gleam in his eye.

DISCUSSION

1. Think of a resident who has dementia. What routines in that person's life have special meaning for him or her?

2. Are there special rituals (e.g., wearing special religious objects, attending worship services, having tea at a special time of day) that add meaning to that person's life? In what ways can you assist that person in maintaining those rituals?

3. What would you do for Tran to enhance his spiritual connections?

HEALING HUMOR

In relating to people and to those with dementia, the gift of humor not only brings joy but is also a great healer and a stress reliever. A profound sense of humor may well be one of the many coping skills that a person with dementia develops. Humor is important to practice for the sake of a person with dementia as well as for staff, friends, and the family of this person. Humor also develops quick and easy friendships and relationships and relaxes the atmosphere between two people. It was Victor Borge who said, "Laughter is the shortest distance between two people" (as cited in Kundtz, 2000, p. 232). It includes the willingness to laugh at oneself for mistakes. It is the ability to kid around with residents when appropriate. Respect for an individual's unique brand of humor and sensitivities to cultural issues that may or may not be interpreted as humor is important.

Humor relieves stress, such as the stress and frustration experienced by a resident with dementia as he or she has difficulty remembering or doing certain tasks, and it relieves the frustrations of caregivers as well. Laughing makes frowning, wrinkling your forehead, or worrying difficult. Everyone needs laughter in their lives each day.

Nursing assistants in secured dementia units of nursing facilities believe in humor. They are constantly "ribbing" each other and doing funny things like wearing weird hats to make the residents laugh. They also show videotapes of Laurel and Hardy, The Keystone Kops, and Charlie Chaplin.

DISCUSSION

1. Do you have a sense of humor? How do you show it?

2. Is there humor and laughter between staff members? How is it expressed? How do staff benefit from humor?

3. Describe to the group a time when humor was present between you and a resident and what difference it made to your and the resident's well-being?

LIVING IN THE MOMENT

Remaining faithful to a resident as a caregiver and respecting him or her as a human being regardless of his or her condition is vital for the well-being of the resident. It is also vital for the well-being of the staff members in that it brings fulfillment and meaning to their lives as caregivers.

Professional caregivers need to adopt the same attitude that a caring family member has. In *I Can't Remember: Family Stories of Alzheimer's Disease,* Esther Strauss Smoller said,

> I am going to keep on visiting her even though I know it is a one-sided visit. As long as my mother is in that bed, I will go to that home; I will visit with her and I will hold her hand and I will look into her eyes and I still tell her how much I love her and what a good mother she has been. I guess you can say this is unconditional love (and) the longest goodbye I will ever have to say. (1997, p. 124)

Wayne Ewing, in his book *Tears in God's Bottle: Reflections on Alzheimer's Caregiving,* talked about his journey with his wife Ann, who had Alzheimer's disease, and told the story of a visit from their granddaughter. The 4-year-old granddaughter wanted Wayne to go away for a while so she could have some private time with Granny. When Wayne returned, he asked his granddaughter what she and her grandmother had talked about during their private time. She responded, "Well, Grandpa, when I was hugging and kissing her, I wasn't talking about anything. I was just loving her" (Ewing, 1999, p. 56). Such wisdom!

When people connect soul to soul, they bring hope to individuals with dementia. There is no way to reverse Alzheimer's disease, but the loving presence and caring acts of staff, friends, and family assist the resident on his or her journey. Love and affection heal the wounds of the body, mind, and spirit. Hope is largely relational. The residents will experience hope if people pay attention to them. A resident may not know who someone is from one day to the next, but his or her experience of kindness is comforting. The situation with a resident is not helpless or hopeless. It is the help of others that brings hope. Do not let others say that life is hopeless. Having dementia is not hell on earth, but knowing that one is not loved is.

One of the basic ingredients of caregiving is to recognize residents as they go down hallways and pass rooms. The lives of residents are always enhanced by this feeling of connection, and they are filled with hope if staff members recognize them with a smile, a wave of the hand, a greeting, a gentle touch, or a nod of the head. Even when a staff member is very busy with another resident or a chore, some form of recognition affirms for a resident that he or she is still a worthwhile human being.

For some elders, remembering people and events from long ago is a lot easier than remembering what happened yesterday. As dementia progresses, a person may remember less and less of the past and have no concern for the future. This is a person who lives in the moment and only for the moment. Many people in this world relive the past over and over again and/or live in apprehension of the future by planning it in an obsessive manner. These people and many others find practicing meditation and mindfulness helpful so they can be attuned to and not lose the experience of the moment by being too busy with the past or future. It seems ironic that only people with dementia really experience living in the moment whereas healthy people without dementia frequently have to work very hard to achieve this state.

Connection to the past, however, is helpful for all elders as they try to find meaning in their lives. One of the steps that family and friends can take to assist a resident with dementia is to place familiar objects on or near the door to the resident's room to help the person identify his or her home. Families can also create a memory book—a photo album with a few pictures—and talk with the person with dementia about his or her past. Both family and staff can use the memory book to help the resident connect to his or her history. If a resident cannot remember something, the staff and family can remember for him or her. An unknown author once said, "To love someone is to learn the song that is in their heart, and to sing it to them when they have forgotten."

ADIE

Adie was 95 years old and in the early stage of dementia. She could not remember how to do simple things, such as tie her shoes, and she was angry. Her anger was a result of the fear of what else would affect her as she began the descent to the last stage of dementia. Her fits of anger were marked with loud cursing and swearing. They were very upsetting to the other residents and staff. Jackie, one of the staff members, knew how to help. Jackie approached Adie, stood in front of her, spoke in a

soft voice, and touched her arm. This got Adie's attention. Because of their long relationship, Jackie could
hug Adie tightly, and Adie's cursing would turn to sobs.
She eventually relaxed and Jackie could lead her to an
activity or to her room to play a CD of jazz, her favorite
music.

DISCUSSION

1. Describe a resident who cannot recall the past and
   does not think about the future but lives only for
   the present. How do you feel about caring for this
   resident?

2. Do you get frustrated when a resident asks the same
   question over and over again and you give him or
   her the same answer over and over again? How do
   you deal with your frustration? Do you think that
   the resident has really heard your answer? Is there
   something else going on with the resident other
   than what the question asks?

3. When have you observed hope in a resident with
   dementia? What have you done to foster this hope?

4. Share ways in which you and others can help maximize the limited cognitive ability of a particular resident with dementia.

EXERCISE

When one of your residents with dementia is agitated
and frustrated, practice the following meditation. Sit still
in a comfortable position, and breathe in through your
nose and out through your mouth slowly and deeply to
relax your body. Imagine yourself at your favorite resting
place (e.g., a mountain lake, the ocean) and reestablish
in your mind the peaceful feeling that you experience in
that place. As all of the different worries and cares of the
day come into your mind, visualize them leaving your

mind on a fast-moving cloud or going into a sack that you give to the divine or toss in an ocean or deep hole. Think about those who love you, and experience the warm feeling of love. Remember your gifts and abilities in gratitude. Then, listen to your breathing and nothing else. See if this doesn't calm and restore you, allowing you to focus more clearly on the present moment, the resident's needs, and what is needed to reduce the resident's agitation.

FAMILY ISSUES

Facility staff contacts and communicates with not just residents but families and friends, too. As a staff member stands shoulder to shoulder with a resident, so does he or she stand with that resident's family and friends. Just as the resident experiences well-being because of a staff member's kindness and care, so does his or her family experience goodness as staff listens to them and acknowledges their pain and grief in relating to their loved one.

Most residents with terminal diseases deteriorate and die and leave family behind. Eventually, the triad of fear, anger, and grief can be processed and overcome. However, a person whose spouse or parent has dementia must face losing the person he or she knew and loved, although that spouse or parent's physical self is still present to relate to. In addition, his or her spirit or soul remains—the inner self. The total self does not disappear. When a person is not able to relate to his or her loved one with dementia at all, the grief he or she experiences, with all of its accompanying emotions, continues as long as the person with dementia is alive.

Dementia has been called a thief of time. A person's memory of the past disappears, as well as his or her sense of future, so family members have a very difficult time relating to the disease. They no longer receive the benefits of communication and the relationship they once did. In addition, people with dementia may or may not respond to hugs, and they may not receive the same physical, emotional, and spiritual well-being from their loved ones as they once did. But the body often retains memory independent of the mind and will react to some situations out of habit. Even if memory, as we understand it, is gone, the resident can respond to longtime conditioning either in a positive or in a negative way. For example, if you raise your voice in anger, a resident may cower and run away because that is the way that he or she always reacted to angry people.

Some family members consider dementia in their loved one to be worse than an early death because of the disease's long and difficult process. Death brings finality and is a natural part of the life cycle. Dementia, however, is not natural and the dying process in which a loved one deteriorates over a long period of time seems to last forever. It is more heartbreaking for family members than death. The grieving process is perpetual until death, which is sometimes seen as a blessing that finally allows a family to move on. The staff's ability to listen, touch, and pay attention to a resident's friends and family is vital to their healing process. Staff and others who support a resident's family also bring well-being to the resident. In addition, friends and family of residents with Alzheimer's disease or dementia should be encouraged to connect with their local Alzheimer's Association and to join a support group that can comfort, guide, and give them hope (see Chapter 13).

Although it is important to consider the necessity for support between families and residents, staff should also be aware of the many spiritual and ethical implications of residents being in an environment separate from their spouses or children. One of the difficult dilemmas for spouses and other family members of a loved one who has Alzheimer's disease or a related dementia is how faithful they should be in visiting the resident and in other aspects of their relationship with that person, especially when they no longer receive anything from the relationship, not even recognition of who they are. What are the responsibilities of a spouse whose loved one has been in an institution for years? Should he or she be able to pursue intimate relationships despite having a spouse in a nursing facility? What are the implications if a wife comes to visit her husband and finds him holding hands with another female resident? Hand holding certainly brings some good feelings to the resident, but what does it do for the wife who may well think that her husband has substituted another resident for her? If the wife finds her husband holding another resident's hand, it will create strong emotional responses such as anger, and she might even try to separate the two and lead her husband away or even push the other resident away. A response could also be one of grief or depression expressed by crying.

In such situations, staff members will want to ensure that they don't impose their own beliefs or value systems on the couple but rather help the couple honor its own. However the wife responds, such as in the previous case, staff may want to provide support in the form of words by saying, "It must be hard to see him holding someone else's hand" or "It must really hurt to see this happening." Then, staff could gently lead the husband to the wife and give them some time alone.

DISCUSSION

1. Discuss what your role and responsibility may or may not be in a situation such as those above. How do your religious, spiritual, and ethical background and beliefs form the basis of your comments? Are you open to other opinions formed by another staff member's cultural and spiritual background?

2. What would you say to the visiting wife in the situation above?

CARING REDEFINED

Each individual with dementia is a precious, unique individual. People are precious because they exist and not because of what they can do or remember. The task of staff is to assist residents so they can live each day to its fullest potential and even find enjoyment and fulfillment. It is the staff's turn to be caregivers and residents' turn to be care receivers, whereas, in previous times in their lives, these residents were the caregivers. It seems that people take turns being givers and receivers of care throughout their lives.

In the realm of dementia, caregiving tasks may be straightforward in terms of physical care but more complex in terms of emotional and spiritual support, for communication is often nonverbal between staff members and residents. A resident can sense the caring attitudes of staff members by recognizing tone of voice and body language more than the words spoken. This is true even for humor. The resident may not even understand a joke or phrase, but laughter and lightheartedness is contagious. It is also essential for staff members to care for themselves and each other so they have the skills and personality to adequately care for residents with Alzheimer's disease or other dementias.

ACTION STEPS

1. Based on the information you have learned in this chapter, including what you have learned from each other, what changes would you make in the pro-

grams of your facility to enhance the daily lives of the residents with dementia?

2. What would change in activities, daily personal contact, meal times, and family visit time?

REFERENCES

Brennan, T. (1999). *A perspective on religion, spirituality and Alzheimer's disease.* Handout presented at the Alzheimer's Association workshop, Spirituality and Dementia, Los Altos, California.

Ewing, W. (2003). *Tears in God's bottle: Reflections on Alzheimer's caregiving.* Portland, OR: First Books.

Gwyther, L.P. (1985). *Care of Alzheimer's patients: A manual for nursing home staff.* Chicago: Alzheimer's Disease and Related Disorders Association; Washington, DC: American Health Care Association.

Kundtz, D. (2000). *Everyday serenity.* Berkeley, CA: Conari Press.

Richards, M. (2000). Communicating soul to soul challenges for care providers. *Southwest Journal on Aging, 15*(2)/16(1), 3–6.

Smoller, E.S. (1997). *I can't remember: Family stories of Alzheimer's disease.* Philadelphia: Temple University Press.

RECOMMENDED READING

Aging and God: Spiritual pathways to mental health in midlife and later years by Harold George Koenig (Haworth Pastoral Press)

The Art of happiness: A handbook for living by His Holiness the Dalai Lama and Howard C. Cutler (Riverhead Books)

The Best Friends approach to Alzheimer's care by Virginia Bell and David Troxel (Health Professions Press)

Ethnicity and the dementias edited by Gwen Yeo and Dolores Gallagher-Thompson (Taylor & Francis)

God never forgets: Faith, hope, and Alzheimer's disease by Donald K. McKim (Westminster John Knox Press)

The light inside the dark: Zen, soul, and the spiritual life by John Tarrant (HarperCollins)

The loss of self: A family resource for the care of Alzheimer's disease and related disorders by Donna Cohen and Carl Eisdorfer (Norton)

Meeting the spiritual needs of the cognitively impaired by Marty Richards in *Generations, 14*(4), 63–64

A path with heart: A guide through the perils and promises of spiritual life by Jack Kornfield (Bantam Books)

Speaking our minds: Personal reflections from individuals with Alzheimer's by Lisa Snyder (W.H. Freeman)

The tao of inner peace: A guide to inner peace by Diane Dreher (Plume Book)

When Alzheimer's disease strikes by James S. Sapp and Stephen Sapp (Desert Ministries)

Wherever you go, there you are: Mindfulness meditation in everyday life by Jon Kabat-Zinn (Hyperion)

RESOURCE

Alzheimer's Association
919 North Michigan Avenue
Suite 1100
Chicago, Illinois 60611-1676
Telephone: 800-272-3900; 312-335-8700
E-mail: info@alz.org
Web site: http://www.alz.org

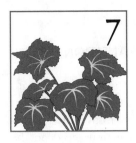

The Impact of Change

Managing Life Transitions

Julie Barton

OBJECTIVES

As a result of reading this chapter and working through the exercises, participants will be able to

1. Appreciate the impact of transitions on all people throughout the life cycle

2. Discover ways to honor and work with those who are going through life-changing transitions

3. Devise practical strategies for easing life-changing transitions

DEFINING AND UNDERSTANDING TRANSITIONS

It may be helpful, in thinking about the concept of life's transitions, to look through two different lenses. One lens shows the larger transitions, such as aging across the lifespan or the gradual change from robust health to growing limitations and frailty. These larger transitions need not be negative: People can also grow away from a life dictated by job and family concerns toward a greater sense of freedom to reflect, enjoy, create, and share their wisdom. Transitions are not unique to old age. Milestones mark all stages of life: birth, starting school, graduation, employment, marriage, children—and then the cycle begins again with a person's offspring.

The second lens shows the smaller transitions that occur under the umbrella of the larger transitions. A person may become a grandparent or great-grandparent, may retire, or may, because of health concerns, have to give up a home of many years to enter some sort of care arrangement. These transitions are not really "small" given the emotional and spiritual impact they can have. Moreover, the people who might help are often going through their own transitions as well. Finally, it is important to remember that the transitions that are forced on a person are likely to have a more negative psychological and spiritual impact than the transitions that are actively undertaken. Transitions appear to have many layers and many facets as well as a certain progression: preparation (if there is time), the actual change (which in itself may have a continuum), and a regrouping following the change. A time of transition is often a time when spiritual support is sorely needed.

There are some questions staff members might ask themselves when they are dealing with transitions or working with others who are. Nancy Schlossberg (1990) outlined some of these important questions:

- What type of change is occurring?
- Does the person see it as positive or negative?
- Does it come at a good time, or perhaps the worst of times?
- Is it premature or "on time"?
- Does it change everything about a person's life, or just certain things?
- Is the change permanent or temporary?

Staff members need answers to these questions if they are to understand residents and be compassionate listeners, helpers, or companions for residents who are negotiating change or transitions. Staff members also need to be aware that a person in transition may not be experiencing just one emotion but may entertain a host of differing emotions (e.g., grief over leaving home, relief in knowing that his or her needs will be met and that fear of being isolated at home is no longer an issue).

FAMILY INVOLVEMENT IN TIMES OF CHANGE

Residents are frequently not the only ones involved in transitions, a point that can be easily overlooked. Family caregivers must relinquish much of their role and come to grips with the fact that their loved one can no longer remain in their care. This is a tremendous change for the caregiver, even though it may also bring physical and emotional relief. The spiritual need to care is still there, and the need for assurance that family members are still important to both resident and staff must be addressed. (See Chapter 3 for more information about family involvement.)

ACKNOWLEDGING AN ENDING

Table 1 outlines the steps necessary for a successful transition. Accepting the end of a life transition is perhaps easier said than done, especially when a person must enter a care facility. A person in this situation may experience an assortment of endings: an end to self-care and complete independence, an end to driving (a big transition!), an end to enjoying the comforts and conveniences of one's own home, or an end to the level of good health he or she has previously enjoyed.

It is not easy to accept a walker when one has always been mobile and independent. It is difficult for a person to accept being cared for or to be dependent on the kindness of strangers when he or she has always been the caregiver. It is numbing to lose a spouse or child. And it is heartwrench-

Table 1.   Steps for successful transitions

1.   Acknowledge that an end has occurred.
2.   Grieve the loss (or the change).
3.   Acknowledge the positive parts of what has just ended.
4.   Notice and acknowledge that your life now has spaces open to be filled with new possibilities.
5.   Welcome new possibilities. Go forward with your life.

Source: Satir (1988).

ing to give up a beloved home, church, pet, or neighborhood in order to be cared for elsewhere. This is a time when physical complaints and symptoms may become exacerbated, almost as a substitute for unspoken spiritual and psychological needs. The task of recognizing the emotional stress underlying physical complaints can be delicate. Care facilities need to find ways to be alert to verbal or nonverbal cries for support.

EXERCISE

Think of a time in your life when you had to stop doing something that you really loved to do, or think about a time when a treasured relationship ended. If you can, write about your experience here.

1. How did you handle it?

2. What were your feelings when this happened?

3. How can this experience help you with a resident who is having difficulty with an ending?

GRIEVING THE LOSS

At first, the idea of grief over transitions may seem a little odd. Grief is customarily associated with particular kinds of losses—the death or absence of a loved one, a cataclysmic event, or a serious accident. However, the experience of grief is also often involved in making transitions, even transitions that might seem small to others. Losing the right to drive, for example, can have a profound impact on a person. A driver's license, for most people, is a symbol of freedom: being able to come and go at will, to travel, and to take care of personal needs. Thus, losing the right to drive can produce a period of grieving over a loss of freedom before the person can begin to adapt to this new limitation.

If an elder in a care setting seems depressed and unwilling or unable to adapt according to expectations, someone may need to ask, "What has happened recently in your life? You seem sad, and I wonder if you'd like to talk about it."

There are even times when depression is diagnosed by a medical professional, when in reality, the person who seems depressed is grieving and should be allowed to do so at his or her own pace. The distinguished therapist, David Freeman, in his lectures, refers to depression as "sadness of the soul"—an eloquent description of grief, indeed. What is required of staff when confronted with grief such as this? Listening, listening, listening; allowing tears, even if witnessing another's tears causes discomfort; and, as Freeman advises, being a safe witness to another's pain. This means repressing the private urge to "fix" the resident in order to put an end to one's own discomfort.

PERSONAL, CULTURAL, AND GENDER DIFFERENCES

Staff can benefit from remembering that personal, cultural, and gender differences affect the way people deal with loss and grief or any strong emotion. The loss of the ability to be in charge of one's home may be very different for a homemaker versus an executive or a plumber! Each will feel loss but very likely will deal with it in quite different ways. Similarly, if a resident has grown up in a family or culture where a show of great emotion is considered unseemly, that still does not mean that he or she is not *experiencing* powerful emotions. These emotions just may need to be acknowledged in a different way. These differences can be noticed in most facilities. A simple phrase such as "I'm sorry for your loss" or "I see that perhaps you are feeling sad" may suffice. It is really not for others to impose their way of handling grief on another person. If a resident, however, seems distraught with grief, a staff member might consult with a member of the resident's clergy who is well-trained in counseling or with a compassionate mental health professional trained in gerontology. And at some point, staff or family might ask the resident if he or she would like to have someone special to talk with.

ACCENTUATING THE POSITIVE ASPECTS OF TRANSITION

Satir's last three steps of transition (see Table 1) have to do with adaptation and with attempting to look on the positive side of transitions. This can be tricky. It requires being able to sit with a resident who is grieving, encourage him or her to share some of the wonderful aspects of his or her former life, without triggering a "cheer up" instinct. It means gently offering, at the proper time, new ways for residents to feel useful and in control, affirming for them that there is still more to their lives, and convincing them that they are valued members of the community. It involves finding ways to do these things within a particular care facility. Discovering the resident's talents and experience may help. Many churches ask new members to complete a "spiritual gifts" inventory in which talents, likes and dislikes, and opportunities to share are uncovered. Perhaps this same device should be tried in care facilities! What a wealth of wisdom and grace staff would find!

PREVENTING CRISES IN DEALING WITH TRANSITION

Transitions can take their toll on an individual, but they need not turn into crises if a few simple guidelines are observed. Correct information about the transition is a necessity for anyone in the process of change, especially a new resident and his or her family. What does the resident think is going to happen, or what is the resident telling him- or herself about the change or transition? Is he or she correct? If not, how can the facts be presented in a caring, compassionate way, especially if dementia is a factor? What information must staff have in order to assist the resident and his or her family?

Support is also of paramount importance at this time. Sometimes just knowing that someone is willing to walk with him or her can make a person's journey easier. Determining a resident's strengths will also help staff evaluate his or her need for support. Too often, residents are assumed to have no strengths because they are in a care situation, an attitude that may make caregivers miss a great opportunity to let residents act constructively on their own behalf! What strengths does a new resident have that staff members can discover and encourage? Sometimes, just chatting with a resident about his or her life will uncover a rich field of experience and strength. Staff might ask, "How have you dealt with transition in the past? What was particularly helpful to you then? How can we help make that available to you now?"

DISCUSSION

1. In Chapter 3, the concept of the community or system that can be created in a long-term care setting is discussed: a mutual presence in a sacred space for the benefit of residents, family, and staff. What better atmosphere could there be for the crucial job of managing transitions, particularly those that take

an emotional, physical, and spiritual toll? What else can we do to encourage residents to contribute to the life of the community?

2. What communities have you been a part of? Describe how you would feel or have felt about having to leave your community or change your role as a professional, a homemaker, a writer, or whatever your chosen work has been.

3. Think back to a recent transition in your life. Why was it necessary? How did you manage it? Who was there to help? Do you feel you were successful? If not, what would have made a difference?

4. Are there residents in your facility (and their families) who have recently negotiated a transition or had one imposed on them? Was it recognized and provided for? What spiritual or emotional support might have been offered? What supports do staff offer if a transition is painful?

LOOKING FOR RECIPROCITY

Residents in a care facility are always on the receiving end, and that can be difficult, even demeaning. Some sort of reciprocity is almost always possible (e.g., asking for a simple prayer or kind thought from a resident). Residents who are physically able can be encouraged to visit others in the facility or share their stories with visiting school children. Staff, when appropriate, might say to a resident, "I have a friend who could use a prayer today" or ask, "A lady at the end of the hall is having a bad day. Could you say a prayer for her?" The concept of "when appropriate" cannot be overstressed. Residents or family members shouldn't be asked to do what is uncomfortable.

The concept of reciprocity, however, also cannot be overstressed: Most people, and perhaps especially those in care facilities, have a deeply spiritual need to *matter* and to help. The idea of reciprocity will be a spiritual benefit to all concerned.

Many transitions are difficult. They become more difficult if a person is ill, is feeling out of control, lacks sufficient information, or is experiencing a sudden and unexpected transition. This does not mean, however, that expected transitions are necessarily easy! It is extremely helpful to be aware of the effects that change and transition have had in one's own life as a way of understanding the difficulties that residents and their families may be having.

ACTION STEPS

1. Is there a plan for welcoming new residents or for helping them move from home? For those who have no family, are volunteers or other residents available to listen, hold a hand, or offer prayers? What training might such volunteers need?

2. Discuss how to obtain important information about a person's spiritual background and preferences in a nonintrusive manner. How can spiritual supports be identified that have been helpful in a resident's past that might be employed in the present?

3. What tools might you use in the future for being aware of the impact of transitions?

Follow this discussion with a role play of transition situations, using good listening and communication techniques. Staff may want to revisit Mrs. Sanchez and her family from Chapter 3, paying specific attention to those things that will ease the transition for everyone, including staff.

REFERENCES

Satir, V. (1988). *The new peoplemaking*. Mountain View, CA: Science and Behavior Books.
Schlossberg, N. (Winter 1990). Training counselors to work with older adults. *Generations,* *14*(1), 7–10.

RECOMMENDED READING

Winter grace: Spirituality and aging by Kathleen R. Fischer (Upper Room Books)

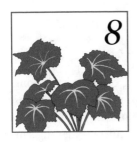

Spiritual Richness

*Celebrations and Rituals
that Give Meaning to Life*

Julie Barton

OBJECTIVES

As a result of reading this chapter and working through
the exercises, participants will be able to

1. Enhance their understanding of the importance of
    rituals and celebrations

2. Identify times and situations in which rituals and cel-
    ebrations would further the sense of community

3. Increase their sensitivity to cultural and religious
    preferences when devising or supporting celebra-
    tions and rituals

THE MEANING OF RITUALS

One of the most important goals in creating a caring community in long-term care is the preservation of meaningful celebrations and rituals. These actions and events provide a sense of safety and belonging; they speak to others about an individual's personal, religious, and cultural identity; and they become an anchor that is relied on to get through rough times. If some important rituals are impossible to continue in a care situation, new ones need to be created to take their place.

Whether traditions or rituals spring from a resident's or staff member's family, culture, or religion, they are often spiritual necessities and can become even more meaningful when shared. A birthday remembered, a man or woman's history honored (a retelling of his or her story and who he or she was or is in a family or community), a holiday tradition celebrated, a death mourned: All of these practices bring a sense of belonging and continuity to a person's life. They must be observed in truly meaningful and respectful ways, in mutual consultation, and honored for what they are: sacred traditions.

DISCUSSION

1. Think back to a tradition that you and your family observed when you were a child. What was it? How long was it observed? What made it special?

2. Think about any feelings you have about that tradition being or no longer being a part of your life. If it is no longer a part of your life, what has taken its place?

3. What traditions, celebrations, or rituals do you hope to pass on to your family?

EXERCISE

Turn to a partner and describe a ritual or celebration that is or has been important to you. Notice how you feel about this, especially if what you are describing is no longer being observed. Now let your partner do the same thing, and notice how you feel as he or she is telling you about an important observance. Then, discuss with the group how this exercise might be helpful to you in your work with residents and families.

TYPES OF CELEBRATIONS

Of course, celebrations and rituals can be divided into certain types or categories. These might include holiday observances, whether religious or civic; birthdays and anniversaries; weddings; graduations; and promotions. Religious services or practices could include baptism, bar or bat mitzvahs, praying at sundown, facing Mecca, anointing the sick, sitting shiva (a Jewish mourning ritual), manhood/womanhood ceremonies, attending Bible study or reading, praying privately, attending services, singing hymns, meditating, and so forth. In addition to these rituals and celebrations, each person's family, his or her more intimate "culture," often invents rituals and reasons to celebrate. For example, food frequently plays a big part in rituals and celebrations. Family home videos display a parade of special meals and birthday cakes emerging from the oven, each made special for the person of honor. Many places of worship use wine and bread symbolically and invite visitors to share in this fellowship. Other traditions may also appreciate being offered traditional foods: a red egg at Easter in the Eastern Christian tradition, herbal teas or healing soups in some Asian traditions. There is no reason why certain traditional feasts can't be prepared for residents in a care facility.

THE NEED FOR BEAUTY

Many cultures have rituals that are feasts for the eyes and ears: flowers and music, decorations and stories. These seemingly simple things are laden with meaning, even for people with memory impairment. In fact, people with memory impairments seem to blossom when they hear familiar music or see something beautiful. Staff members can encourage residents and their families to share treasures—such as ornaments, pictures, music, memories, and special holiday clothing—at special holiday times. A holiday bazaar featuring ornaments, costumes, books, and food would be a way to encourage residents to contribute to the holiday mood.

CULTURAL SENSITIVITY

It is useful to remember that not everyone shares the dominant traditions and celebrations of a particular society. Certainly, it is important to invite people to share in traditions that are not their own as long as the staff does not demand their participation or encourage them inappropriately to participate in a ritual that would perhaps seem a violation of their own traditions. By the same token, in a country as richly diverse as the United States, individual horizons can be expanded by learning about the customs of friends, neighbors, and the residents in nursing facilities; however, cajoling a Buddhist or Jewish resident to celebrate at a Christmas party, for example, is not respectful. Instead, it could be time well-spent perhaps to sit with them to learn more about their own comparable traditions. It may be unrealistic to expect a recent Asian immigrant to understand American Thanksgiving or Halloween decorations and feasts. Perhaps staff could tailor Halloween traditions to include the religious customs of the Day of the Dead for Hispanic residents or All Saints' Day for Catholic residents. What a great learning (and artistic) opportunity that might be!

The staff also needs to remember that even within similar faiths and cultures, rituals and celebrations have important differences, often depending on personal or family traditions. For example, some Catholics say the Rosary daily, if not more often. Others may have abandoned that practice in favor of more personal prayer or different forms of meditation. Orthodox Jews observe the Sabbath in one way, reformed Jews in another. Some Protestant worshippers want to receive Communion; for others, Communion is not as central to their faith. Muslims and Buddhists may differ in how they read and interpret key tenets of their faiths. Some people will be open to learning about or sharing in new traditions; some will not. For still others, times of celebration that typically bring joy may be filled with painful memories. Those who are mourning need not be urged to take part in celebrations, even if the reason for their grief occurred a long time ago.

INVENTING CELEBRATIONS OF AGING

Other than retirement parties or 50th wedding anniversaries, aging affords few celebrations. Only recently did a Grandparents Day tradition begin, and this has not become a fully established part of American culture.

Perhaps it is time to invent some new celebrations or rituals that have to do with aging, wisdom, and honored positions within today's families, communities, and institutions. Kathleen R. Fischer, in her book titled *Winter Grace,* suggested that we "open the album of our lives" (1998, p. 51). She referred to the joyful and sorrowful "mysteries" of people's lives, comparing them with the mysteries of the Rosary, a tradition among many Catholics. She said that memories are to be not merely "recalled," but "reawakened" with all of the accompanying feelings. In this way, healing can happen. One way to encourage residents to reawaken memories might be to create a "memory hour" once a week and encourage family and staff to participate. Songs, poetry, and art can bring memories alive, and tears can be part of a healing process.

EXCHANGING THE RITUAL OF BLESSINGS

The ritual of giving and receiving blessings is also honored among some cultures and traditions. Rachel Naomi Remen spoke of this in her book, *My Grandfather's Blessings: Stories of Strength, Refuge, and Belonging,* noting that "We can bless others only when we feel blessed ourselves" (2000, p. 18). What would happen in care facilities if staff freely exchanged blessings with each other on a daily basis? In some cultures, it is very important to receive a blessing from a dying mother or father in the biblical tradition of Isaac and Jacob, who blessed their families before their deaths. For others, it is important to bless the children before sleep each night. For still others, the reverence paid to an elder in the family or to ancestors is certainly in the realm of blessings. Creating a sacred space for residents, staff, and family to truly feel blessed could allow grace to overflow and transform these residences.

So many traditions and rituals are based on religious beliefs. Leaving the milieu or community in which they are celebrated is difficult. Most facilities ensure that clergy are provided and that Sabbath or Sunday services are available at least monthly, but what else could nursing facilities provide? Some ideas might include prayer groups, Bible studies, exercises such as tai chi, journaling (dictated or recorded, if necessary), and a special space dedicated to prayer or reflection. Staff can identify the religious rituals that are important to residents and add this information to their charts, especially whether a resident would like access to particular religious rituals. Perhaps staff would volunteer to organize a religious committee to handle finding religious resources requested by residents.

DISCUSSION

1. Think about a celebration or ritual that is most meaningful to you. How could you openly share it in a ritual or celebration with fellow staff members or residents and families?

2. Brainstorm possibilities for generating celebrations that will create a feeling of community in your facility such as honoring a home town; featuring residents' careers or families; inviting residents to share memories of holidays, friends, and family; throwing a welcome party for a new resident; or holding a memorial service when someone has died. The possibilities are legion, and the events do not have to be complicated or time consuming: a flower on the breakfast tray (with an extra flower for a birthday!) or the dedication of a garden, with everyone given a chance to plant or select a favorite bloom or vegetable.

In a garden at a private home near one of the facilities in Cupertino, California, each plant or flower represents a member of the family, 20 in all, and this provides family members with an opportunity to pray for each other as they water the plants. Because each person chose his or her own bloom, family members often check each other's plants to see how they're doing. A grandchild may call and say, "How's my yellow rose today, Grandma?" Might there be a way to develop a personalized garden in a care facility? The beauty and fun of plants and animals add so much to the meaning of life, as The Eden Alternative program (see p. 13) has shown.

It is difficult to imagine what life would be like without celebrations to look forward to, without traditions or rituals to treasure, and without someone with whom to share memories. It is less difficult to imagine care facilities being sacred spaces in which residents, families, and staff can reclaim the joy of sharing and honoring not only events of the past but creating memories for the future.

ACTION STEPS

1. Identify what rituals and/or celebrations of aging might be appropriate within your care setting.

2. How would these be implemented? (Some answers might include the use of favorite sayings and quotations; residents' life experiences and careers; memories, especially those tied to regional, national, or world events; and mentoring advice for future generations.)

3. We have no trouble saying "Bless you!" after someone sneezes. Can you think of other ways to create a ritual of blessings?

REFERENCES

Fischer, K.R. (1998). *Winter grace: Spirituality and aging.* Nashville: Upper Room Books.

Remen, R.N. (2000). *My grandfather's blessings: Stories of strength, refuge, and belonging.* New York: Riverhead Books.

RECOMMENDED READING

Green winter: Celebrations of later life by Elise Maclay (Henry Holt and Company)

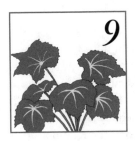

9

The Pleasures
of the Table

*Fostering
Healthy Food Experiences*

Marita Grudzen

OBJECTIVES

As a result of reading this chapter and working through the exercises, participants will be able to

1. Understand the multilayered significance of food and eating

2. Identify the risk factors for older adults related to malnutrition and undernourishment

3. Relate to the importance of the social and cultural dimensions of eating

4. Appreciate the important role of food and eating in many religious observances and rituals

5. Appreciate the issues of autonomy related to eating and nutrition

6. Utilize interactions with residents at mealtime as opportunities for better understanding and nurturing residents

A HOLISTIC APPROACH TO FOOD

In an effort to guarantee nutrition and safety for residents in long-term care, nutritionists have relegated the functions of food and eating to the realm of medicine and dietetics. And yet, the dietary and medical aspects of eating represent only a small part of people's deep and complex relationship to food. Members of a family and community have gathered together from time immemorial to eat. Meals are among the important daily rituals guaranteeing time with family and friends, and they become an intimate place for contact and sharing. Many religious and cultural practices involve special foods, as well as abstinence from foods (fasting). Bonds of all kinds are formed in the sharing of food. Some of the finest art has been created for and been inspired by what happens at the table. Experience teaches that the more pleasant the conditions surrounding meals, the greater the satisfaction derived from them and the better the digestion.

EXERCISE

Part 1: Sharing Positive Memories

Think back to some of the special meals you have had with family and friends—times that are still vivid because they were characterized by good company, relaxation, pleasure, a lovely or endearing environment, and familiar food. What do you remember of these sights, sounds, smells, and conversations? What were the social occasions around some of these meals? Ask for a volunteer or assign a recorder to make a list of some of the characteristics of the memories that participants describe. The list should include specific favorite people (e.g., aunts), places, celebrations, and foods. Try to list 20–25 characteristics to awaken the group's sensual memories.

DISCUSSION

1. Discuss your experience with preparing food. Is it different at different times (e.g., weekdays, Sundays, holidays)? What are your intentions and concerns in feeding yourself, your family, or friends?

2. Do you eat a main meal alone? If not, would you prefer to eat alone? Why?

Part 2: Envisioning Residents' Dining Experiences

Use the preceding discussion to gain a fresh perspective on the experiences of nursing facility residents. What do you observe about residents' eating practices? List the sights, sounds, and smells associated with their dining experience. Are these comforting or disruptive? Nurturing or impersonal? Social or isolating? Now, try to re-envision the dining scene in a way that supports residents' physical well-being and serves their social, sensual, emotional, and nutritional needs in ways that engender respect both for autonomy and social needs and for the residents' history with food, including their cultural and religious practices. Share some of your ideas that emerge from this visualization exercise.

DISCUSSION

1. Think of difficult times in your past relationship with food and eating with others (e.g., illness, emotional or financial difficulty). Were there any particular foods that you wanted and could not have?

2. Did anyone prepare food for you? If so, what was that experience like? Did it enhance the relationship between you and the preparer?

3. Whether you had social contact or support at the time, do you remember how you related to food and eating?

In both conscious and unconscious ways, food often represents much more than simple nourishment. M.F.K. Fisher (1990), the well-known food writer, says that when it comes to food, "nourishment, comfort, and love are indistinguishable" (p. 678). Fisher highlights the powerful connections around eating. Even in institutional settings, mealtimes can be maximized in many ways to provide meaning for the residents. Having staff or family members present is one way, creating a social context. Another is to accommodate residents' former mealtime patterns (e.g., provide a newspaper for a resident who used to read the paper during breakfast; stroll around with a resident who used to go for a short walk after meals).

Many older adults experience a great deal of loss and isolation in nursing facilities. Mealtimes provide a familiar structure, one that provides a vehicle for addressing loneliness and disconnection with oneself and others. Even a facility's more frail elders, or those who need to be fed, might be placed around a table *together* to create their own dining society.

Too often, residents' energy patterns are considered static, without any connection to time. Staff who observe residents closely, however, notice different levels and patterns of alertness, such as whether a resident desires to communicate and whether a resident is willing to participate in activities. Relating a resident's energy levels and the cycle of the day's light to the resident's activities at mealtime is another way to build a healing rhythm into his or her days.

THE EFFECT OF HEALTH CONCERNS ON NUTRITION

Certain medications can affect elders' eating habits by altering their sense of taste or appetite. This can create disinterest in eating and even dehydration. Disinterest in eating is also a cardinal sign of depression. Residents whose eating patterns change dramatically should be assessed for depression as well as for dehydration and compromised nutritional status. About 50% of older adults in hospitals and nursing facilities are malnourished and may be malnourished at the time of discharge (Nutrition Consortium of New York State, 1997). Most of these elders are discharged to nursing facilities. Weight is not the only way to assess nutritional status. Physical assessment (focusing on skin, muscle, hair, and the mouth), blood tests, and functional assessments can reveal nutritional deficits as well as other health concerns. Undernourishment can result in fatigue, muscle weakness, infection, hip fractures, anemia, and pressure ulcers. Nutritional clinical strategies can include specific suggestions for the family and a checklist for a nurse to provide to a physician for medical considerations, food considerations, and environmental considerations (Morley, 1999).

The purpose of this chapter is not to provide clinical assessment and treatment strategies. These are mentioned to underscore the importance of successfully including food in the life of frail elders and of doing so in a way that enhances all aspects of their quality of life, individually and communally.

It is important to respect that some individuals may choose to eat in private, but wherever a meal is taken, it should be normalized by removing a tray, if present, and assisting the resident into an armchair (as opposed to the resident eating in a wheelchair), if possible. An occupational therapist can adapt seating or eating implements. It may be possible to provide smaller and more frequent meals for some residents. In addition, staff can offer pain medication prior to meals for individuals with severe arthritis or pain-producing illnesses.

SOCIAL AND CULTURAL DIMENSIONS OF EATING

The African proverb, "If you eat alone, you will die alone; if I eat, my brother will eat," highlights the basic social dimension of eating. All cultural festivities have food at the heart of their celebrations. Staff should gather information from residents and families about events important to their culture and, as much as possible, include them in the dining and activity programs.

Food plays an essential part in maintaining ethnic identity. In the Muslim culture, the Eid festival, held during the Eid-al-Fitr, a 3-day Islamic holiday, occurs at the end of the month-long fasting period of Ramadan. This is expressed in religious, familial, and cultural activities. James Sinclair, in his reporting of the Eid festival in Ottawa, Canada, described families praying and relaxing together, enjoying games and activities, and participating in "an international halal food fair offering a mix of cuisine from Lebanon, India, and Afghanistan" (*The Ottawa Citizen*). Another culture-specific eating practice is seen in most Asian American elders, who are accustomed to having rice with every meal. Noodle soups and porridge are also preferred by many older adults. Residents need to be asked, however, about their preferences. Staff must be cautious about making generalizations since cultural and ethnic practices vary within ethnic groups as well as between groups.

Families are a great resource for gathering culturally relevant information. In addition, current nutrition science programs include information about various cultures' dishes so that dieticians are well-versed in multicultural foods and diets. Making mealtime interventions successful requires taking this interdisciplinary approach, which also includes families.

Food has symbolic meaning in various ceremonial and social functions. On the Day of the Dead (El Día de los Muertos) in Mexican culture, people celebrate a meal at the graves of their loved ones. It is a symbolic way of entering into communion with deceased family members. Another example can be seen in a Christmas tradition in the Mexican culture.

Women gather to make tamales for extended family to enjoy on Christmas Day. Two films that portray the role of food and eating in the family are *Tortilla Soup* and *Like Water for Chocolate.*

Food is also believed to treat and prevent certain diseases. Ethnic elders who follow Chinese medicine have a long tradition of preventing and treating disease with herbs in traditional teas and soups, which is an expression of the yin-yang philosophy and belief system that classifies all foods and other everyday experiences (McBride, 1996). Sometimes this is called *kitchen medicine,* which is also what C.K. Jeong called his Chinese cooking classes. Jeong discussed the philosophy and practice of kitchen medicine for prevention, early intervention, support, and recovery from disease in a presentation titled "Kitchen Medicine" at a medical conference in San Francisco in April 2001, "Enhancing Communication and Clinical Understanding of Chinese American Elders."

In addition to soliciting family support for celebrations involving food, facilities can often tap into local schools, churches, temples, and community organizations for contributions. A nursing facility in San Diego highlights the place of nativity for each resident. Every month, a particular city, state, or country is the focus of a celebration. Pictures of the chosen area, as well as other information, are posted prior to the event. Families are invited to attend the celebration. Dance, song, and food from that region are all components of the celebration. These celebrations have been a great success and have generated interest and involvement from the larger geographical community, which adds another layer of connection for the residents in the facility.

RELIGIOUS RITUALS AND FOOD

Certain religious groups observe rituals regarding preparation, blessing, and serving of meals (e.g., providing communion, saying grace, blessing food, serving kosher food). These religious rites typically hold a great deal of meaning for residents. It is important for staff to educate themselves about any food-related religious practices of residents and to make an effort to have them available.

Dayle A. Friedman, a rabbi in a skilled nursing facility in Philadelphia, facilitated a weekly Shabbat (Jewish Sabbath) service and meal with staff and residents. Because of the ceremonial participation and regularity of the Shabbat every week, residents felt connected to that "sanctuary in time," a holy place where they perceived their lives to be counted and to have purpose and meaning (Friedman, 1995). Friedman pointed out that religious rituals give rhythm and context to time when the rituals are part of the regular schedule of the facility and involve the residents in ways that are significant. For residents in a facility, time and the days of the week have no context outside of the facility's schedule. The Jewish elders who participated in Friedman's weekly Shabbat, in fact, spoke of the days of the week in relation to the past or upcoming Shabbat. This activity literally framed their existence in time:

> In religious life, time is divided into cycles of the week (Sabbath to Sabbath) and month (new moon to new moon) and year (festival). Each moment has its *location* in time—today is not just Tuesday, which looks like Monday and Wednesday, but...it is the third day after the Sabbath.... Ritual time creates a sense of continuity that is woefully absent from much of nursing home life. (Friedman, 1995, pp. 365–366)

EXERCISING AUTONOMY ABOUT MEAL CHOICES

People who live independently, irrespective of their socioeconomic differences, exercise their autonomy every time they eat something. Eating, which is so fundamental to existence itself, is often the last arena in which a person can exercise his or her autonomy. Every day people choose what and where they eat. Even a homeless person exercises some choice about what he or she eats. The older adults in nursing facilities, however, have notably fewer choices about what, when, and where they eat. It should be noted that residents can request food or refuse to eat; through an advance directive, they can also choose to have or not to have a feeding tube should they become unable to eat by other means. Generally, however, what they eat, where they eat, and even the time of day when they eat is controlled by others.

One way of supporting independence and choice in eating is to actually involve residents in the production of food. The following case study is an example of an intergenerational project that draws on the experiences of elders who have had vegetable and flower gardens. The project engages elders in the outdoors (something that often increases appetite), gives them some choice about what is planted, involves them in the harvesting (and possibly in the food preparation), and gives them a forum for sharing their experience and expertise, as well as for focusing on problem solving.

VALLEY HIGH SCHOOL

The Valley High School art class took as a project the design and creation of a garden at a local nursing facility. A local construction company and two garden nurseries donated materials. The finished garden included a water fountain, birdbath, raised flowerbeds, and beds containing herbs and vegetables. Vegetables were planted in season and harvested for the residents' meals. Broccoli and three types of lettuce were grown in the winter months. In the spring, more lettuce was planted, as well as strawberries, beans, tomatoes, and squash. Sufficient quantities were planted so that all residents (whose diets allowed) could partake in the experience. The planting beds brought many residents outside to inspect the garden for snails and weeds and to select ripe fruit and vegetables for the kitchen. The space was designed so that residents could easily move their wheelchairs through the garden, and students tended it with the elders twice each week. The students also participated by moving garden beds into the sun, purchasing seeds and small plants, getting garden books from the local library to share with residents, and joining a weekly gardening group to share gardening "secrets." The nursing facility provided a horticulture class for residents and distributed small plants (particularly African violets) to participating residents. The class included sessions for elders to reminisce about trees, plants, and gardens.

EXERCISE

Assign participants to roles either of feeding residents or of residents needing to be fed; have the participants rotate so that each participant experiences each role. Have the participants practice their feeding or eating roles in dyads. The food used for the exercise will be whatever the residents are being served that day. Each participant should pay attention to all aspects of each experience, which might include emotional feelings or associations (e.g., intimacy, embarrassment, joy, shame, interdependence or dependence), physical experiences (e.g., having or not having time to eat or taste, being forced to eat, being injured [e.g., by fork or spoon]), social experiences (e.g., associating with others).

Have participants debrief with their partner after the exercise, describing the experience. Then, have participants discuss their experience with the entire group. Was the exercise useful? What did participants learn? Finally, have participants discuss what, from this exercise, can be applied to resident feeding. Invite participants to develop an action plan for implementing one of the suggestions. Follow up after 2 weeks to evaluate participant implementation efforts and address any barriers. One important goal is to empower the direct-care staff with both suggesting change based on their own experience and values and evaluating the process.

COMMUNICATION ISSUES

Nursing assistants can make a significant contribution to the mealtime experience as well as expand their understanding of their role in the facility. For the nursing assistant, mealtime can be seen as an important venue for interaction with the resident, regardless of a resident's functional ability (i.e., whether a tray of food is delivered to the resident or the resident is fed by the nursing assistant). Staff can observe and engage in meaningful ways with residents while encouraging a genuine connection and exploration of each resident's personal identity through storytelling and reminiscence during eating or feeding, as well as by opening the door for expressions of concern.

Communication is essential for identifying residents' food preferences and for maintaining positive dining experiences. Just how important is communication? Table 1 provides questions that nursing facilities can ask about their mealtime services as a way to discover methods of fostering the pleasures of the table.

Table 1.   Staff discussion for fostering the pleasures of the table

1. How could mealtimes be made more nourishing (nutritionally, emotionally, socially, culturally, and spiritually) at our facility? What methods are in place but are not working?
2. Describe any general food preferences of residents that are known.
3. Can the elders use any of their own tableware for eating?
4. How might residents' stories about food preparation, family, celebrations, and food preferences be elicited and incorporated into mealtime experiences?
5. What changes would foster a connection between residents and/or staff at meal-times? Would it be possible for staff and residents to eat together?
6. Is it possible for staff members to eat with residents and take longer breaks at times other than meals?
7. How can residents be involved, if only on an occasional basis, in food preparation (e.g., setting the table, arranging flowers, providing afternoon tea, baking bread)?
8. How could staff be involved in investigating and enhancing this daily activity of resident life? Could a certified nursing assistant have a special role in this goal and work collaboratively with dietary staff and families to meet resident prefer-ences and needs?

SUSAN AND ROSIE

Susan was a very dedicated, experienced, and highly trained dietician working at a nursing facility. She was responsible for preparing meals for the residents who were confined to their rooms. Everything she prepared was pleasing to the eye and within the residents' dietary requirements. After a few months of serving residents, she observed that two of them were sending back their trays untouched. This offended the dietician. She had never visited the residents to get acquainted and inquire about their preferences. She had even less desire to do so after her culinary creations had been rejected. The facility's administrator asked Rosie, one of the nursing assistants, if she would be willing to work as a dietary assistant. Rosie was chosen because of her communication skills, and she successfully provided the missing link with the residents, who were quite com-fortable expressing their complaints and wishes to her. The residents who had offended the dietician, it turned out, had no family in the area and therefore no one to communicate on their behalf; for them, the tray was the only new thing that came into the room each day.

When Rosie began providing feedback from these residents, Susan found creative ways to respond to their requests while maintaining their dietary requirements, and the residents began taking pleasure in their meals again.

EXERCISE

1. Identify some typical gaps or breakdowns in communication specific to resident eating. List as many specific situations or issues as possible in a column on the left side of a chalkboard or on a piece of paper. No names are necessary; just describe the characteristics of the communication issue.

2. Elicit from the group any ideas, resources, or possible solutions for addressing each of the communication issues related to resident eating. Encourage all responses without evaluating their implementation. See Table 2 for additional resources for improving residents' mealtime experiences.

3. Select one or two issues for discussion of implementation and evaluation. Identify committed participants to participate in implementation. Once there is agreement and issues are prioritized, one of the participants in the in-service discussion can be involved as part of the implementation team in making specific recommendations, evaluating them, and ensuring their success.

Table 2. Resources for improving mealtime experiences

Dietary staff to assist with interdisciplinary training

Residents' families and personal networks

Cultural experts who reflect the resident population and can offer important cultural information and resources

Religious representatives who reflect the resident population and are willing to provide religious blessings and services that are appropriate for the residents

Culinary schools and departments of nutritional science in the area

The repetitive and frequent rhythm of meals creates a range of experiences from stressful to nurturing. An activity as frequent as eating, it seems, could be either a positive or burdensome experience. If it becomes burdensome (i.e., representing irritation or effort with no positive gain), in fact something to be recovered from, it will inevitably wear a resident down. If, in turn, it becomes a respite or pause from effort, worry, and preoccupation, it can encourage a resident to recall familiar sensual pleasures, personal engagement, and possibly his or her ethnic identity, as well as another's company. A common daily event becomes *healing medicine.*

ACTION STEPS

1. If you were king or queen for a day, and your every wish could be fulfilled, what would you change about meals served to elders in your facility?

2. What would you change about food preparation or eating arrangements if your parents were residents at the facility?

3. Brainstorm ways in which these changes might be brought about in your facility.

REFERENCES

Fisher, M.F.K. (1990). *The art of eating.* New York: Collier Books.

Friedman, D.A. (1995). Spiritual challenges of nursing home life. In M.A. Kimble, S. McFadden, J.W. Ellor, & J.J. Seeber (Eds.), *Aging, spirituality, and religion: A handbook* (pp. 365–366). Minneapolis: Fortress Press.

Jeong, C.K. (2001, April). *Kitchen medicine.* Presentation at the Enhancing Clinical Understanding and Communication with Chinese-American Elders conference, San Francisco, California.

McBride, M., Morioka-Douglas, N., & Yeo, G. (1996). *Aging and health: Asian and Pacific islander American elders* (2nd ed.; working paper #3). Stanford, CA: Stanford Geriatic Education Center.

Morley, J. (1999, Spring). Nutritional clinical strategies in long-term care. *Aging Successfully,* 9(1), 1, 7, 19.

Nutrition Consortium of New York State. (1997, November). *Nutrition programs.* Retrieved from http://www.meals.org/meals/nutrition.htm

Sinclair, J. (2000, December 30). Festival of food and games marks end of Ramadan. *The Ottawa Citizen.* Retrieved March 17, 2003, from http://www.ottawamuslim.net/ Newsarticles/feature_sinclair.htm

RECOMMENDED READING

"Ethnicity and nursing homes: Factors affecting the use and successful components for culturally sensitive care" by Gwen Yeo. In C.M. Barresi & D.E. Stull (Eds.), *Ethnic elderly and long-term care* (Springer)

Food and culture in America: A nutrition handbook (2nd ed.) by Pamela Goyan Kittler and Kathryn P. Sucher (West/Wadsworth)

Nutrition and health of ethnic elders: Curriculum guide, course outline, instructors manual by N.J. Downes (Stanford Geriatric Education Center)

"Position of the American Dietetic Association: Nutrition, aging, and the continuum of care" by the American Dietetic Association (2000) in *Journal of the American Dietetic Association, 100*(5), 580–595.

RESOURCES

Cultural and Ethnic Food and Nutrition
Education Materials: A Resource List for Educators
Web site: http://www.nal.usda.gov/fnic/pubs/bibs/gen/ethnic.html

Slow Food
Web site: http://www.slowfood.com

10

Nurturing the Mind, Body, and Soul

Recovering the Self Through the Arts

Marita Grudzen

OBJECTIVES

As a result of reading and working with the material in this chapter, participants will be able to

1. Understand the potential of the arts for enriching the lives of nursing facility residents

2. Understand the power inherent in beauty to provide joy and peace

3. Identify new ways of including the arts and nature in the lives of nursing facility residents

4. Identify resources in the community that provide additional access to the arts for nursing facility residents and staff

5. Celebrate the ethnic diversity of staff and residents through sharing of traditional cultural dress, food, crafts, music, dance, story, and rituals

6. Use specific art therapies to increase engagement and build confidence

EXPERIENCING LIFE THROUGH THE ARTS

One way to think about human existence and spirituality is to view each person's life as a work of art that has innate integrity, wholeness, wisdom, and beauty. Art, in its classical roots, was defined as a human reflection of the eternal qualities of beauty that transcend space and time. The Greeks made aesthetics, or the study of beauty in human experience, an essential part of philosophy. The Neo-Platonic Academy of Florence, during the 15th century, had a profound impact on many of the great artists of the Renaissance period. Today, it can be said that the arts and beauty have a humanizing effect on life, making people more sensitive to the deeper meaning of human culture as expressed in various forms of literature, music, drama, and dance. In a wider sense, each human life can be considered an artistic project insofar as people's lives reflect the eternal qualities of beauty, truth, and goodness. In order to perceive life as a work of art, people need experiences of beauty and the arts, the opportunity to enrich their interior life, and a community with which to share these experiences. Each generation has its own cultural, religious, and secular experiences of art. How can these essential experiences be included in a nursing facility and in care plans?

Understanding both the profound significance of the arts for residents' well-being and the spiritual dimension that art can offer for exploring meaning, self-expression, and intergenerational communication will enable staff to use the arts to enrich residents' lives.

THE ARTS IN THE NURSING FACILITY ENVIRONMENT

Studying the arts is considered an important part of the education of young people because it helps expand their awareness of cultural values and increases their intellectual creativity and reasoning ability. The same can be said for the role of the arts in the lives of older adults. This role has yet to be fully explored and developed in most nursing facility environments, however.

Participating in the arts is particularly important for continued stimulation of creativity in older people. Creativity is an important factor in continuing intellectual vitality at all stages of one's life. Professionals are beginning to explore whether the early onset of intellectual dysfunction can be mitigated through the active use of one's intellectual powers throughout the life cycle. For example, would providing regular, active cultural stimulation draw on the reserves of creativity that older adults possess? Intellectual powers include perceptual and kinesthetic abilities that are stimulated by the arts, such as the mental grasp of color, sound, movement, shape, and the position of objects in a physical environment. Neurophysiological coding of information gained through artistic experiences stimulates mental processes and provides topics for additional thought and conversation. Creative artistic expression provides many residents with an opportunity to integrate their life experiences.

Brain functioning is similar to a body's other physical capabilities. The brain works best when it is used frequently. Just as muscles lose tone when they are not used, so also do our mental capacities become weak and inefficient when they are not used regularly. Stimulation and involvement can be encouraged with many different materials and through a broad range of creative activities. Following are some examples of activities that can be incorporated into the life of a care facility to provide new learning opportunities and help residents develop skills:

- Show a film on a Saturday afternoon or evening for residents and families, with snacks and a follow-up discussion.

- Establish a knitting or crocheting group for those who are physically able that includes family and friends of residents and staff.

- Have residents compose floral arrangements for the dining area, other common areas, or individual trays; flowers could be provided by a local florist or by friends or family of a resident.

- Provide an art cart for residents' self-expression and activities such as making cards, bookmarks, and table decorations.

- Let residents decorate areas with themes such as sports or tea time that might attract men or women to gather together.

- Invite students from local high schools or college literature classes to pair with interested residents to share poetry and other forms of literature.

- Invite a local high school vocational class to collaborate on the design of a flower and vegetable garden that could be tended by both residents and students.

- Invite a local shop or church to sponsor an intergenerational fair featuring arts and crafts made by elders in nursing facilities or the surrounding community and by children's groups such as the Young Women's or Men's Christian Association (YWCA/YMCA) or Girl or Boy Scouts of America.

- Invite a local bead shop to sponsor an intergenerational jewelry-making event in which residents and families can make necklaces, bracelets, or pins for each other.

- Invite a local Scout troop, boys' or girls' club, pharmacy, or herbalists to help plant an herb garden that would be a healing space and that residents and their families could help design.

- Designate a music listening area with a CD and tape player and comfortable headsets.

It is noteworthy that many of the suggested activities are intergenerational. Interaction between children and elders can be beneficial to both generations. Art exhibits are one of the most straightforward vehicles for stimulating communication between elders and school children, but as the examples just given demonstrate, the possibilities are endless for implementing program ideas and visions generated by facility staff as well as through private, community, and academic partnerships.

Everyday Ways of Celebrating the Beauty of Art

Access to the arts, especially enhanced by conversation, can provide avenues for pleasure, enriched cultural experiences, deep connection, and an expanded view of life. How does exposure to art and discussion about it take place? Connecting with beauty in the nursing facility setting and improving residents' lives with the arts is not difficult. The following are ways of accomplishing this connection to the beauty of art with very few resources:

- Many residents have brought with them from home articles of special significance. To be sure, these are sources of beauty to them and are important pathways of connection for residents to the meaningful experiences from their prior life history. Staff should inquire about the story that lies behind the objects in an elder's room. Each object (e.g., a photo) tells a story that provides a unique perspective on the life of the resident. By asking questions about these special items (e.g., "Who is in the photo?" "Where was the photo taken?"), the staff can develop a meaningful relationship with the resident and create unique opportunities for deeper levels of communication.

- The beauty of nature's art is always available. Encourage residents to find a spot in which they can enjoy sunlight or an area where they can see and experience nature's beauty and rhythms.

- Facilitate the creation of an interior garden in a common room by encouraging families to contribute plants.

- Encourage residents to create their own sense of order and beauty in their living space by helping them select and arrange items they want in their surroundings. Staff can help residents choose, for example, the preferred type of bureau, shelf, or cabinet for their room. This can often be done in conjunction with the visit of a relative who will purchase the item and arrange for its delivery. The resident should be able to have a well-organized space that gives him or her easy access to the objects that are needed for everyday use as well as those objects that are artistic in nature and may be for display only or not be needed every day. This type of organization gives the resident a sense of personal control and emotional security.

- Ask a resident about his or her favorite musical pieces. If the pieces are not available, ask the family to supply them along with a CD or tape player. Note on the resident's care plan to ask about his or her music preferences. Playing the preferred music in a common area can draw the resident out of his or her room.

- Encourage families to engage with their loved ones in the presence of the arts. Residents may be able to attend a favorite performance, cultural event, or religious ceremony outside of the facility.

DISCUSSION

1. What forms of beauty bring you joy and peace?

2. What are your favorite art forms? Which ones might you want to explore in the future and why?

3. How do these experiences of beauty and art relate to spirituality for you and/or for others?

4. Do others' interests or experiences surprise you? Are there any new interests or talents that you want to experience based on what others have shared?

Music as an Art Form

Special rituals, such as birthdays or anniversaries, can often become opportunities for celebration through song. If a resident is confined to his or her room, other residents can visit with staff to celebrate special occasions. Just as a restaurant's staff often gathers to sing a birthday greeting for a patron, so can members of the nursing facility staff utilize song to memorialize and ritualize a special occasion for a resident. Here are some other ways to bring music into a facility:

- Staff and/or residents who have been part of a singing group such as a church choir, or part of an instrumental group such as a string quartet, could perform a song to celebrate an event.

- A local choral group can be invited to "adopt" a nursing facility for performances.

- A program could be developed with a local school's choir to give students community service credit for their involvement with a nursing facility.

- The choral group from a local church, synagogue, or temple could become part of a monthly birthday ritual for a nursing facility.

Meditative music or visual art forms that are symbolic in nature can help provide a context for exploration of the interior self. Music and art forms are generally symbolic in that they do not attempt to represent reality in a purely rational sense. They attempt to explore the emotional and spiritual qualities that elude rational discussion. For example, the symbolism of the cross can be very rich for a person of Christian faith, the third eye is the visual representation of human oneness with the universe in Hindu practice, and the yin-yang symbol carries deep philosophical meaning in Taoist beliefs.

Religious music is another expression of faith that can be used to create a meditative setting. Music such as Gregorian chanting or nature sounds can be provided during certain hours of the day for residents who are interested. A meditation room or small chapel offers a place for listening to music and reflecting on one's rich and diverse inner self. Staff should also be permitted to use this space for personal renewal as well as to understand how the space can benefit residents.

Writing and Other Art Forms

Any written or physical expression can be a basis for personal or interpersonal discovery. Journal writing, especially during a recovery or transitional period, can at the very least validate a person's existence. Something important can also be said for moving the pen across paper without being concerned about what is expressed. This physical act of writing typically creates emotional and mental movement. When personal care is being offered staff could inquire if the resident wishes to write a letter, an article for a local newsletter or newspaper, or a private journal entry (which could include experiments in poetry, watercolor, drawing or pressing flowers and leaves from the garden, or recording dream images). The facility can also foster expression through writing by hosting writing groups or writing classes. Kiku Funabiki, who began autobiographical writing in her late sixties, is an elder who has taught that writing can draw one into an inner stream of creative expression that is deeply satisfying and can distract a person from physical pain.

Another therapeutic art form for older adults in long-term care is drama. Maria Scaros Mercado, drama therapist at the Jewish Home in Valhalla, New York, has encouraged residents to enact their participation in a future public community event (e.g., attending a family wedding). This role playing can transform a routine physical therapy session into a live performance, with volunteers and staff assuming the role of witnesses and participants in the event. Drama in this context builds confidence and prepares residents for activities outside of the facility.

Finally, in addition to leaving written and other verbal legacies (described in Chapter 14), some individuals want to make an object to leave behind for their loved ones. Because of the frailty and fatigue that these individuals experience in their dying process, commitment to an art process requires a great deal of support and work on the part of an activity director, volunteer, family member, and/or friend. Nonetheless, this process is rich with meaning that people can only bring to a creation in the last days of their lives. This may also be the most significant spiritual expression of the individual's legacy.

Artistic experiences usually involve more than the rational self. Music, drama, and dance capture our imagination, sensual self, and spiritual values. Aristotle spoke of the aesthetic sensibility as bringing on a catharsis in the human psyche. Artistic experiences draw on every aspect of our human psyche and provide a means for self-transformation; we become more whole human beings by entering the universal dimensions of both tragedy and comedy expressed in the arts.

Many times, residents will bare their souls with the staff who provide care for them. Staff need to be respectful and nonjudgmental and need to maintain the privacy of residents' disclosures. Should these confidences be troubling or become burdensome, staff should seek the advice of a supervisor.

The Inner Landscape of Meditative Reflection

As people age, they feel the need to reconcile the unfulfilled parts of their lives with those aspects that have reached fulfillment and maturity. As a result, their spirituality becomes ever more central. For example, residents who have accomplished many achievements through family, career, business, and community life often have not had the opportunity to explore the creative dimensions of their psyche.

Carl Jung argued that the latter periods of life were most conducive to *soul work* (Singer, 1994). For Jung, the soul was the seat of the major universal archetypes that influence the relationship of the unconscious to the individual life. Soul work, for Jung, was the process of individuation through which an individual integrated the major life attractions, interests, and desires into a unified and coherent life project. In Jungian thought, soul work is a process similar to the artistic process. The exploration of the soul dimension is best understood in the language of the arts. Poetry, drama, and music are part of the landscape of the soul because they do not exhibit a purely rational or technologically based understanding of human existence.

The writings of Thomas Moore (1992) have helped to popularize the importance of soul work as part of the relatively new field of *transpersonal psychology*. Transpersonal psychology acknowledges a transcendent dimension of human experience and incorporates this aspect of life into its psychological system. Transpersonal psychology seeks to discover the spiritual values and symbols that are reflected, for example, in the dream work of each individual. Moore's work could provide a framework for long-term care staff's exploration and implementation. Chapter 7 (Gifts of Depression) and Chapter 8 (The Body's Poetics of Illness) of Moore's (1992) *Care of the Soul: A Guide for Cultivating Depth and Sacredness in Everyday Life* are particularly appropriate for staff exploration and implementation.

Soul work can best be illuminated in an environment that is sensitive to the many layers of people's lives. Life experiences include both events that are quickly forgotten and some that lead to deeper questioning about the meaning of life. Some such events may include spiritual experiences of enlightenment, relationships that become passionate attachments, and tragic events. Layers of meaning often unfold when people explore these significant events after periods of meditation and interior silence.

Dreams also can be a window into nonrational, intuitive dimensions of human experience and will be discussed in the following section.

Dream Groups Dream groups can be facilitated to explore the emotion-laden images that arise from the unconscious or subconscious of older adults when they enter a dream-like state of mind. Dream groups can be avenues for exploring the interior lives of residents in which skilled counselors in dream work provide a safe place for residents. The recollected dreams often contain rich symbolic content that can be explored with a facilitator in a group setting. A skilled facilitator who has training in this area (e.g., psychologist, marriage and family counselor, clergy member) can help residents to explore their subconscious self as manifested in the symbolic content of their recollected dreams or images, which often becomes more accessible in the latter part of one's life through day or night dreams.

Day dreams are sometimes called *twilight imagery*. Some people can recall their dream life better through "waking dreams" whereas others remember their night dreams better by recalling them as soon as they awaken. Carl Jung's work with patients indicated that older adults tend to have a richer dream life partly because of the variety of life experiences that they have access to through dreams.

A trained facilitator can read a poem and/or play a piece of music as a backdrop for exploring the symbols that arise in the group members' dreams and during meditative reflection. Many mental health professionals (e.g., psychologists, clinical social workers, pastoral counselors, chaplains) have some training in Jungian psychology and can successfully lead dream groups.

Dreams often explain the workings of our inner self through symbolism. For instance, a woman in her seventies dreamed that she opened an empty refrigerator. Before she was a resident in a nursing facility, she had hosted all of her family's holiday meals and cooked daily for her husband who had severe rheumatoid arthritis. The empty refrigerator symbolized a major transition in her life.

Dream groups can help residents to explore potent images from dreams, such as the empty refrigerator, either through the prism of their own experiences or through the experiences and insights of peers and the dream group facilitator. Jung felt that these images usually had a connection to universal archetypes that resonated with every human being. For example, the heroic journey is something common to all ages and cultures. Journey dreams can have multiple levels of meaning, but they are rooted in the journey experience we make from our birth to our final passage from this world at death.

Oral History   Residents can be encouraged to share the richness of their lived experiences by creating an oral history in a group setting or in a video- or audiotaped encounter with a staff or family member. The taping sessions can serve as both a resident's oral history and as a map of the resident's spiritual journey. An oral history helps elders to recollect the significant events of their lives and explore the meaning of those events. The most meaningful events will usually resonate with many images that can be explored as a "map" of the trajectory of a person's life. Usually, the central passions of a person's life are revealed in an oral history.

Oral history has often been limited to the "outer" events of a person's life, but it is just as important for residents to record the "inner" events that have moved them forward on the path of life. The arts help people get in touch with their inner self, that part of the self which is often elusive to rational thought. Inner events are characterized by the manner in which people respond to certain life-changing experiences. An example of this type of intra-psychic event could be the emotional transformation that occurs when people "fall" in love. "Falling" in love is not just an outer event; it changes the interior processes of people's thoughts and emotions. The intersections of the events of one's inner life can act as an important fulcrum for understanding the processes of an individual's journey through life. Jung called this the *process of individuation.*

Individuation is the process by which an individual selects the major thematic content of his or her life and chooses a path for incorporating this content into the people and projects that characterize his or her life direction. Individuation is also the unique path that plays out these life themes and can be explored for many levels of meaning. For example, an individual who loves the outdoor life and camping incorporates the mythic theme of "wilderness" into his or her life. An oral history helps residents articulate these life themes.

It becomes especially important to older adults to record the events of their life in order to pass on their living tradition or family history. Human life does not begin at point zero. Each person is part of the ongoing stream of history. People can only understand their identity and meaning by viewing the larger framework of their extended family history, their ethnic or cultural history, and the spiritual or philosophical meaning they find in life. For most human beings, this is a project that evolves from the experience of extended family and cultural influences over time.

EXPLORING ETHNICITY AND CULTURE THROUGH THE ARTS

Nursing facilities have many different cultural cohorts, and it is important for staff to continue to increase their knowledge and appreciation of the ethnic and cultural variations and heritage in the community. Each culture expresses its own symbolism in multiple art forms (e.g., ethnic or cultural music). Each generation in each ethnic group has a different set of historical experiences that greatly affect that generation's sense of identity and interests.

For many ethnic minority elders, these historical experiences have included racism and discrimination. Although the arts are a relevant way to share these histories, a strong multicultural environment of respect and appreciation for the pain and struggle that these elders endured on their life journeys is necessary. Artistic representations and resources that are brought into the nursing facility need to reflect the cultural composition of residents and staff (e.g., ethnic or cultural music such as mariachi, gospel, jazz, or country/western; celebrations such as the Posadas festival for Mexican Americans or Chinese New Year for Chinese Americans).

A *cultural audit,* which takes into account age cohorts, can be an important tool for understanding the cultural framework within which staff could develop an artistic program. Cultural forms such as ethnic festivals, holidays, or religious rituals can become the vehicle through which staff, volunteers, and consultants learn to enrich the lives of residents. Cultural programs (e.g., performances by religious or social choral groups, chamber music groups, or folk singers; poetry readings coordinated by local poetry societies; small drama productions; art exhibits) speak to both the historical events of a resident's life and his or her interior life that has been a guide through many difficulties and dangers.

Culture provides a natural vehicle for celebration, affirmation, and community building. The nursing facility community has a richly diverse staff as well as diverse residents. Regular opportunities to celebrate ethnic cultures through food, music, dance, dress, crafts, pictures, and stories often create new interactions, strengthen bonds, build bridges of understanding and appreciation, and increase pride for members of cultural groups. In addition, different artistic groups in the community represent the artistic heritage of each culture found in the nursing facility.

International celebrations held annually could demonstrate the facility's commitment to diversity by honoring staff and residents from particular parts of the world. For these celebrations, families of residents and staff from those regions could bring various expressions of their culture such as clothing, food, music, stories, pictures, maps, dances, songs, and crafts for the celebration.

Ethnic-specific arts groups (e.g., Ballet Folklorico of Mexico) could be invited to perform in the nursing facility. If that is not possible, facilities might be able to obtain audio- or videotapes of their performances and play them for the residents of that particular ethnic or cultural heritage. Almost every arts group records at least some of their performances and makes them available to the community for promotional purposes. In some cases, it may be possible to interest one or more cast members from a drama group to come to the nursing facility for a community event in conjunction with the opening of their show or to show a videotape of their performance. These activities can be a way for an ethnic or cultural group to explore the unique historical aspects of their culture. Each person's life is rich with his or her own culture and can be shared through storytelling. Some residents may even have been part of cultural performances (e.g., powwows, drumming circles, church choirs, folk dance groups) earlier in their lives but are now too infirm to participate. The viewing of the performance and its discussion can be a form of participation.

Long-term care staff members can be most effective in their mission when they realize all of the dimensions of human culture that are important to residents and focus on delivering more than just a medical model of care. A more humanistic model of care emphasizes human communication and interaction as important dimensions of the "care" plan for elders. The western medical model relies more on technology and pharmacological treatment of ailments, often ignoring the healing power of human understanding and the building of meaningful relationships. Without this kind of care, elders often lapse into depression, leading to even more physical and mental problems. To this end, a facility's administration needs to incorporate the arts in its mission statement (see Figure 1) and begin to promote opportunities for, and expressions of, this commitment.

DISCUSSION

1. Which ethnic groups predominate among your staff and residents? How can you include artistic expressions from these ethnic backgrounds in the lives of your residents?

2. What cultural holidays can you identify? Which of these might be good for international celebrations?

3. In what ways can the arts be integrated into the planning processes of your facility?

EXPLORING ART EXCHANGES WITH THE COMMUNITY

The arts can become a central focus in a long-term care setting with support from the surrounding community. (Nursing facility leaders can see Relationships in the Arts Community at the end of the chapter.) Many of the arts become more prevalent during the holiday season when, for example, Christmas carols are sung for the benefit of residents. For increased variety throughout the year, however, consider encouraging the presence of other forms of artistic expression by individuals or groups in the community.

Remember first that many residents have had very active lives and possess a wealth of talent and experience upon which to draw for artistic expression. Some residents may have extensive creative talents in the visual arts from having worked in the fields of commercial art or design. Others may have had prior experience in advertising, floral design, musical training or appreciation, or singing. Many residents also have literary talents

---

It is the goal and objective of this senior facility to incorporate the arts and artistic experiences into the life of our senior residences. We will include experiences that assist residents to express their own artistic sensibilities through programs adapted to their physical, mental, spiritual, and emotional capabilities. We shall also make every effort to involve local arts groups that draw from many ethnic and cultural backgrounds to sponsor artistic performances within the environment of the senior facility or a facility accessible to our senior residents, accommodating the residents' needs (e.g., wheelchair accessible). A member of the senior center staff will be appointed to coordinate artistic programs and experiences for the residents in our senior care home and an annual arts plan developed with input from both residents and other staff. Just as the humanities are considered essential for the education of our youth, we feel that cultural experiences are essential for the mental, spiritual, and emotional well-being of our senior residents.

Figure 1. Example of a nursing facility's mission statement.

that can be expressed through storytelling and many forms of writing such as editorials, fiction, poetry, memoirs, and plays.

The arts need not be limited to activities in the nursing facility, however. Residents are capable of high levels of artistic expression deserving recognition in the larger community. Some residents may be willing to be part of a talent show, and the staff could invite members of the wider community to take part in the event. Holidays are particularly appropriate for this type of event. Residents who often feel isolated during the holidays then have something to look forward to.

The arts function as an important connecting mechanism to involve the nursing facility in the activities and life of the larger community. Some arts groups seek live audiences for the preparatory stages of their presentations, or for preview performances. Amateur drama groups, community college choral and dance groups, and high school drama clubs are just some of the arts groups that could be invited to share an upcoming presentation with a nursing facility's residents. Arts groups can also partner with nursing facilities to seek new avenues to fund their work. Many funding agencies like to see community involvement and participation as part of the design for a proposed arts project.

Musical and/or dramatic tableaus with seasonal themes involving staff and residents are another creative option for exploring the arts. These displays can help older adults participate in the seasonal rhythms of spring, summer, fall, and winter and can also draw from their experiential wisdom. Each season may have special meaning because of the symbolism it contains for residents (e.g., renewal of the human spirit in spring, gathering the fruits of labor in autumn).

Each resident's reminiscence of different events in his or her life can be used as a rich vessel for exploring the arts through photography. Residents' personal photos can become the content for an artistic tableau that re-enacts scenes involving family and friends from the life of a nursing facility resident. Selected photos of the resident and his or her family members can be prominently displayed in a resident's room or on a public bulletin board. With the growth of Internet photograph "albums," it is possible for residents to share their photographs with relatives who live far away. High school and community college students involved in photography classes could be recruited to assist residents in such projects and could participate in photograph exhibits at local nursing facilities.

The most prominent national program to foster the relationship between life story and creativity is Elders Share the Arts (ESTA), now part of the National Center for Creative Aging (NCCA) in Brooklyn, New

York. For 20 years, ESTA has provided many art mediums and intergenerational collaborations for working with the raw material of one's life experience. Founder Susan Perlstein, Executive Director of the NCCA, was funded in 1998 by the National Endowment for the Arts to develop a national database and national resource center.

Here are some other ideas for using the arts to intermingle nursing facility and community life:

- Invite school children to the nursing facility to share holiday art projects and inspire the holiday spirit in residents.

- Inquire if a floral designer would volunteer to design a holiday floral bouquet for the facility's foyer or cafeteria.

- Commission a muralist to design a mural for one of the community rooms.

- Solicit local government or civic groups (e.g., Rotary, Kiwanis, Optimist) to provide funding for arts projects that provide a service to older adults.

- Ask local high school literature or drama teachers to encourage their students to perform a creative reading of a play or series of poems.

- Investigate if instructors from a community college can offer courses on-site or through a cable television broadcast.

- Provide space for local arts groups to rehearse and perform in a nursing facility.

- Inquire if area painters and watercolorists will volunteer to provide artistic expertise, mentoring, and materials to residents and staff.

- Locate a potential host from area museums, churches, businesses, or schools who is willing to exhibit residents' work, such as intergenerational projects, in his or her establishment. In connection with such an event, encourage social interaction for residents with an open house that allows them to interact with other age groups in the community and not feel limited to members of their own age group.

An example of a successful facility–community collaboration is Art with Elders (AWE), a program of the Eldergivers organization located in San Francisco. AWE provides art classes for older adults and hosts an annual art exhibit at a major museum in San Francisco featuring the art of elders who live in senior housing, assisted living facilities, and nursing facilities. Artists-in-residence from the AWE program can visit nursing facilities for a fee to encourage residents to explore the arts through one-to-one teaching of painting and watercolor. In 2002, the Eleventh Annual AWE Exhibition debuted 87 works of art created by older adults; each work was framed and accompanied by a picture and brief biographical sketch of the artist. It is quite moving to see buses full of culturally diverse elders, many of whom are in wheelchairs, arriving for an event honoring the artwork that most of them have just begun creating in this later period of their lives. Attendance for the event draws largely from the arts community and the gerontological community.

Volunteers in Arts Programs

The role of volunteers as *animators of the arts* in the nursing facility cannot be underestimated. Volunteers, particularly enthusiastic volunteers, can offer a level of commitment and love for their art or craft that is infectious, inspiring residents to try something new. In this sense, they are animators, encouraging a kind of artistic license to create what might be lacking without their presence. These volunteer groups will often become sponsors of performances by local arts groups that may need some funding to take their performance on the road. Local churches, synagogues, and mosques often want to do community outreach, and the arts are a way to do this in a nonsectarian way. In this sense, such volunteer groups offer a way for everyone in the community to participate. These volunteer groups may be enlisted to participate in the arts programs of a nursing facility as well as act as sponsors for arts programs that are brought to the nursing facility. In many cases, certain arts activities are not within a nursing facility's budget. However, animators of the arts can often raise the funds necessary to sponsor an arts program and to purchase the materials that are needed for projects such as needlework or oil painting. All such projects also require volunteers to mentor the residents and to provide an audience for viewing residents' work. Animators of the arts can also arrange for a display of the artwork in a local religious institution in which a reception could be held for the resident artists.

Partnerships with Local Schools

More and more school districts throughout the country are requiring senior high school students to earn community service hours as part of their graduation requirements. Almost all high schools have drama and music groups that could earn their community service hours in conjunction with a local nursing facility. Any partnership through the arts with a school community would need the guidance and coordination of the nursing facility's activity director.

Many nursing facility residents love to have young people visit them. If a local school becomes involved with a nursing facility through the school's arts program, the residents and youth often become a part of each other's lives. Youth and elders have much in common because they often have the freedom to explore dimensions of life and learning that are often not available to those immersed in their middle years in the daily responsibilities of raising a family, earning a living, and meeting the multiple requirements of society. The vulnerability of youth and elders also gives them a common bond and interest in each other's lives. This sense of mutual interdependence can become a vital source of community when youth and elders have the opportunity to interact with each other. The arts become the medium through which this exchange can occur.

Poetry readings given by student volunteers or as part of a class requirement offer a good example. Poetry expresses the deeper mysteries of life that seem to elude rational analysis. Elders are more open to the transcendent dimension of life and often have an expanded aesthetic sensibility based on their mature life experience and greater understanding of and appreciation for life's transience. An activity such as a poetry reading can help students and residents become part of each other's lives and awareness within the context of the arts. In many cases, the nursing facility can become a venue for a live audience for poetry readings, dramatic readings, or musical performances during the school day when others are not available because of work and family obligations.

Schools can also benefit from the feedback that residents can give to students who participate in such programs. Discussion groups can be formed at the nursing facility to discuss the works of literature that students and residents have read or seen performed. In addition, cable television arts programs provide opportunities for students and older adults to watch major arts performances together. The students earn community service credits in addition to participating in an intellectual discussion with residents.

DISCUSSION

1. Are you or other staff members part of a community arts group that might be interested in participating

in an arts enrichment program for your nursing facility?

2. What is your perception of residents' interest and potential involvement in these programs?

3. What types of arts programs do you think would generate the greatest interest and engagement among residents?

In this chapter, various methods for bringing an artistic awareness and artistic experiences into the life of a long-term care community have been explored. A variety of strategies and partnerships need to be established with community groups and arts groups (see the appendix, Relationships with the Arts Community) for elders to gain access to these types of enriching artistic programs. Staff training can facilitate this awareness and awaken an interest in the arts. Actual arts programs can be made a part of the long-term care facility with sufficient planning, outreach, and coordination with the local arts community.

ACTION STEPS

1. Think of the types of artistic activities and programs that would be appropriate for the common area of your facility or one-to-one activities in residents' rooms. What type of research would be needed to develop or locate suitable activities and programs? Who could begin this process?

2. What particular areas of your facility might be enhanced with color, flowers, music, or prints of famous paintings? Could a particular space be used for meditation or religious art that represents the diversity of traditions in the facility? What steps or approvals would be necessary to make these changes?

3. Consider ways you could share your artistic interests or experiences with the residents and your co-workers.

4. Make a project of identifying staff members who are connected with community groups that could enhance the presence of the arts in the nursing facility.

5. Discuss forming a committee charged with outreach in the community to make this vision a reality. A rotating committee, with new members every 6 months or more, could help to identify new opportunities as well as to balance the work involved.

6. Assemble a list of potential intergenerational projects. Then, discuss possible youth groups with which to partner.

7. Consider having one or two international days for a festive celebration of staff members' and residents' cultural traditions. What ideas do you have about implementing such events? When and where could the festivities take place? What should be included in the events? What costs would be incurred? What foreseeable barriers might need to be addressed?

REFERENCES

Moore, T. (1992). *Care of the soul: A guide for cultivating depth and sacredness in everyday life.* New York: HarperCollins.

Singer, J. (1994). *Boundaries of the soul: The practice of Jung's psychology. Revised and updated.* San Francisco: Anchor.

RECOMMENDED READING

Beyond the tunnel: The arts and aging in America by Joan Hart (Museum One)

Where people fly and water runs uphill: Using dreams to tap the wisdom of the unconscious by Jeremy Taylor (Warner Books)

RESOURCES

Eldergivers

Web site: http://www.eldergivers.org

Includes information about the AWE program

**American Association of Homes and
Services for the Aging (AAHSA)**
Web site: http://www.aahsa.org
Represents nonprofit approaches to caring for and serving older adults

National Center for Creative Aging (NCCA)
Web site: http://www.center-for-creative-aging.org
Includes information about ESTA

Lutheran Services in America
Web site: http://www.lutheranservices.org

A faith-based organization that provides a number of caregiving services, including nursing facility services

Appendix

Relationships with the Arts Community

Every connection with the community can benefit residents of long-term care facilities as well as the facilities themselves. Some tangible benefits of community involvement for a facility include easier recruitment of volunteers; more access to fund-raising activities; scheduling of shared events with other community groups such as churches, synagogues, schools, or civic groups (e.g., Kiwanis, Rotary); and opportunities for development of joint programs with other health or elder-related institutions in the community. For residents, tangible benefits include many different opportunities for making art, being exposed to new expressions of art and beauty, and, most notably, increased attention and stimulation. Intangible benefits for both parties can include increased visibility in the community, improved image of the long-term care facility, greater awareness of the needs of residents living in long-term care communities, and greater public acknowledgment of the important role of the long-term care facility in the life of the larger community.

Some of the biggest challenges in the long-term care industry are finding ways to overcome residents' feelings of isolation and boredom and finding funding for supplemental programming. The long-term care community can gain greater access to private and public funding sources by becoming more visible in the community and developing strategic partnerships with schools, churches, and civic groups. Each community has key leadership groups that set the tone for that community. Usually, such groups like to reach out to elders and people with disabilities in the community for special projects, particularly during holidays. With good planning, the staff of long-term care facilities can develop links with these groups and gain support for meeting their facilities' social and financial needs. Following are some ideas about creative programs or collaborations to pursue and ways to finance them.

143

FUNDING

Individual nursing facilities usually do not have the leverage to obtain major grant support for arts projects. More likely they receive small donations made by individual donors or small businesses in their neighborhood. They can bolster this support and reduce the cost of a project by obtaining needed materials through community donations rather than by direct purchase by the facility. Beyond that, however, the arts community can be an important partner in developing funding proposals for the nursing facility community. Funding agencies, both private and governmental, usually develop requests for proposals based on some demonstrated need for services in a particular community. Because funds are often in short supply, part of the criteria for receiving any funding for a particular project may be the ability of the program sponsor to link with other community groups and leverage the private or public funds with those of other agencies in the community. Most grant developers actually like to see arts groups enter into partnerships with other community service agencies. Moreover, residents in nursing facilities are an important focus of service for many foundations and government grants agencies.

Long-term care facilities need to become aware of the demonstrated needs of elders in their local or regional community. Usually, the local Area Agency on Aging (contact the National Association of Area Agencies on Aging for a local agency) can provide an overview of the needs identified for elders in a particular community. With the assistance of the local Area Agency on Aging and other community health or cultural planning groups, facility staff can determine potential areas of community concern that are eligible for funding. The facility can then determine which group or groups may be logical partners for helping to secure such funding.

Long-term care facilities are frequently very committed to fostering educational and intergenerational activities between older adults and youth. Local educational facilities can therefore become ideal partners in seeking funding for innovative learning programs with children, teenagers, and adults. In these programs, older adults get to share much of their wisdom and youth learn how to interact and share with the older generation. Elders can also learn how to use new technologies such as computers and cell phones that help to relieve their sense of isolation from the larger community. Of course, cultural activities can also provide a bridge between older adults and the neighboring community.

Partnerships build community and a sense of shared responsibility for the well-being of a community. Funding agencies like to see cooperation rather than competition among community agencies so that each agency provides a portion of the service delivery needed for a healthy community. Older adults are becoming a larger and larger sector of almost every community in the United States. The population of older adults will continue to grow rapidly in the years ahead with continuing advances in health care and the entry of baby boomers into their "golden years." Funding agencies will likely be targeting a portion of their grant money to service this growing sector. A coalition of elder care delivery systems can illustrate to funding agencies the links that are already in place among them. Cultural groups can also benefit by linking with an older adult consortium because elders can provide a stable population of interested "consumers" during times when the rest of the population is at work or otherwise unavailable. Elders can, for instance, attend daytime matinees or Sunday evening performances when many other age groups are too busy to attend.

Arts groups in almost every community across America depend heavily on foundation and government support for their programs. Ticket sales make up only a small portion of the funding for arts groups' projects. Private corporations also like to support the arts and any partnerships with other community groups are an additional bonus for their charitable donations. Nursing facilities can also form a consortium with each other and with the local arts community to benefit from United Way funding and other corporate charitable activity. Many funding agencies want to see their funds dispersed to the most neglected members of a community; this is the principle behind programs such as Head Start, which aids young, disadvantaged children. Agencies, whether private or public, that fund programs for older adults should be educated about the under-representation of elders residing in nursing facilities as beneficiaries of the grant funds dispensed for elder projects.

More ambitious partnerships can be formed with the arts community or funding agencies that support arts projects by collaborating with other long-term care facilities for elders. Such grants can include performance subsidies for the residents, artist-in-residence projects, the subsidization of arts instruction, and arts materials for use by the older adults.

ARTIST-IN-RESIDENCE

The artist-in-residence concept can provide great benefit for both the artist and the residents of a nursing facility. The artist receives a grant to make the nursing facility a place in which to develop his or her art and perform or display it for the benefit of the long-term care community. The artist-in-residence could be a poet, painter, sculptor, graphic designer, musician, or actor/actress who works in an area that is accessible to the residents of the long-term care community and also takes regular opportunities to interact with residents and share insights about the artistic process. The residents have the opportunity to interact with the artist-in-residence, who spends one or more days each week in the nursing facility working on arts projects. Usually, the artist also teaches some aspect of his or her specialty to residents who are interested in acquiring these skills and using them in making their own art. In some cases, the residents can actually participate in an arts project with the artist-in-residence. With the opportunity to collaborate over several months, the residents and the visiting artist form a close relationship and enjoy each other's presence while being involved in an artistic process.

WEB SITE DEVELOPMENT

Constructing a web site can both assist in the recruitment of resources outside of the nursing facility and benefit those residents who have the capacity to understand and appreciate the web site development process.

A web site for a long-term care facility could serve to represent the quality of care and the value of members in a long-term care community. With the consent of the residents, the home page of such a web site could provide information about residents, such as their historical backgrounds. These descriptions give an institution a more human quality that is often overlooked. In addition, a web site could link to the nursing facility's strategic partners so that people can easily find the facility via more than one link (e.g., schools and art programs that partner with a facility).

A web site can be used for outreach such as recruiting individual volunteers from the community, collecting donations for projects, and displaying art that is generated by either residents or an artist-in-residence. Volunteer positions, as well as opportunities to collaborate with other community groups that serve long-term care residents, can be listed on the facility's home page. Volunteers can be recruited to help residents with arts-and-crafts projects and to help residents learn how to use computers to send e-mail to relatives and friends or to communicate with people in the community who have similar backgrounds or interests. A request can also be put out for volunteers to help decorate a facility for special events or holidays.

COMMUNITY ART GALLERY

One way to make the nursing facility more visible to the community is to construct an art gallery within the facility environment. Many local artists want a public place to hang or display their artwork. Certain common areas can be designated as part of a gallery. Community volunteers or even a local art gallery owner can be enlisted in this effort to mount art displays by local artists on a periodic basis. The community can then be invited to view the art displays and interact with the artists and the residents. In addition, local art associations can be enlisted to jury the shows and award prizes for the best art.

There are several benefits to providing a community art gallery. The arts community benefits by having a free space to hang artwork that might not be exhibited at commercial galleries but that still has great artistic merit. If any art is sold in the public display, a portion of the proceeds can go to art classes and activities that are conducted within the nursing facility. These public art displays become another method for connecting the long-term care staff and residents with the wider community. These events can also garner public support for the nursing facility when the facility applies for grants or foundation support.

COMMUNITY ARTS PARTNERSHIPS

A partnership model can be developed that links nursing facilities with organizations or institutions that support the arts, such as major art schools or museums that exhibit the work of professional artists. If successfully established, these partnerships provide access to major funding sources (e.g., wealthy patrons) that support art schools and museums.

Nursing facilities can explore becoming part of existing programs already funded by art institutions. Professional art students can be recruited to do work for a nursing facility for which they can obtain credit. An art museum could sponsor special visits by professional artists during times when residents can visit the museum to view exhibits and interact with museum staff and artists. Such events can be held annually or semi-annually and be co-sponsored by a nursing facility association (e.g., American Association of Homes and Services for the Aging, Bay Area Ministry to Nursing Homes, National Center for Creative Arts), a local art school, and/or a local museum. Specific donors may also consider sponsoring these types of "high visibility" events that may be heavily publicized in the local media.

The public relations benefit of such events for both the long-term care community and the arts community cannot be overlooked. Both communities struggle to secure sufficient public or private funding. Such collaborative events help both entities become more visible to the overall community, particularly if they are covered by local media. Articles in the press are just one more tool for demonstrating the merits of a program and obtaining grant support for an ongoing program that links the arts community and a long-term care community.

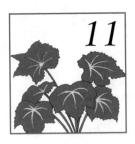

Pathways
to Comfort

The Importance of Self-Care

Ron Zielske

OBJECTIVES

As a result of reading this chapter and working through the exercises, participants will be able to

1. Reaffirm their value and worth as human beings

2. Identify those things that contribute to caregiver fatigue

3. Identify and learn new ways to care for the whole self

4. Understand the spirituality of work

THE VALUE OF STAFF

Wellness has to do with body, mind, and spirit. If the staff can perform the physical aspects of care but not the emotional, or if staff members are angry or irritable, the residents' wellness will be affected. Residents feel as well in any one day as the caregiving staff feels well. When staff members are exhausted or preoccupied with personal and family problems, they may have difficulty performing care duties and in the nursing facility environment may not be truly present to the residents.

Practicing self-care allows individuals to reach their own potential and find meaning in life. In spiritual terms, each person is unique, for not even identical twins have the same personality. Each person has special gifts, many of which are different from other staff members but are necessary for the care of residents. One person will accomplish a task very differently from a colleague but each staff person will be trying to contribute to the well-being of others. Everyone shares a commonality of body, mind, and spirit, but the specific desire of some to care for others is what brings them to a profession in long-term care.

For some people, recognizing their own self-value may be a stretch, but gaining that insight for oneself and assisting residents to see their own value as human beings is vital to a sense of well-being. By assisting others, a person also assists him- or herself. Although the mission of a nursing facility will emphasize that the care of residents is primary, part of the task of a caregiver is also to show support and concern for others—family and friends—connected to the residents. Before staff members can effectively meet others' needs, however, they must be caring toward themselves.

IDENTIFYING AND MANAGING STRESS

Staff in long-term care can experience many kinds of stress, including the exhaustion of working more than one job, the responsibilities of child raising, and working effectively while experiencing physical problems. Stress very often exacerbates problems in parts of the body that are already having difficulties. For example, a person who has a bad back or stiff neck will experience worse pain in those areas when stressed.

DISCUSSION

1. What internal and external stresses affect you and other staff members and contribute to caregiver fatigue?

2. How many of you are among the many long-term care facility staff members who work more than one job, put in many hours, and also have family responsibilities? How does this feel?

3. Do you get days off? For what reason are you and other staff members absent from work?

4. Do you get any time away from kids? Are you financially able to have a social life?

5. Are you experiencing difficulties in your home life? Who or what makes you frustrated?

6. Do you have access to health care, counseling, or continued education?

7. What are your self-expectations?

8. Think about what messages you have been taught about your worth and value. Share with the group if you feel comfortable.

People are constantly faced with adversity in life, which naturally causes stress. How they react to it is key. Even the most gifted people will have a difficult time in life and have their gifts stunted if they are unable to function or face trouble or criticism, or if they experience flagging confidence.

A nursing facility also experiences difficulties and stresses that get transferred to the staff, for example when a staff has to function with a shortage of employees, especially for a long period of time. Even though the staff gets extra pay in such times, it does not compensate for the lack of sleep, the irritability, or the inability of staff members to perform at their best. Other factors that can create a great amount of stress are residents who require a great deal of care or residents who are dying.

A wise facility allows for support groups. When the staff carries heavy stress loads, it is easy for individuals to forget to carry out ordinary daily tasks of resident care. A stress test can be very helpful in assisting staff members to identify their internal and external stressors (see Resources at the end of the chapter for an Internet link to a stress test).

DISCUSSION

1. Who or what has helped you face hard times in the past? How would you like to deal with hard times in the future?

2. Identify the ways that you and other staff can overcome adversity and carry on, to the fullest extent, with life.

3. What coping skills do you want to develop and how can you develop them?

MARIE

Marie, a nursing assistant, came to work hurt, angry, and frustrated because her boyfriend had walked out on her the night before and had given her a black eye. She had been depending on his paycheck to help support her two children. At work, she could not concentrate and was irritable and unkind to the residents. At break time, she was mad at herself for not being in better control of her emotions, for she truly loved her residents. In addition, she had been yelling at other staff. The staff developer, Pam, who was on the floor training new assistants pulled her aside and asked what was wrong. After listening to Marie's story, Pam assured Marie that she was a valued employee and loved by the other staff and residents but told her that she could not take out her frustrations on them. After asking what Marie's immediate needs were, Pam hugged Marie, who was crying, and referred Marie to Jane, the human resources specialist who was in charge of employee assistance. In turn, Jane referred Marie to community services, where she could obtain food on a temporary basis and explained how Marie could receive temporary assistance from an advance in pay. Jane also referred Marie to the facility chaplain, a skilled counselor who could help her grieve her losses and find new direction in life, and to a support group for single mothers. In addition, the counselor gave her resources for an affordable after-school program so she could work extra hours when the facility was short staffed.

DISCUSSION

1. How do you recognize when you are under stress? What are the physical, emotional, and behavioral signs and symptoms that your stress presents?

2. Are you able to see stress coming, recognize it only after it affects your work or other life matters, or only when someone else alerts you?

3. How do you deal with negativity in your life? How do you react to positivity?

STEPS TO SELF-CARE

One way to practice self-care is to identify personal values and purpose in life and how these are demonstrated every day in thought and action. MVP usually stands for *most valuable player*. Long-term care workers are the most valuable players in their nursing facilities as they strive to identify, seek, and/or change their *m*eaning, *v*alues, and *p*urpose in life. It may be a great feat for someone to change attitudes about him- or herself and to practice self-care. In finding one's own MVPs, a person will find it easier to assist residents in finding their meaning, values, and purpose in life and to help them recall how their ideals have shaped their lives.

Human beings were created to live in communities and are designed to be interdependent. Rather than thinking that life choices are either independent or dependent, it is hoped that staff members can turn to each other or friends for assistance when help is needed to keep a balanced life.

EXERCISE

Throughout life you have taken and will take turns being caregivers and care receivers. Think of how infants are dependent on their caregivers, of your need for care when you are sick, and of the many times you have cared for others in their need. Assist each other in identifying the various support people and agencies that are available, such as clergy, psychologists, family counselors, and social service agencies that can assist with food and housing. Make a commitment to encourage other staff to pursue one of these supports in the next week.

Rachel Naomi Remen (2001), in her book *Kitchen Table Wisdom,* indicates that the first healing task of burnout or fatigue is to grieve—in this case, to grieve the loss of a balanced life and of well-being. Grieving is the beginning of self-care. One of the important ingredients to self-care is the ability to let go of unrealistic expectations.

Everyone has hopes and dreams, but being able to distinguish between unrealistic expectations and those that can reasonably be expected to happen is often difficult. A dialogue with another person, such as a counselor or friend, can be essential to gain a realistic perspective on who one is at a particular point in life and what abilities one has or has been failing to utilize. Letting go of unrealistic goals can relieve a lot of pressure. Recognize, however, that letting go of these goals may involve grieving. Friends can be a help in this time of need and grief.

Another important ingredient to self-care is rest. Rest means not just sleeping, but relaxing, meditating in silence, and enjoying pleasurable sensations such as listening to music, watching TV, and having conversations. Being alone can be healing and renewing but too much of it can become uncomfortable. Different people require different amounts of solitude. Some people need to be alone to reflect and feel renewed, others find that being with friends helps them experience renewal; perhaps both help at different times. It is important to learn to recognize for oneself what is needed at a given time and how that desire will be fulfilled.

Much has been written about the physical and mental benefits of exercise, which is also important to self-care. The best way to reap the benefits of exercise is to practice an exercise regimen faithfully. Exercise can relieve a person of the energy that anger, frustration, and disappointment can produce. Forcing oneself to exercise when depressed or stuck can often provide relief from the depression. During exercise, the body is functioning at its best, which helps a person easily meet the physical and emotional tasks before him or her. A sense of courage, determination, and even joy can be a byproduct.

Equally important is developing the ability to play. Some kinds of play, such as participation sports, take the form of exercise. In the midst of laughing at a good joke, seeing a comedy, enjoying good times with friends, or participating in a social club or special-interest group, people's worries in life are suspended.

DISCUSSION

1. What are the tools that help you practice self-care and how can they become a vital and continual part of daily living?

2. How can you be more in tune with stressors and quickly identify your need for self-care?

3. How do you grieve? What form does it take? How do you grieve the death of a resident? When another staff member leaves? How do you grieve any losses in your life? Who and what help you?

4. List the things that you do that are renewing physically, mentally, emotionally, and spiritually. Share your list with others in the group.

5. If you look at how you spent time in the past month, would you say that your life has been balanced between mind, body, and spirit (e.g., rest, work, play; alone time, family time, friendship time)?

CARING FOR THE PHYSICAL, MENTAL, EMOTIONAL, AND SPIRITUAL SELF

There is an old saying: "Be good to your body. Be careful what you do. Be good to your body, and it will be good to you." David Kundtz (1998) in his book, *Stopping: How to Be Still When You Have to Keep Going,* says he hands out green stop signs in his workshops on stress reduction to indicate to staff that they should slow down. He suggests placing them on the telephone, for instance, to remind people to take two deep breaths before answering the telephone or posting them in a visible area as a reminder to relax before beginning a new project. Staff members need to think about similar ways to remind themselves to take momentary breaks.

EXERCISE

What do you do that harms your body? That is good for your body? Commit to one new thing to care for your body during the next week. What one thing will you stop doing that harms your body? Discuss the results of your efforts with other staff at the next in-service meeting.

DAN

Dan, a nursing assistant, was doubtful that exercise would do him any good but decided that exercise was worth a try to make his life better. It was very difficult for Dan to motivate himself to use the exercise bicycle that he purchased a year ago and had used only once. But, he did do it—for a few minutes at a time and then a few more minutes each subsequent time. He was sore after the first week, but strangely enough, he was beginning to feel good about himself for being in a little better shape. The following week he worked out only twice and for the next month his routine was up and down, but the more he exercised, the more he realized he was less angry and frustrated. Somehow, all of the energy behind his anger dissipated when he worked out. He was beginning to feel good about his physical self and his growing emotional stability. As his exercise routine became more regular, he began to use this time to think about his favorite fishing stream and could picture himself in that place of serenity. His mind drifted to thoughts of what he wanted to do with his life and what was really important to his future. Dan was beginning to experience total well-being, and he discovered that he enjoyed his work and really was present and involved in the residents' lives.

In this example, Dan uses exercise to enhance his physical self and soon discovers an improvement in his emotional and spiritual self. Dan could have started with emotional well-being or spiritual well-being practices and the results would most likely have been the same. Body, mind, and spirit affect each other, and growth in one area leads to growth in total personhood. Each individual must use the method that best fits his or her lifestyle and personality type for improving the physical, mental, emotional, and spiritual self.

DISCUSSION

1. Do you have a social life? Are there times when you can get away from work, kids, and other responsibilities for a few hours or even a whole day for rest and renewal?

2. Are you willing to try something new? If you always go to the movies for rest, would you be willing to go to a play or the symphony? What would expand your interests and perhaps help you to discover other ways of learning and relating to the world?

3. What can you do to grow in knowledge about any subject you are interested in?

Some spiritual practices encourage the concept of *mindfulness* to reduce stress. Mindfulness is similar to living for the moment in a way that makes people totally aware of what is happening and to whom they are relating in their present situation rather than having their minds in some other place, borrowing the worry and stress from that other place. Equally important to mindfulness for the self is being mindful of residents, staff, and family members.

Being mindful is to recognize that one of the great gifts that one person can give to another is to be fully present (i.e., to pay attention without interference). When others are fully present to each other, they feel a sense of belonging, health, and well-being. Being truly present with another person helps that person find healing in the sense of well-being. Healing is not always about curing the physical or mental illness but about experiencing support and love and hope to survive difficult times.

Most people can identify a special place that gives them a sense of peace and rest in life. The place may be a room in their house that is a refuge, a beautiful mountain scene, the ocean, or a place they have read about. Thinking of this place even when it is not possible to go there during the day will help alleviate stress. The first assignment for anyone who cannot identify an actual or imagined place is to find one. This exercise is called *visualization* and can be used to induce a relaxed state of mind in the midst of physical or emotional confusion.

Staff, in addition to practicing visualization themselves, can encourage residents to do the same. A staff member who knows from conversations with residents the places that they visited on a vacation or the locations that held special meaning for their family can use this knowledge to help soothe a resident. Speaking to the resident in a calm, soft voice, the staff member can encourage him or her to visualize this place, take several deep breaths, and experience the feelings that he or she had in this special place. Guided images can greatly benefit residents, especially those in chronic pain. Another relaxation method to try is described in the exercise on pages 40–41.

Perhaps the most important physical, emotional, and spiritual healthy act is loving touch (e.g., hugging, holding hands). Any form of loving touch helps people get through hardship and is a way to demonstrate compassion. Staff will want to be sensitive to various cultural perspectives on this subject because touching in this way may cause a negative reaction for some people. The safest way to ensure someone's comfort with physical contact is to first ask permission to touch or hug.

DISCUSSION

1. What makes life meaningful for you? When do you feel good about yourself?

2. How do you solve problems when they arise either in your private life or at work?

3. Who and what helps you when you feel tense, upset, grief-stricken, or guilty?

4. What are the religious or other spiritual practices that can help you focus on healing the self?

5. Do you want to deepen your religious faith, and if so, how can you do that? (Perhaps you can take religion courses or learn meditation, journaling, or different forms of prayer.)

6. If your spiritual life is not specifically religious, what practices or what exercises about your values and

meaning in life can you perform that would enhance self-care?

7. List the things that you need to do to have a better-balanced life? Who can help you accomplish this? What do you need to ask for?

8. How can you make this "new you" appear every day?

9. How will you encourage your fellow workers to live the "new them" each day?

SERVING AND HELPING

Staff in long-term care facilities work in positions that are classified among the *helping professions*. However, it is better to think of the work they do as *serving* rather than *helping*. The concept of help often implies that the helper is superior to the person being helped and that the person being helped is indebted to the helper. The word *service* implies that people are equals—residents receive some assistance for a fee and staff will be of service to residents at other times. Residents often give the gifts of life, advice, example, and kindness in return for the service they receive from the nursing facility. Residents express joy and congratulations at a staff member's special event or graduation and sorrow and concern for deaths in the family, as well as other difficulties that staff members experience. Just listening to the life stories of residents can be a source of encouragement for staff members who may be able to relate to the stories in the context of events in their own lives. The residents are survivors and can show staff, through their stories, how to become survivors. Of course, some residents may be good examples to staff of how not to grow old and deal with physical problems, but there are more positive examples than negative. By expressing words of thanks, residents can also help staff feel great satisfaction and fulfillment about who they are and what they do.

People in helping professions, because they are so used to providing services for others, sometimes accept too much responsibility or provide too many services for others. In the Christian Scriptures, Jesus tells the story of the Good Samaritan who discovers a person who has been beaten and robbed alongside the road and takes him to an inn to care for him. The next day, the Samaritan gives money to the owner for further care and then leaves to go on his way. The point is that the Samaritan allowed his life to be interrupted in order to care for another person, but he eventually went on his way again. He did not let the needs of the injured person dictate his life forever, nor did he take over responsibility for that man's well-being. Taking control over someone else's life prevents that person from growing, having a unique personality, and fulfilling a unique purpose in this world.

DISCUSSION

1.   Identify the ways that you overdo yourself physically, mentally, and/or emotionally?

2.   Identify signs that one person has taken over responsibility for another person.

3.   Identify and share with other staff members what can be done to prevent taking over control of another person, particularly one who, like the residents of a facility, has many needs and limitations.

FACILITY CONTRIBUTIONS TO WELL-BEING

An organization can do many things to alleviate stress and contribute to the well-being of its staff such as fostering an environment that promotes praise and compliments and provides rewards and recognition. Parties, picnics, and other celebrations of staff diversity and cultures will contribute to staff well-being. Exercise equipment, support groups, and chaplaincy services assist the physical, emotional, and spiritual well-being of staff. Offering classes on English as a second language can help staff cross communication barriers with non–English-speaking residents. Educational growth can also be found in opportunities for staff to attend workshops that develop technical skills, provide knowledge of gerontology, and give insights to the spiritual lives of residents. Finally, competitive salaries and benefits are essential basics of staff appreciation.

Facilities need to seek the input and suggestions of staff through written comments or focus groups. Appropriate responses to these comments are also important. It is vital to honor staff members as human beings. One way is to keep them informed about what is going to happen and about any and all changes. Staff members have wisdom and insight into the needs of the facility, whether the needs be new equipment, remodeling or redecorating, and so forth. The staff also feels valued when its members are able to contribute to the strategic planning and development of new ways of delivering daily services and activities to residents. The staff, in a sense, belongs to the facility and has a need to be part of planning processes that affect the future of individual members as well as the facility as a whole.

THE SPIRIT AT WORK

The staff is comprised of human "beings" first and human "doings" second. Most people, however, are evaluated and rewarded at work for *doing* their jobs and doing them well. Newer management books (e.g., Conger et al., 1994; Marcic, 1997) recognize that in order for people to *do* well, they have to *be* well, and a management's task is to treat employees well. Dorothy Marcic (1997), in *Managing with the Wisdom of Love: Uncovering Virtue in People and Organizations,* talks about the need to create community to manage well. She also describes the new management virtues as trustworthiness, unity, respect and dignity, justice and service, and humility. Although there is a lot of talk about how to treat residents with dignity, the staff also needs to be treated with dignity.

DISCUSSION

1. Describe how you are valued and how you value other staff. How have you been deprived of dignity or not treated others with dignity? Discuss what can be done to increase respect for each other.

2. Identify what you need from your supervisors and upper management in order to feel valued.

3. People's spirituality is nurtured in relationships, so a staff's work environment needs to be hospitable. How do the people at work—staff and residents—practice hospitality?

In *Spirit at Work: Discovering the Spirituality in Leadership,* Jay Conger (1994) says that people bring with them to work their needs for family, community, and spirituality. Leaders who focus on the vision, mission, and values of the organization need to be providing for the fulfillment of these needs.

When the mission of the organization and the personal missions of staff members coincide, then both the staff and the organization can be well. In John C. Haughey's (as cited in Conger et al., 1994) summarization of Vaclav Havel's views about spirituality, he states that people long for being and being connected to the BEING (i.e., a higher being). To connect with the BEING, people need to take responsibility for themselves, be attuned to what the conscience is saying, and be engaged in an endless pursuit of meaning. In *The Stirring of Soul in the Workplace,* Alan Briskin (1998) states that people must always confront the questions of meaning, which he lists as: Who am I? Where am I headed? What have I become? The Golden Rule says, "Do unto others as you would have them do unto you." The mature spiritual person knows that loving others comes from love for his or her self (a healthy appreciation of one's gifts and abilities). Successful companies are those that help workers answer the "questions of meaning" in a positive way.

ACTION STEPS

1. List the benefits of belonging to your nursing facility. What do you like best about being at this facility?

2. Do you consider your presence at your nursing facility as work or a job? People need work, not jobs, for work comes from the inside and is an expression of the inner self. How could a job be transformed to work?

3. Discuss times at your facility when you felt as though you were at work and not at a job, or at a job and not at work. Identify ways that each is different and how the facility can promote a positive work environment.

4. What would you like to see offered that would help you as a human being and to assist you in performing your work? What procedures could be followed to request assistance?

5. What one new thing can you agree to do to promote your well-being—physically, emotionally, and spiritually—in the next week? Discuss these goals at the end of the week with colleagues. How effective or ineffective were they in helping you? How will you encourage each other to maintain your new way of living?

REFERENCES

Briskin, A. (1998). *The stirring of soul in the workplace.* San Francisco: Jossey-Bass.

Conger, J., et al. (1994). *Spirit at work: Discovering the spirituality in leadership.* San Francisco: Jossey-Bass.

Kundtz, D. (1998). *Stopping: How to be still when you have to keep going.* Berkeley, CA: Conari Press.

Marcic, D. (1997). *Managing with the wisdom of love: Uncovering virtue in people and organizations.* San Francisco: Jossey-Bass.

Remen, R.N. (2001). *Kitchen table wisdom: Stories that heal.* Thorndike, ME: G.K. Hall.

RECOMMENDED READING

Care of the soul: How to add depth and meaning to your everyday life: The illustrated edition by Thomas Moore (HarperCollins)

Complete idiot's guide to journaling by Joan R. Neubauer and Kathleen Adams (Alpha Books)

Counting on kindness: The dilemmas of dependency by Wendy Lustbader (Maxwell MacMillan International)

Everyday serenity: Meditations for people who do too much by David Kundtz (Publishers Group West)

Meditation for dummies by Stephan Bodian (IDG Books Worldwide)

"Spiritual well-being of staff, board and care" by Ron Zielske and Marita Grudzen in *Quarterly Forum* (2001, November/December), Volume 4, Number 6.

RESOURCES

"The Serenity Prayer" at http://open-mind.org/Serenity.htm

"Slow Me Down, Lord" prayer at http://www.poeticexpressions.co.uk/Prayer.htm

"Take the Stress Test" at http://www.balancetime.com

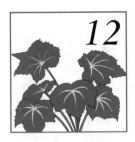

12

Compassion in Action

Pain Management and Palliative Care

Marita Grudzen

OBJECTIVES

As a result of reading and working with the material in this chapter, participants will be able to

1. Recognize the symptoms, types, causes, and effects of pain common to nursing facility residents

2. Understand the philosophy and practice of palliative care as it applies to frail elders

3. Learn methods for improving pain management protocols

4. Identify the role of culture in pain assessment.

5. Discover ways of effectively assessing pain as the fifth vital sign

6. Utilize resources for implementing nonpharmacological pain management modalities for residents, families, and staff members

COMMON AND INDIVIDUAL EXPERIENCES OF PAIN

Everyone has experienced pain. Although people don't like to think about it, when they are able to anticipate pain, they are often able to manage it. Consider, for example, why people choose to have surgery or dental care. Before discussing the relief of pain, however, it is important to discuss what pain is. First thoughts about pain usually turn to sensations of distress or hurting on a physical level. A broader concept, however, is that of *total pain* (Twycross, 1999), which is used in palliative care and can also be applied to the care of frail older adults. This concept acknowledges the combined effect of different types of human pain: physical, psychological, social, and spiritual.

Many familiar physical symptoms, which can also include fatigue and insomnia, fall under the category of physical pain. Psychological pain relates to emotions such as fear, anger, and helplessness. Social pain results from isolation, loss of independence, and certain perceptions about social roles and status. Loss of meaning or purpose; of access to religious rituals and resources; or of communion with God, nature, or of other sources of spiritual nurture often are sources of spiritual pain. For many residents, total pain includes all, if not most, of these four types.

EXERCISE

The following exercise encourages participants to relate to their own experiences of pain. Make sure that the participants understand the distinctions between the different types of pain. The facilitator should relate these different types of pain to examples found in the nursing facility in which the training is being held.

1. Begin by writing *total pain* and the four distinct types of pain discussed above in columns on a large paper pad or board. Collect 5–10 examples of each distinct type. Include ethnic-specific aspects of loss (e.g., not hearing one's language spoken).

2. Think back to your own experiences of pain. Select three vivid experiences of pain to write about and/or draw using writing and drawing materials provided

by the facilitator. Next, label the different types of pain that comprised the *total pain* experienced in each situation.

DISCUSSION

1. Share some aspect of your personal experience with pain (e.g., a severe migraine headache, a sporting accident that resulted in a bad sprain or broken bone, the pain of loss or separation from a loved one).

2. Identify the differences and similarities of each type of experienced pain.

3. Reflect on the personal, subjective nature of the diverse experiences or perceptions of pain that emerge from this discussion.

What do staff need to know about pain? The probability of having physical pain increases with age and with the body's decline. Most common causes of physical pain among older adults in long-term care facilities include (Hughes, 2001)

- Arthritis (osteoarthritis and rheumatoid arthritis)
- Osteoporosis and associated bone fractures
- Neurological pain (multiple sources)
- Cancer
- Contractures
- Headache
- Ischemia
- Other medical causes

Untreated pain is an important national public health epidemic among nursing facility residents (Teno, Weitzen, Wetle, & Mor, 2001). Dr. Teno and her colleagues at Brown University conducted a nationwide study of pain in nursing facilities during 2001. They found that 41% of nursing facility residents who were in pain at the time of the study still experienced moderate to severe pain when evaluated 2–6 months later. Physical pain affects mobility, appetite, and general quality of life. When untreated, it frequently causes depression. Facilities need to evaluate themselves using Minimum Data Sets (MDS), an assessment instrument that evaluates a resident's functional limitations and strengths. These data sets are important for people entering Medicare- or Medicaid-certified nursing facilities and can help to improve pain assessment and management for residents. Direct-care staff members are an important part of the team when it comes to assessing pain levels in residents. Nursing assistants are often in the best position to ask questions or carefully observe when a resident is suspected of being in pain. This important information needs to be communicated to and valued by the charge nurse. When a resident is known to have pain, for example, that person may need to be medicated before he or she is moved by staff members for personal care and feeding.

Not all residents are willing or able to complain verbally about pain. Some useful signs of discomfort to observe and report include crying, moaning, wincing, or frowning, as well as guarding or protecting any part of the body (Teno et al., 2001).

DISCUSSION

1. **What might be barriers to residents reporting pain?**

    Suggest the following barriers, if they are not raised:

    -   Fear that the pain may represent a worsening of their condition

    -   Fear of becoming addicted or being viewed as an addict of pain medication

    -   Fear of drug side effects; wanting to be alert and not over-medicated

    -   Acceptance of pain as punishment for past actions

    -   Belief that pain must be borne because it comes from God and "God will give me the grace to endure it"

    -   Fear of becoming weak or immobile

    -   Ignorance that a particular pain can be treated with medication

- Acceptance of pain as a normal part of aging
- Stoicism
- Inability to communicate (e.g., language barriers)
- Result of cultural beliefs and expectations (e.g., designation of family member to communicate with staff)

2. What are the barriers to recognizing pain from the perspective of the nursing facility?

    Suggest the following barriers, if they are not raised:

    - Inadequate assessment
    - Discrediting a resident's report of pain
    - Language barriers
    - Misconception that older adults do not tolerate opioids
    - Lack of pain management and palliative expertise
    - Cultural beliefs and expectations about treating pain
    - Poor team communication

CONSIDERATIONS FOR IMPROVING PAIN MANAGEMENT PROTOCOLS

What is needed to accomplish effective pain management for residents is a well-informed, interdisciplinary team of facility staff that also includes the resident, family, and a certified nursing assistant (CNA). It must be remembered that the most accurate information about the pain comes from the resident. Getting this information may require the use of an interpreter or the presence of a family member. The resident and family need to be empowered with the expectation of receiving good pain management and having their pain reports and suggestions honored. CNAs need to be affirmed in their role as coordinators of personal care and as important resources of valuable information. The commitment to compassionate care and effective pain management requires a systems approach. Implementing this approach requires an owner/administrator who endorses and supports this goal with

- Adequate staffing
- Required education and competency of nurses in pain management

- A medical director who is knowledgeable and skilled in pain management and palliative care
- Hospice services available for any terminally ill resident who requests the service after being informed of eligibility
- Consultation with and education by hospice care workers
- Language and cultural resources

Accomplishing these goals takes time. It is therefore important to keep the vision intact through a strategic plan that encompasses all of the above components and that contains an action plan detailing the implementation, time line, and vision statement of the facility, thus demonstrating its commitment to compassionate, skilled, and effective pain management.

Regular assessment and appropriate follow-up interventions by nursing staff are the most critical strategies for controlling pain and providing comfort in any facility. They should be the first line of intervention.

PAIN AS THE FIFTH VITAL SIGN

One of the most effective ways to assess and monitor pain is to recognize it as a fifth vital sign, together with pulse, temperature, blood pressure, and respiration. This means that when staff members check residents' vital signs every 4 hours, they include an assessment of the residents' pain levels. A simple approach is to use a scale of 0–10 with 0 representing no pain and 10 being the highest level of pain. A visual chart can also be an aid, showing facial expressions that correspond on the pain scale with *pain free* (0) through *experiencing severe pain* (10). Pain scales need to be placed in clear view of the resident when assessing his or her pain level.

Any resident who reports pain should be brought to the attention of the nurse on duty, who will need to follow up with a comprehensive assessment and treatment plan. This assessment should include the resident's condition, a full description of his or her pain, how long it has been experienced, and the goals of treatment for diminishing pain (e.g., increased activity, side effects willing to be tolerated) (Hughes, 2001). It can be helpful to ask residents what improves or worsens their pain and to explore their explanation for the pain (e.g., What do they believe may be causing their pain and what would relieve it?) (Kleinman, 1988). Having a working relationship between the nursing facility and a hospice agency is invaluable for consultation on dealing with all aspects of pain assessment and management.

MR. GONZALES

Jorge Gonzales, a 73-year-old Mexican American, was admitted postsurgery to a subacute unit of a skilled nursing facility. When the licensed vocational nurse asked Mr. Gonzales to identify his pain on a scale of 0–10, he always engaged in conversation and avoided responding to the queries. One morning, shortly after Mr. Gonzales's admittance to the facility, it was clear that he had been in pain for some time. Because he did not respond to the nurse's assessment of pain based on a numbered scale (0–10) relating to his pain level, pain medication had not been administered.

DISCUSSION

1. How could this situation be remedied so that it does not occur again?

2. Identify issues and strategies for dealing with other pain treatment problems, such as refusal to take pain medication based on religious belief or because of undesirable side effects such as unsteadiness or bowel impaction.

RELIEVING SUFFERING

Bartlow said, "Illness and death are the soul's last attempt to be recognized and honored and achieve its goals" (2000, p. 6). Suffering affects people both as individuals and as families. As individuals, it can threaten people's sense of identity (Cassel, 1982). Suffering can cause a personality change in an individual who does not have the inner resources to cope with this pain. Such personality changes can cause an individual to revert to earlier periods of his or her life or to express inappropriate emotional states of mind. Suffering can also affect how families feel about not being able to offer relief (e.g., inadequate, guilty).

Prolonged illness can lead to various types of depression, which is another form of suffering. Depression leads to a deadening of emotional and sensory experience and the will to live. Emotional pain can affect an individual just as much as physical pain, and although it often goes unnoticed, it may be the more prevalent type of pain in a nursing facility environment. Until physical pain is under control, however, dealing with any other form of suffering is difficult.

DISCUSSION

1. What do you notice about the presence of pain in residents? What helps residents get through this pain?

2. Can you recommend some cultural resources in the community for helping residents deal with cultural isolation?

3. What are some religious resources that can aid residents who have emotional and/or spiritual pain?

4. What information is needed to refer a resident to the appropriate resource for pain management?

Genuine presence and active listening, as nursing facility staff members know, offer tremendous healing to residents. It is not uncommon for residents to feel abandoned, even though many of their families are devoted and visit them often. Staff members' attention, presence, concern, and skilled care do a great deal to relieve residents' suffering, but some forms of emotional, social, or spiritual suffering may not be resolved despite what staff members and facilities are able to offer in the way of compassion.

NONPHARMACOLOGICAL
APPROACHES TO PAIN MANAGEMENT

The medical treatment of physical pain has already been discussed, but pain management can be further enhanced through nonpharmacological approaches. As Chapter 11 points out, some of these modalities (e.g., relaxation, imagery techniques) can be taught and applied within a group context by trained nurses, therapists, and wellness instructors. These methods typically focus attention on breathing and use the potential of people's intuition and imagination to relax and evoke healing energies for

the mind, body, and soul. Harold Benson (1992) was the first to popularize these quieting modalities through his work at Harvard University on
relaxation and its effects on many disease conditions. He helped to highlight the healing power of meditation as a pathway to stress reduction and
better health. The connection between high levels of stress and disease has
been well documented. Benson's work has been expanded by Jon Kabat-
Zinn (1990) and his use of mindfulness meditation for chronic pain and
Dr. Joan Borysenko's (1988) Mind/Body Clinic at Harvard Medical
School's New England Deaconess Hospital. For more than 25 years, Dean
Ornish, M.D., and his colleagues at Preventive Medicine Research Institute have shown that through comprehensive lifestyle and diet changes
coupled with yoga and social support, heart disease can, in some instances,
be reversed. The same research is now being done with men who have
prostate cancer.

Chapter 2 discusses breathing exercises for releasing pain or stress as
well as for relaxation. These breathing techniques and other mind-atten-
tion strategies can be used by residents to manage stress, transfers (e.g.,
from bed to a chair), and insomnia. Healing techniques such as these can
be taught to residents or staff members in a group setting, with music
and/or a guided meditation by a group leader (e.g., hypnotherapist, nurse,
chaplain) that encourages participants to discover their healing images.
Therese Schroeder-Sheker has promoted the prescriptive use of music alone
(typically the harp) as a holistic approach for alleviating the spiritual and
physical pain experienced in the dying process (Horrigan, 2001). Essential
to palliative care practice is the role of a trained musician-clinician who is
skilled in working with diverse patients and uses music in specific
response to an individual's dying processes (e.g., breathing, physical pain,
emotional pain, withdrawal). The Chalice of Repose Project reports being
effective with pain associated with cancer, infectious diseases, respiratory
distress, and Alzheimer's disease (Horrigan, 2001). This knowledge and
skill has become available in hospitals, nursing facilities, and private
homes across the country. These strategies are not substitutes for pain or
sleep medication; they are tools to give the resident another level of control. (See the section in Chapter 2 called Toolkit for Healing, pp. 39–42).

Staff members need to identify respectful and nonthreatening ways of
asking about ethnic-specific healing practices, traditional healers, and
medicines. This information ideally could be obtained at the time of
admission. Traditional beliefs, customs, and practices, although they need
to be evaluated for any medical contraindications, can be adapted to the
nursing facility environment with the support of ethnic liaisons, families,

and volunteers. Chinese medicine, for example, focuses on nonpharmacological approaches to health and pain management through the use of herbal remedies in teas and soups and the practices of acupuncture and acupressure, whereas American Indian elders are traditionally more concerned about eliminating the cause of an illness than with symptom management. Many older American Indians do not ask for pain medication or may ask only once and "are more likely to use internal resources" (Hendrix, 2001, p. 30). As a result, they are undertreated for pain. In such cases, extra care is needed to elicit the person's pain level, explanatory model of the illness, and resources for a healing process. Consulting traditional healers and including ritual and ceremony as well as family and community members in interventions as appropriate can provide the cultural framework that is needed for improved health and total wellness, as well as for the integration of Western and Indian medicine (Williams & Ellison, 1996). Aspects of personal care that need provision and/or attention have been identified for Navajo Indian people and include personal space, touch, modesty, and cleanliness. The Navajo Nation nursing facility in Chinle, Arizona, provides an integrated model (Mercer, 1996).

Many elders practice some form of prayer or meditation and may desire a healing ceremony, chanting, or communion by their minister, rabbi, or priest. Healing rituals can also be performed by friends and family. Sometimes, a small altar or religious image affords peace and comfort. For example, an altar can be constructed with the help of families or a cultural liaison in recognition of the Day of the Dead. Residents and staff members can place pictures of departed loved ones and other tokens of remembrance on the altar. Residents are comforted by the sense of communion they feel with their relatives and friends on this special occasion.

VERONICA

Veronica was a Caucasian woman in her eighties who had devoted many of her adult years to environmental issues and interviewing American Indians for her book about living between two cultures. After she was given a diagnosis of cancer and consulted with medical personnel about her options, she asked 10 close friends (women and men) to spend an evening with her in a healing circle. Veronica asked each person to spend some time in nature that day (as was her intent) and to bring some of nature's healing energy to the circle. One person assumed responsibility for preparing a space and for opening and closing the ritual. Friends brought shells and driftwood from the sea, feathers, leaves and flowers from gardens, and other specially selected sources of life and energy. Her friends' feelings of helplessness were transformed into acts of healing, connection, and strength, as each individual approached Veronica and intimately touched and spoke to her, bringing their gift of healing. Some sat beside her on the bed; others knelt next to her, moving their hand in a blessing on her forehead. Another friend massaged her feet, sending her strength to walk through her experience. Each expressed endearment through gentle movements. Veronica was relaxed and emotionally open to receive each gift. A deep sense of intention and unity permeated the circle and seemed to grow as each person approached Veronica. Veronica's facial expression mirrored the joy and peace that had grown in her body as she absorbed the love and blessing communicated to her during the ceremony. Her friends described how the ritual had changed them, deepening their capacity to be present, be a companion to one another, form a community, and communicate healing energy. The isolation that characterized Veronica's diagnosis of cancer and her life in a skilled nursing facility had been forever pierced with gentle touching, prayers, and the display of flowers. This had a profound effect on Veronica.

Distraction is an important function of healing rituals. Residents look forward to certain activities that can be perceived as ritualistic including reminiscing with family pictures, watching television programs, visiting with family and friends, reading books, or listening to music. One resident was typically unaware of pain while watching *Jeopardy!* every weeknight. Her family observed this and arranged to join her whenever possible at this time to share her pleasurable experience. Creative activities can serve as distractions as long as they effectively capture attention and imagination and the resident is capable of participating at a level that is satisfying for him or her.

MASAKO

Masako, a Japanese elder with severe rheumatoid arthritis, wanted to limit her pain medication. She said that her creative writing, which she composed on a word processor, was a marvelous distraction. She became so completely engrossed in her writing that many times her medication was not needed.

SHINJI

Shinji was admitted to a hospice unit in a large long-term care facility. In addition to being treated for his terminal illness, he was being treated with psychotropic drugs for his emotional and mental imbalance. One day, the hospice social worker on the unit, who had purchased an inexpensive calligraphy set, sat down next to Shinji and attempted calligraphy. Within minutes, the Japanese elder, who hadn't done calligraphy in years, was showing the social worker how it "ought" to be done. Before long, Shinji became deeply engaged with his former talents of calligraphy and Japanese painting. The facility's activity director held an art exhibit for Shinji's family and guests of the inpatient hospice, displaying the several works he had completed on the unit. During his hospice stay, he was taken off of the psychotropic drugs that were necessary at the time of his admission. Now, beyond his death his transformation continues to be a source of life, as his paintings and calligraphy bless the walls of the hospice and those who enjoy them.

EXERCISE

Ask participants to gather in small groups of no fewer than four people to discuss the case of either Veronica, Masako, or Shinji. The cases can be assigned, or the groups can choose the case they want to review. Ask each group to select a recorder who can compile the group's answers to the following questions and share them with the larger circle.

1. Which aspects of the case person's story do you identify with? Have you observed anyone with a similar experience?

2. What meaning does the case have for you?

3. Does the case remind you of a resident who might: a) be open to using an art form (e.g., writing, painting) as a way of finding relief from pain; b) welcome a healing circle facilitated by a chaplain, family member, friend, or healer; or c) benefit from prayer (e.g., the Psalms, a prayer phrase said repeatedly)?

4. Can you recommend any next steps for fostering positive outcomes similar to those illustrated in the scenarios?

As the considerations on compassion and pain management come to a close, there is evidence of cornerstones to an edifice of compassionate care for older adults. One of the cornerstones is *knowledge and skill in pain management,* which includes knowledge of the common types and extent of pain experienced by older adults, especially in nursing homes, and knowledge and skill in the art of palliative care and in the management of total pain.

A second cornerstone is *practice of assessment, management, and ongoing monitoring of resident pain.* This requires a commitment of the facility as well as of all members of the team. There needs to be adequate staffing, a supportive and cooperative team, and good assessment and communication tools, including language resources. A staff member can be identified who would receive state-of-the-art training and oversee the goals and implementation of pain management and palliative care in the facility. One option would be to hire a palliative care consultant (e.g., clinical nurse specialist) as well as to seek support from the affiliated hospice team (Zerzan, Stearns, & Hanson, 2000). Clearly, someone needs to champion the development, assessment, and implementation of a pain management and palliative care program, and that individual needs the support of the facility's administration.

Nursing assistants are an essential cornerstone of compassionate care in any nursing facility. Acknowledging and supporting their contribution and their well-being is of great importance. Such support inevitably enhances their presence and engagement with residents. It is preferable for nursing assistants to be assigned to care for the same residents over time. This provides opportunities for connecting with and knowing the resident's strengths, vulnerabilities, sources of pain, daily rhythms, preferences, social history, interests, sources of meaning, and coping styles, as well as spiritual and cultural healing practices in some detail. The nursing assistant is often an important link between the resident's family and friends whom the nursing assistant typically gets to know over time. Nursing assistants can foster interactive activities with the resident and provide a welcoming presence for visiting family members. They are an invaluable resource for resident care meetings. If their perspectives on residents are elicited and valued in this context, it is expected that their self esteem and engagement with residents will continue to improve.

Finally, palliative care and pain management in older adults require an engaged commitment. The application of palliative care and pain management needs to be *personal* and *holistic,* acknowledging the multifaceted and complex nature of each human being. Owen Lum, M.D., a Chinese American psychiatrist who frequently visits nursing facility residents, seeks to establish a relationship with residents and to balance the residents' needs and medications, providing, when possible, a waking presence wherein a person's "soul can shine" (personal communication, December 13, 2002).

ACTION STEPS

1. Research the resources that are available for dealing with the emotional, psychosocial, and spiritual pain of residents in your nursing facility?

2. Review the different types of pain and the signs and symptoms for emotional, social, and spiritual pain. What are some potential resources (e.g., psychologist, chaplain, hypnotherapist, acupuncturist, family) for helping residents cope with emotional, psychosocial, and spiritual pain?

3. Identify in-house resources, hospices, and family and pastoral networks that can aid residents. Identify ethnic and religiously diverse resources to address cultural isolation and spiritual pain. Discuss forming a committee to identify several untapped services in your community and prepare a plan for gaining access to them.

REFERENCES

Bartlow, B.G. (2000). *Medical care of the soul: A practical & healing guide to end-of-life issues for families, patients and health care providers.* Boulder, CO: Johnson Books.

Benson, H. (1992). *The relaxation response.* New York: Wings Books.

Borysenko, J. (1988). *Minding the body, mending the mind.* New York: Bantam.

Cassel, E.J. (1982). The Nature of suffering and the goals of medicine. *New England Journal of Medicine, 306*(11), 639–645.

Hendrix, L.R. (2001). Health and health care of American Indian and Alaska native elders. In G. Yeo (Ed.), *Curriculum in ethnogeriatrics: Core curriculum and ethnic-specific modules* (2nd ed.). Retrieved on March 17, 2003, from http://www.stanford.edu/group/ethnoger/index.html

Hughes, A. (2001, June). *Pain management: Improving end-of-life decision-making in nursing facilities.* Paper presented at Improving End-of-Life Care in Nursing Homes conference, California Coalition for Compassionate Care, Sacramento.

Kabat-Zinn, J. (1990). *Full catastrophe living: Using the wisdom of your body and mind to face stress, pain, and illness.* New York: Delacorte Press.

Kleinman, A. (1988). *The illness narratives: Suffering, healing, and the human condition.* New York: Basic Books.

Mercer, S.O. (1996). Navajo elderly people in a reservation nursing home: Admission predictors and cultural care practices. *Social Work, 41*(2), 181–189.

Teno, J.M., Weitzen, S., Wetle, T., & Mor, V. (2001). Persistent pain in nursing home residents. *JAMA, 285*(16), 39.

Twycross, R. (1999). *Introducing palliative care* (3rd ed.). Oxford: Radcliffe Medical Press.

Williams, E.E., & Ellison, F. (1996). Culturally informed social work practice with American Indian clients: Guidelines for non-Indian social workers. *Social Work, 41*(2), 147–151.

Zerzan, J., Stearns, S., & Hanson, L. (2000). Access to palliative care and hospice in nursing homes. *JAMA, 284*(19), 2489–2494.

RECOMMENDED READING

Cultural issues in end-of-life decision making by Kathryn L. Braun, James H. Pietsch, and Patricia L. Blanchette (Sage Publications)

Dying well: The prospect for growth at the end of life by Ira Byock (Riverhead Books)

Facing death and finding hope: A guide to the emotional and spiritual care of the dying by Christine Longaker (Doubleday)

Full catastrophe living: Using the wisdom of your body and mind to face stress, pain, and illness by Jon Kabat-Zinn (Delacorte Press)

Healing and the mind by Bill Moyers (Doubleday)

Improving care for the end of life: A sourcebook for health care managers and clinicians by Joanne Lynn (Oxford University Press)

RESOURCES

California Coalition for Compassionate Care
Web site: http://www.finalchoices.calhealth.org

Center for Advanced Palliative Care
Web site: http://www.capc.org

Chalice of Repose: A Contemplative Musician's Approach to Death and Dying [video] by Therese Schroeder-Scheker (Available from Sounds True, Post Office Box 8010, Boulder, Colorado 80306; 1-800-333-9185)

End of Life/Palliative Education Resource Center (EPERC)
Web site: http://www.eperc.mcw.edu

Growth House
Web site: http://www.growthhouse.org

Healing and the Mind: Healing from Within [video] with Bill Moyers (Available from Ambrose Video at http://www.ambrosevideo.com/displayitem.cfm?vid=376)

Last Acts
Web site: http://www.lastacts.org

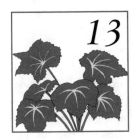

Letting Go

*Coming to Terms
with Death and Dying*

Ron Zielske

OBJECTIVES

As a result of reading this chapter and working through the exercises, participants will be able to

1. See how life is a series of gains and losses (hellos and good-byes) and that rituals ease major life transitions

2. Become aware of the importance of listening as a caregiving measure

3. Be aware of some of the cultural variations in dealing with death and dying

4. Understand how survivors grieve over the loss of their loved ones

5. Realize the importance of resolving life's issues and letting go

6. Explore ethical issues on the subject of dying

LIFE AS GAINS AND LOSSES

Although there are many transitions in life, dying is the final transition. During this time, the resident will face many different emotions and may finally ask, "Was my life worthwhile?" It is healthy to view all of life as a series of transitions, of hellos and good-byes. All hellos need to be celebrated, and all good-byes need to be grieved. Moving from one town to another or one house to another is an example of a major life transition. Part of the process is usually a remembrance of all that took place in the previous home and neighborhood as well as the memories of neighbors themselves. People who move residences need to remember this part of their history and experience their feelings of joy from happy memories and their sadness over leaving them behind in order to move ahead and create a healthy life. In addition to this process of remembrance, the excitement of a new home with new neighbors and perhaps a new job can be celebrated with the feelings of eager expectation that newness brings. It is very possible for people to feel the emotions of excitement and sadness only moments apart.

Creating rituals for good-byes and hellos for residents moving to a nursing facility helps them process feelings and make a healthy transition. For example, before a prospective resident moves into a nursing facility, someone could take him or her through the home that he or she is leaving for a final remembrance ritual such as lighting a candle, stopping in each room, and encouraging the elder to remember major events that took place in the room. This ritual can become a religious observance with prayers and hymns for those of a particular faith. If this cannot be done physically, it can be done mentally. Likewise, a ritual of welcoming with presents, balloons, cards, a party, and perhaps prayers and blessings can assist the resident in claiming the new space as his or her own.

As a person journeys through life, he or she begins to lose some of his or her former abilities and does not function in ways that he or she formerly could. Older adults experience physical changes such as loss of limbs, arthritis, stroke, and impairments of hearing and eyesight. Caregivers and residents alike need to recognize that these losses and challenges need to be grieved and residents need to work through their limitations and adapt to new ways of functioning. In a sense, all losses prepare people for death, the ultimate loss. Whether a person believes in life after death, death can be frightening, perhaps even for those who, in their illness, wish death to come. Elders will ask many questions: Will it be a good death? Can I just go in my sleep quickly? Why do I have to linger? Why doesn't God take me? Why do I suffer so much while others do not? They will also ponder the larger question: Was my life worthwhile? These are all spiritual questions that are part of the great mysteries of life. There are no answers, or at least no easy answers.

As older adults lose some of their former abilities and begin to react to their fears and challenges in a number of ways, the people near them may try to alleviate their fears and frustrations by advising them to "pick yourself up and go on" or "get out and socialize." A spouse may even say, "You cannot let the kids see you cry." Although well intended, these suggestions do not allow residents to grieve or to find their own meaning in life. Nursing facility staff can be most helpful by being there to listen much and talk little. It is not necessary to supply life's answers but to help residents reflect and draw on their own spiritual resources. The one assurance that staff can give to residents is that their life has meaning. That meaning mostly has to do with *who* the resident is more than *what* that person has done. The dying live on in the memories of families and friends because of the relationship they shared with the family or friends, not because of their social status. The late U.S. politician Paul E. Tsongas once stated, "No one on their deathbed ever said, 'I wish I had spent more time on my business.'"

FLORENCE

Florence was recently admitted to a nursing facility from the home she had lived in for 35 years. She had osteoarthritis and could walk only short distances with a walker or with assistance, and she was in the middle stages of Alzheimer's disease. Her husband, who had been her caregiver, seldom left the house during her care and died shortly after Florence's admittance. One of her daughters has been keeping Florence company since her husband's death. Florence was very depressed, wept a lot, and was angry with anyone who approached her, including all staff, her family, and her daughter. Devoutly religious, she was also mad at God.

DISCUSSION

1. How would you approach Florence to welcome her to the nursing facility? What would you say?

2. Can you identify the losses she is going through?
    Who or what resources could help her?

3. How did any of the residents you care for say good-
    bye to their homes when they moved to your nurs-
    ing facility? Did any rituals help them say good-bye
    to their old home or say hello to their new home?
    Did they have the chance to say good-bye or hello?

4. How do residents grieve their losses (e.g., physical,
    mental, and other abilities), and how do you assist
    them in the grieving process? Who else has given
    them comfort (e.g., families, clergy, volunteers)?

5. Have you had the experience of grieving over the
    loss of any of your abilities?

LISTENING AS CAREGIVING

Rabbi Cary Kozberg (1998), the Director of Rabbinical and Pastoral
Services at Wexner Heritage Village in Columbus, Ohio, likes to say that
the most important reason why people are unwilling to go to a nursing
facility is because they are unsure that there will be really good caregivers.

A great caregiver is one who can be with residents throughout their
dying process; who can listen to residents (not only their words but their
body language as well); and who will ensure them love, care, and com-
panionship in their journey. Real listening means paying attention to the
resident, making eye contact, and being positioned so the resident can see
the other person or feel his or her presence. It also means being available
for touching, holding hands, or hugging when it is culturally and otherwise acceptable. Listening means giving the dying or grieving person the
opportunity to talk without interruption. It also means fully accepting the
choices and lifestyle of the person without judgment or pushing him or
her to change. Listening is sacred work. It must be remembered that residents who are dying or grieving are still alive and need to be exposed to
whatever life has to offer them.

DISCUSSION

1. Can you recall a time when a friend or family mem-
    ber created a sacred space for you so you were com-

fortable and able to let go of your emotions? What was it about that person and what did that person do or say that created this sacred space? Think about your relationship with one of your residents and reflect on whether you could do or say the same things to create a sacred space.

2.   What things can you do to become a better listener? What and/or who can assist you?

BEING PRESENT IN DYING

People who are dying experience many emotions. Sometimes they experience outright shock and denial (This is not happening to me). Quite frequently there is anger (Why is this happening to me?), which can result in emotional explosions or be kept inside and result in depression. People who are dying may bargain with a higher power for more time (If I'm spared, I vow to do some particular thing or give up some particular vice), eventually followed by acceptance or anticipation of the inevitability of death. Not all dying people experience all of these emotions nor always in the order described.

The grief experienced by those who are dying is not only sadness over the loss of oneself but grieving over no longer being with loved ones. In addition, dying people are faced with the emotional and relational task of handling the grief of their loved ones.

Hurrying residents through various stages of death is not helpful. The task of the staff is to show support by holding a resident's hand and listening. Residents have the right to die in any stage they choose. The very insightful social worker Marty Richards (1999) lists the rights of the dying as

1.   The right to be in control

2.   The right to have a sense of purpose

3.   The right to be in denial

4.   The right to choose death

5.   The right to touch and be touched

6.   The right to be spiritual

7.   The right to hear the truth

8. The right to reminisce

9. The right to laugh

It is important to be alert to the spiritual needs of a dying resident and to solicit from him or her or from others of the same religious or cultural group the special thoughts about his or her faith and belief system that are most helpful. The spiritual needs of a dying person, from a Christian perspective, are

- The need for a God who is present. This is a God who loves and cares about the person and whose compassion can be imagined through images such as lying in the hand of God rather than in a bed, or talking with God under an oak tree in a green pasture. Any image that promotes warm feelings of love from God is important.

- The need for a sense of identity and meaning in life, of being connected spiritually with God and with all other living beings.

- The need for that which is spiritually familiar: prayers, hymns, poems, and other forms that have provided comfort in the past.

- The need for relief from guilt as well as the giving and receiving of forgiveness so as to experience peace with God and others.

- The need to know that one's God is stronger than one's fear of death, an assurance that can be conveyed in part by an experience of caregiving so powerfully positive that the person can die in peace.

- The need to know that God will not punish someone who questions or is angry with God for the suffering, pain, and impending death that is experienced. This reaction is often a way for people to come to terms with the realization that life is not fair and that their God and other spiritual people are with them on the journey through dying and that death does not mean failure and is not the enemy.

- The need to have a companion along the journey, a person who is sensitive to the dying person's needs and can be a loving, listening, and hugging presence.

Death is the final, natural experience (perhaps the most important experience) of all living things. The resident can review his or her life, make meaning of his or her life, and experience satisfaction about the contribution that he or she has made to family members and others in society.

DISCUSSION

1. What is your earliest experience of a loved one dying? How did you feel? Was there a memorial service? Who and what gave you comfort? How did you and others express your grief?

2. Were you or others in your family taught not to express grief around others? If so, how has that affected you in life?

3. In considering your own end, how would you like to die? Do you know where you would like to be and who you would like to have present? What would you like to say to those who are grieving about your impending death? What rituals would you like to have?

4. Have you thought about what medical treatments you would want and not want? Who would you choose as a surrogate to make decisions about life's end if you cannot?

5. What do you think would help you cope with your own death?

GRIEF OF THE SURVIVORS

A grieving survivor often goes through similar emotional feelings as a person who is dying. The grieving survivor needs to talk through emotions and needs a nonjudgmental listener. The grieving survivor also needs to express emotions and needs to know that tears are okay. However grief is expressed, it is an expression of love and attachment. Finally, the grieving survivor needs to begin daily activity and participate in special events that will give new meaning and purpose to life. People who are grieving do not find comfort in phrases such as "Remember, everything is God's will," "It was a good way to die," "Your loved one is better off," "You are lucky to have had so many years together," "Time will heal," or "Count your blessings." These are all well-intended but moot points. The best support in times of grief is providing a comforting presence.

As for the dying person, rituals can bring hope to survivors through the various stages of dying and grieving. Rituals, both cultural and religious (e.g., anointing with oil, funerals or memorials with special hymns and sacred words, family gatherings), can be greatly comforting to those who grieve. Rituals can assist people through the grief process and help them establish a new life without their loved one and at their own pace. Families can create their own rituals separate from established spiritual or cultural ones. Many families have existing traditions that can become part of remembrance and the grief process.

THE LAZO FAMILY

In the Lazo family, people who die are always buried in an inexpensive casket. The family gathers with the clergy at the graveside for a committal service. A memorial service is held within one week at a time when most of the family and friends can come. After the memorial service, family members join for a meal to talk with one another and the immediate survivors. After the meal, the participants gather, bring out old pictures, and talk about the one who died. They traditionally stay together for 2 or 3 days. At the end of that time, each member of the family shares how the person who has died influenced him or her, then a candle is lit and prayers are offered by all. At the next family reunion, a brief time of remembrance and a moment of silence are observed for each family member who has died since the last gathering.

It is important for staff members to recognize that they, too, may be grieving the loss of a resident and need assistance with handling their grief. Recognizing one's own grieving process prevents projecting one's needs and feelings on others who are dying or grieving. Death often evokes profound emotions. It is healthy for staff members, in their interactions with family, friends, staff, and other residents, to recognize why they are crying, feeling depressed or irritable, or displaying other intense emotions.

HOWARD

Howard was in his seventies and dying from cancer. He and his wife were faithful members of their local Catholic church, but his children did not attend that church and seldom went to any other congregation. Throughout the family's history, Howard had at times been estranged from all three of his children. As he was nearing the end of his life, his wife Alice convinced the children to gather one last time as a family and have the pastor perform the Eucharist. This was Howard's great wish before he died. The Scripture readings, prayers, and bread and wine tied the family together in a deeply spiritual way, connecting them in love one last time. It brought peace to Howard and comforted the others in their grief.

DISCUSSION

1. What have you been grieving over lately? How have you expressed your grief, or how did it show itself in your daily life? What and who helped you cope?

2. Can you recall a time when the family of a resident gathered around that person toward the end of his or her life to celebrate a tradition or devise a ritual that was beneficial to all? Did that event have an effect on the staff?

3. Can you describe both the simplest and the most elaborate rituals that are part of your family's traditions and that you continue to practice?

CONCLUDING LIFE'S TASKS

As life draws to a close, a resident may be dealing with unresolved issues and need to express him- or herself to others. The resident often feels a deep need to be forgiven or to forgive or say final words to family and friends. The staff members of a facility are often in a unique position to hear these needs and bring the appropriate person (e.g., clergy, family member, friend) to a dying resident and/or encourage the resident to fulfill his or her end-of-life tasks in whatever way he or she is able.

Many times, residents hang on to life for the sake of a family member even though they wish to die. For family members to let a loved one go and to give him or her permission to die is a true gift.

HENRY

Henry was 98 years old and had been in his nursing facility for 9 years. In addition to ambulation and incontinence problems that initially brought him to the facility, he had developed colon cancer and soon was in the final stages of dying. Hospice workers had been called to assist the staff in providing comfort care only. The hospice volunteers and chaplain talked with Henry about his life and what meaning it had for him and others with whom he came into contact. During those discussions, Henry admitted that he had never forgiven his grandson Sam for fleeing to Canada to avoid being drafted to fight in the Vietnam war. Henry had served in the Marines for 4 years in World War II. Henry had been very close to dying but was struggling to stay alive, and now the staff knew why. Henry desperately wanted to forgive and be reconciled with Sam before he died. The chaplain called Sam, who agreed to come. The nursing facility staff witnessed the tearful reunion and reconciliation of grandfather and grandson, and Henry died that very night, 2 hours after Sam left.

DISCUSSION

1. If there had not been a chaplain, what could you have said or done to help Henry die in peace?

2. Have you worked with any residents long enough to hear them review their life and find meaning in it? If so, provide an example of a life review to assist others in the group.

3. Have you known of a resident who died not making peace with others or of family members who visited a resident but never made peace with their dying loved one? What effect did that have on the dying process or on the family members after the death of the resident? What was the effect on you and your co-workers?

CULTURAL SENSITIVITIES

In order to respect those who are dying and grieving, the staff needs to be aware of both the cultural and religious customs and beliefs of the facility's residents and the residents' families. In some ethnic groups, such as the Chinese, one does not touch a dead body in order to allow the soul appropriate time to leave. For some people, the presence of the body at a funeral is important, whereas for others a graveside service is held for the immediate family as soon as possible and a memorial service is held for other friends and relatives some time later. Some people within various religious and cultural groups cremate the body of the deceased instead of providing a burial. In addition, some families will not want the bodies removed from the facility before they visit, and others would prefer not to come at all after the death. In all issues relating to death, dying, and grieving, it is hazardous to assume that one culture will share the same value system as another, or moreover that members of a cultural group will share the same religious beliefs or customs as other members of that group.

As a resident nears death, the staff needs to review his or her social history, his or her chart, and any notes made by nursing or chaplaincy staff to see not only what the resident's end-of-life wishes are but whether there is a religious preference or clergy person listed. Staff members should notify any relevant clergy and pay special attention to any indications noted in the resident's chart or gleaned from family members about what should happen after death. The issue of dignity should be paramount during the time after death before the body leaves the facility. A helpful in-service training program for the staff would be to invite representatives from various religious and cultural groups to speak about their typical rites and customs of death.

DISCUSSION

1. Have you been to a funeral or memorial service other than that of your own religion or culture? Share with other staff what you learned from that experience.

2. Share the customs of dying of your own religion and family with other staff.

3. What resident's family custom relating to death has surprised or impressed you the most?

END-OF-LIFE DECISIONS

Many ethical dilemmas surround the end of life, including whether to insert a feeding tube, whether to transfer the resident to a hospital, or whether to use antibiotics for pneumonia. In the United States, individual wishes and choices are prized highly. Thus, the durable power of attorney option for health care was developed to enable dying people to have their wishes fulfilled. The facility staff is often in a position to encourage residents to express their wishes. It can be emphasized that doing so is not only for their own sake but for the sake of family members, who often agonize over end-of-life decisions.

One of the most difficult decisions that a family needs to make is whether to use mechanical support systems such as respirators or feeding tubes to prolong a loved one's life. Even more difficult, once such supports are in place, is the decision to turn off respirators, withdraw feeding tubes, or discontinue other treatments. Making these decisions can cause internal family conflicts and feelings of guilt and shame for those who are part of the decision making. Some residents in the dying process linger for a long time at the end of life because family members are unable to make any kind of decision.

The durable power of attorney eliminates potential conflict between families and friends and prevents guilt or uncertainty over end-of-life decisions. This is a great gift that a dying person can give to those who survive. When families are in conflict about end-of-life treatment, if the physician is at odds with the family or the dying person, or if staff members are in conflict with the resident or with each other, the issues should be presented to an ethics committee.

Many facilities have an ethics committee that can hear and mediate such conflicts. It should help all of the parties involved to understand and reflect on each other's positions, and moreover, raise issues that have not been considered by any group. Ethics committees are composed of various staff and consultants and usually include the resident's physician, nurses, the nursing facility administrator, a nursing assistant, a social worker, clergy, and others who can give insight into the wishes of the resident.

The ethics committee does not make decisions but provides a systematic way of examining the resident's issues and wishes and thereby provides the insights by which the resident and family can make an informed decision through durable power of attorney.

MAI

Mai was a 95-year-old Vietnamese woman who had cancer. Her son and daughter insisted that her physician not tell her of the diagnosis or the side effects of the chemotherapy. In their belief system, being told of the diagnosis and harmful side effects would be an invitation for them to happen. After the first oral chemotherapy, Mai was so sick that she refused to take any more medication. Neither the family nor the woman told the physician that she had stopped taking the medication. After a few months, the woman was admitted to the hospital in a very advanced stage of cancer. The son and daughter still insisted that their mother not be told of the diagnosis or the side effects of the chemotherapy. Some of the staff wanted to tell the mother anyway, and others were unsure about how to proceed, so they asked for an ethics consultation.

DISCUSSION

1. If you were on the ethics committee, what facts would you like to know to help you decide the best course of action?

2. How would you discover more about Mai's religious and cultural beliefs and practices?

3 Who else would you invite to be part of the ethics consultation?

The only thing certain in life is change, and how all of us live life to the fullest depends on how all of us respond to change. Some changes are planned and anticipated, and others just happen. It is the way the spirit is nurtured by oneself and by the spirit of others that determines how life can be meaningful. Again, being present, listening, and touching are the practical ingredients in supporting those who are dying and grieving.

ACTION STEPS

1. Learn about the end-of-life rituals of all of the ethnic and religious groups represented by the residents
   in your facility. Establish some procedures for finding
   out more about the essential cultural and religious
   beliefs of each resident. Discuss how your facility
   honors these beliefs.

2. If you were facing inevitable death, what would
   matter most to you? What would make the process
   less painful? What would you do to prepare for your
   own death? Have you filled out a durable power of
   attorney health care for yourself? Investigate the
   answers to these questions for several residents in
   your facility.

3. Do you know if the residents you care for have a living will to take care of their estates? Do you have
   one?

4. Think about the main thing that you have learned
   from the last three people to whom you have given
   care who have died. Let these lessons inform your
   caregiving efforts.

REFERENCE

Kozberg, C. (1998). *Running a unique race.* Workshop presented at the American Society for
   Aging conference, San Francisco.
Richards, M. (1999, June). *Connecting soul to soul.* Workshop presented at the Center for
   Gerontology, Spirituality and Faith, Cupertino, CA.

RECOMMENDED READING

A cry of absence: Reflections for the winter of the heart by Martin E. Marty (W.B.
   Eerdmans)
A grief observed by C.S. Lewis (HarperSanFrancisco)
All our losses, all our griefs: Resources for pastoral care by Kenneth R. Mitchell
   and Herbert Anderson (Westminster Press)
Dying well: The prospect for growth at the end of life by Ira Byock (Riverhead
   Books)

How we die: Reflections on life's final chapter by Sherwin B. Nuland (Alfred A. Knopf)

Journal of Religious Gerontology published by The Hayworth Press, 10 Alice Street, Binghamton, New York 13904

Living with grief: Loss in later life by Kenneth J. Doka (Hospice Foundation of America)

Questions and answers on death and dying by Elisabeth Kübler-Ross (Maxwell MacMillan International)

The path through grief: A compassionate guide by Marguerite Bouvard with Evelyn Gladu (Prometheus Books)

Tuesdays with Morrie by Mitch Albom (Wheeler Publishing)

We live too short and die too long by Walter M. Bortz II (Bantam Books)

RESOURCES

California Coalition for Compassionate Care
1215 K Street, Suite 800
Sacramento, California 95814
Telephone: 916-552-7573
E-mail: loneill@calhealth.org
Web site: http://www.finalchoices.calhealth.org/

Last Acts
Partnership for Caring
1620 Eye Street NW, Suite 202
Washington, DC 20006
Telephone: 202-296-8071
E-mail: lastacts@aol.com
Web site: http://www.lastacts.org

National Hospice Foundation
1700 Diagonal Road, Suite 625
Alexandria, Virginia 22314
Telephone: 703-516-4928
E-mail: nhf@nhpco.org
Web site: http://www.hospiceinfo.org

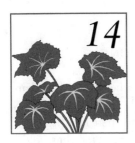

14

Spiritual Legacy

Passing on
the Spirit of a Life

Marita Grudzen

OBJECTIVES

As a result of reading this chapter and working through the exercises, participants will be able to

1. Understand that most residents in long-term care are bringing their lives to completion and realize the significance of this endeavor

2. Understand the need to assist elders in their efforts to hand on their legacy

3. Identify psychological and spiritual processes for older adults to articulate and pass on life legacies

4. Appreciate cultural variations in the practice of handing on knowledge and wisdom

5. Identify ways for families and communities to honor the spiritual legacy of their elders

THE SEARCH FOR LIFE'S MEANING

Every person has a desire to find meaning in his or her life and to share that with others. Approaching the end of life, people are faced with many questions concerning what they have contributed to their families, their friends, and the wider world. This is particularly true for those older adults who find themselves somewhat incapacitated within a nursing facility environment, with little ability to influence the exterior world. By necessity, nursing facility residents often look inward for understanding of how they have impacted others and how well they have lived their lives.

Victor Frankl, noted author and Holocaust survivor, referred to a person's search for understanding about his or her life as a "search for ultimate meaning" (1992, p. 104). He used the term *tragic optimism* to describe the kind of existential approach that can characterize even the most unforgiving situations that ultimately lead to death. Tragic optimism is "an optimism in the face of tragedy and in view of the human potential which at its best always allows for 1) turning suffering into a human achievement and accomplishment, 2) deriving from guilt the opportunity to change oneself for the better, and 3) deriving from life's transitoriness an incentive to take responsible action" (Frankl, 1992, pp. 139–140). This, in turn, presupposes the human capacity to creatively turn life's negative aspects into something positive or constructive. In other words, the key to life is making the best of any situation.

Frankl's words are apropos for older adults in a nursing facility. In many cases, older adults are faced with debilitating illnesses and loss of functioning that can make life seem tragic. Many older adults have defined their identity through a profession or role that no longer exists or gives meaning to their lives. They also reflect on past failures and regrets, some of which are buried in their subconscious or unconscious and are manifested only as a sense of sadness, futility, or loss. The suppression of feelings of regret and failure associated with past memories may be part of the reason for increased memory loss in many older adults. The pain of remembering may be too much to bear. Helping these men and women face their memories with greater confidence and self-respect is both worthwhile and possible. The process of creating some form of legacy to pass along to others can be a powerful way for residents to express Frankl's search for ultimate meaning.

DISCUSSION

1. What are some of your sources of meaning and strength? Have these resources changed over time?

2. What gives meaning and purpose to the elders in your family?

3. Has aging added meaning and purpose to or diminished the lives of elders in your own extended family?

4. How does aging affect your family relationships?

The meaning attributed to one's life is also tied to a societal context that carries ambiguities associated with each historical epoch or a given ethnic or cultural heritage. Staff members must recognize that in the United States increasing numbers of older adults have originated from other native lands and that a blending of worlds is part of their personal history. Having adopted the United States as their homeland, immigrants often carry regrets and sadness about family members who stayed behind in their country of birth, particularly if their lives seem very harsh. Immigrants who have successfully acculturated to their new communities may nevertheless adhere to former cultural beliefs, values, and practices. Many elders believe that younger generations have abandoned the ethnic and cultural traditions that helped to create and define them as human beings. Understanding such residual feelings and attitudes is useful for staff members who wish to help residents explore their spiritual legacies.

DISCUSSION

1. Describe some aspect of your family's immigration history. How is it similar or different from those of other families?

2. What stories can you tell about your family's immigration to the United States of America? What do you know about your relatives who first came to this country?

3. Who has the best knowledge in your family about your descendants? Has someone in your family done genealogical research on the family's history?

LIFE RECOVERY THROUGH THE IMAGINATION

Exploring cultural diversity in the context of one's spiritual legacy can be approached as an exercise of creative imagination. Diverse cultural experiences can be included in a spiritual legacy in many ways, but imagination is one of the most important tools for identifying what is most meaningful to each resident. It can be challenging to assimilate diverse cultural experiences into one spiritual legacy when individuals have lived portions of their lives in various cultures or been married to someone from a culture distinct from their own. Within the imagination, however, people can move easily from one world to another without conflict. If it's helpful, residents can use meditative experiences to picture their different worlds.

Usually, a person's imaginative faculties will focus on important images that express deep meaning. Many elders learn to draw on this rich heritage of images from their interior life. Often, the images are evocative and come from nature—perhaps a pond or lake that the person visited as a young child. An image may also be symbolic, such as a boat that brought the person from one culture to another.

With the help of a facilitator, nursing facility residents can go through a process of life recovery that taps into the cultural heritage that has helped form their historical experiences. The facilitator might provide props and materials that evoke memories for the residents, who in turn can build a collage of images representing the symbolic forms of their lives. Using memory and imagination, residents can identify the types of activities that gave the most meaning to their lives. For some residents, these experiences might be related to child care or domestic activities. Symbolically meaning-laden activities, such as preparing a meal or setting a table, can be simulated for residents in the nursing facility environment without great difficulty. Another trigger for recollecting key events, memories, and images can be watching a television program that relates to the history of a resident's life.

Using the imagination for life recovery can be compared with the existential meaning described by Frankl in his logotherapy treatment. Logotherapy refers to the primordial human drive to find meaning in one's experience of life even when that experience may lead to diminishment and suffering. Memories present themselves to people in symbolic forms, and people need to explore and understand the significance of these symbols to find their meaning. The symbolic content of one's imagination carries with it the hidden sources of optimism about one's life.

Elders often have rich conscious and subconscious experiential content that can be explored through writing, art, sculpture, and drama.

Many older adults will have to integrate their diverse cultural experiences, if not prior to admittance to a nursing facility, then within the walls of the facility. Cultural symbolism can take many forms, and one such form is food. In many cultures, food provides emotional and intellectual nourishment as well as physical replenishment. It is over the daily breaking of bread that a family often partakes of the meaningful activities of the day by sharing significant events; discussing issues about home, school, or work; requesting support in one form or another; and expressing solace when a family member is distressed. The same symbolic context continues to surround mealtimes for residents in long-term care facilities. They can have easier access to the symbolic context of a meal when they are surrounded by a loving, supportive community.

The American experience is unique in that immigrants and many of their subsequent generations have had to adapt to more than one cultural heritage in their lifetime. This has led to many benefits (e.g., an older adult who has had exposure to various cultures throughout his or her life will adapt more easily to new experiences), but it also makes the work of life integration (the process of recalling and reconciling one's diverse life experiences) more challenging.

SOUL PASSAGES

Creating a spiritual legacy is often a process of spiritual healing. Spiritual healing takes many forms but its focus is always on preserving the integrity of the soul. The legacy, once created, captures the central values that have sustained a person throughout his or her lifetime and provides seeds of hope and nourishment for future generations.

In ancient cultures (African, Native American, and aboriginal cultures of Australia), shamans helped people unite the inner and outer worlds of their experiences. The shaman was usually the one person in a tribe who could mediate contact with the world of the spirits, which included deceased ancestors and animistic powers and personalities that controlled various aspects of the physical and psychological world that human beings inhabited. The shaman did this through rituals (rites of passage such as birth, death, or coming of age) that would allow for passage between the physical world of ordinary daily experience and the spiritual and symbolic world of the imagination.

Jeanne Achterberg (1985) has documented the unique nexus between imagery and healing in her study of shamanism. First and foremost, avoiding death is not the purpose of medicinal practices in the shamanic traditions. The typical Western mistrust of shamanic healing systems often stems from observations that they often do not result in a cure or extension of life. Healing for the shaman, however, is a spiritual rather than physical affair. Disease is considered to have origins in and gain its meaning from the spirit world. The purpose of life in this tradition is to maintain oneself in concert with all things on earth and in the sky, which requires becoming imbued and initiated into the visionary regions of the spirit. Since the spirit world is pervasive and powerful in so-called "primitive" cultures, an individual only attains man- or womanhood through initiation rites, often carried out by the local shaman, that enable the initiates to understand more fully the spirit world that they inhabit in order to maintain the health of the tribe. To lose one's soul is the gravest occurrence, according to shamanism, because it eliminates any meaning from life, now and forever. Thus, the purpose of much shamanic healing is primarily to nurture and preserve the soul and to protect it from eternal wandering.

Encouraging imaginative recall in nursing facility residents can be a contemporary form of shamanic healing because it allows elders to better understand their own psyches instead of leaving issues unresolved or buried. Imaginative recall becomes a kind of initiation to the world of the soul (spirit) through symbolic imagery. Healing can occur for residents insofar as they are able to integrate all aspects of their psyche, and especially the elements of shame, guilt, or grief. Everyone has regrets about the events in their lives that have diminished them or distracted them from their core life purpose. The Taoist teaching about yin and yang, darkness and light, is built on a similar belief that dis-ease often occurs when people fail to allow suffering or sorrow to become part of their psyche.

DISCUSSION

1. Have you experienced any form of spiritual healing? If so, what form did this take?

2. Are there any individuals in your community recognized as healers? What principle or principles seem to make them effective in their own healing work?

UNLOCKING DIMENSIONS OF THE PSYCHE

Carl Jung's work delved into the substratum of the psyche and helped to reveal a deeper level of symbolic content beneath the surface of human consciousness that has an immense impact on people's daily existence (Singer, 1994). Jung spoke of the *shadow* as those elements in the psyche that are somewhat beyond the horizon of waking consciousness and that contain the negative or self-destructive elements of each persona. Many of the negative elements of the psyche come out of unrecognized personal traumas.

Jung saw the shadow as a potential ally in the unfolding of an individual's higher calling because the shadow often revealed some unfulfilled dimension of *soul work* (Singer, 1994; see also Chapter 10, pp. 281–315). For people who have been very goal directed in their lives, for example, their shadow could pull them toward laziness and a sense of boredom; it could also cause them to question the meaning of their active life. This shadow helps to shift the soul toward a more contemplative approach to existence, which might be the soul work of an elder's time in a nursing facility environment. A resident who can no longer rely on any work or project to fill his or her days will need to turn inward to a period of inner reflection to find the center of his or her being and accept the fact that eventually the ability to do most activities diminishes (Singer, 1994). A person can, however, learn to find a real meaning to this diminishment in the sunset of his or her physical life.

As mentioned earlier, elders should be encouraged, with the help of a facilitator, to visualize scenes from different points in their life history. These scenes are a kind of dramatic tableaux in which the richness of a resident's life experiences can be explored. The scenes, whether from present or past experiences, often become part of the archetypal imagery that Jung believed derived from the universal consciousness (the collective psyche of all ages and cultures) underlying all individual consciousness (each person's psyche).

For Jung, the personality, or persona, was a mask that needed to be unveiled. Imagery and symbolism help people to move beyond the superficial layers of consciousness to those deeper layers that connect them to the *soul* level of being (Singer, 1994).

Imaginative scenes become more real if they have details attached to them. Residents often imagine important scenes associated with the lives of their children: birth, first steps, the first day of school, graduation, prom, and marriage. These events can help a resident explore the relationship that he or she had with other people and any problems that may have occurred in those relationships. These details will often reveal important imaginative structures that can be explored. The facilitator can orchestrate these themes into an oral or written testament of the elder's life. The elder resident can then reenact certain "scenes" that need completion or new interpretations.

Reenacted stories become part of the elder's spiritual legacy. It is the meaning of the scenes that is important. Merely reviewing the scenes is not a sufficient method of developing a spiritual legacy, according to Frankl (1992). It is important for the facilitator to draw out and uncover the meaning of the scenes. Any negative dimension or shadow that becomes present in a visualized scene deserves more attention and consideration.

A resident may bring up examples of a rupture in a core relationship such as with his or her spouse or a child. The facilitator should encourage the resident to explore the context of this relationship when the rupture took place and how it might be healed today. It is possible to heal the relationship even if the spouse or child is incapable of interacting with the resident whether because of death or absence from his or her life. The facilitator could draw a picture for the resident or role-play a situation that represents how he or she might express him- or herself to that person if the loved one were actually present today. This imaginary dialogue can become part of the healing process. In addition, the staff member can enter more fully into the life of the resident, and the resident may be able to express deep emotions about the person that he or she loved and lost. A healing process will occur that benefits the resident and gives the staff member a concrete tool for working with other residents.

DISCUSSION

1. Think about a resident who has shared information with you about past or present relationships. How were the relationships important to the resident? How did he or she feel about having or losing those relationships?

2. Does this resident become agitated when certain experiences are brought up involving significant people in his or her life?

3. How does the staff explore the underlying meaning of the resident's relationship in order to help the

resident come to terms with having or losing this relationship?

4. What are some ways to engage this resident in dialogue in order to heal his or her feelings about a relationship that has been troubling him or her?

THE SOUL AS A CONTAINER FOR LEGACY

In the right situation, each person has reminisced about the rich and colorful events that are part of his or her life experiences, but the invitation to express such musings is not often presented. People tend to think that no one is interested in their past experiences. These past events are very much alive, however, within the realm of each person's psyche, having made their imprint. A spiritual legacy is actually formed by the way a person has processed the manifold events of his or her life, particularly those that have forced the person to integrate diverse spiritual and cultural experiences, those that have caused suffering, or those that have caused a person to open his or her heart to transform suffering and conflict.

These experiences tend to become part of each person's subconscious or unconscious psychic life, and they need some prompting to be revealed. For the purposes of this discussion, the *soul* is referred to as the central processing system within one's psyche and *spirit* is a kind of external principle of inspiration that guides the operation of one's soul. The psyche has many layers and, like an onion, must undergo a process of peeling away various layers to find the layer that can be called the soul. The soul represents the spirituality-organizing principle of a person's life, and it silently does its work throughout life.

Making manifest that which is inner and silent—the inner life of the spirit—can often only be accomplished through symbols. Even those who do not recognize the "soul" as a distinct spiritual life force understand that every human being has an interior life that is uniquely his or her own. This interior consciousness needs the same attention as a person's exterior physical self. People are, in fact, a composite of how they perceive themselves as well how they project themselves to others. Elders have a "storehouse" of interior images, memories, and reflections within them that deserve to be expressed and symbolized in words, actions, and creative endeavors.

To assist older adults with the explanation of their inner lives using historical memory and reflection, facilitators should look for those symbols that seem to recur in the residents' visualizations. These symbols can be explored in a group or communal setting for their inner meaning. If an elder's imagination constantly brings up themes dealing with life-changing directions, nursing facility staff can explore the symbols of change and transformation that seem to dominate the resident's consciousness. The elder may be doing soul work that allows him or her to connect the many changes that have occurred in his or her life as well as ones that will occur in the future. Often, for example, physical changes of *place* represent interior transformations that are occurring in the person's spirit or soul. The challenge for nursing facility staff is creating a communal environment that supports such self-revelation as well as finding a skilled therapist to guide this process.

The soul can be viewed as a kind of microprocessor of each person's human experience from the standpoint of his or her ultimate human destiny. Each individual has a specific destiny that is a combination of choice, chance, and providential synchronicity (the marriage that occurs when chance events seem to combine with individual choice to seal a person's life direction or major life choices). Throughout life, people are attempting to use their rational faculties to put all of these elements into their proper frame of reference. Usually, however, the flow of life is too fast for anyone to consciously and clearly process every event. It is only near the end of one's life that a life path becomes more evident and an individual is able to embrace its full meaning. This historical and existential life path is the very core of each person's spiritual legacy. It is not so much a set of spiritual principles as it is a life story that is filled with rich symbolic content. Each elder's life story can become part of the rich legacy of any nursing facility.

Too often the concept of spiritual testaments is treated as a kind of moral testimony, but this is only a very small part of the testament that a person leaves to posterity. The life of each elder has had many ups and downs, tragedies, and comedies. By sharing historical anecdotes, elders can delve more deeply into the symbolic levels of their experiences. As they do this interpretive work, it is important to allow each nursing facility resident to give his or her own meaning to this personal life history. The interior life of the resident should be the core of his or her spiritual legacy, for it is that dimension of the psyche that often contains an unfolding of spiritual riches.

SPIRITUAL STEPPING STONES

One approach to writing or recording a spiritual legacy can be accomplished by drawing from the key spiritual experiences of an elder's life and encouraging him or her to explore the imaginative dimensions of those experiences. Sometimes, the experiences can be as simple as a walk in the woods or a vision of the night sky. Usually, spiritual experiences begin with a sense of wonder and awe about the nature and beauty of the physical universe. A person can also have a spiritual experience within his or her specific religious culture; however, many older adults have not had their most profound spiritual experiences in any organized religion. In many cases, a relationship that has unfolded over a lifetime or a particular mission or vocation may have formed the person's life. Each person should fully explore his or her life path to reveal this spiritual legacy. Staff members need to be very open to the breadth of residents' experiences and to help residents find out what became the core meaning of their lives.

Linda Spence described the act of writing about one's life as a process of legacy:

> It is the everyday joy and sorrows as well as the "big events" that provide the fertile connecting ground between the generations. And today, as we realize our losses, few of us find the journal or stack of letters that might have helped us to piece together the insight or real life story we seek. (1997, p. xii)

The exercise of writing a spiritual legacy is a book waiting to become each resident's story. Parts of the residents' lives may already be known to others, but residents should be reminded not to assume that what seems obvious to them will be familiar to others. Here, too, are questions that may not have yet been asked. If no one has asked, someone someday will, and this written record could be the chance to uncover the elder's answers. Through the process of creating a legacy, elders are invited to share their experience, insights, and the wisdom and humility of their years.

A spiritual legacy is far more than the more familiar *last will and testament*. Most often, people think of someone's last will and testament in purely material terms. The Jewish tradition promotes the creation of a complementary document called an *ethical will* that states a person's values and wishes. A spiritual testament is a written form of spiritual legacy that is generally a declaration of one's spiritual values and the influence that these values have had on the person and those whom he or she loves. An ethical will can be a part of this testament, not only documenting the values a person wants to share, but how he or she wishes to see the legacy carried out by heirs. (For more information on ethical wills, see *Ethical Wills: Putting Your Values on Paper* [2002] by Barry K. Baines, M.D.)

The spiritual testament can include the major stepping stones that influenced one's life and the gifts that emerged over a lifetime of service. Spiritual gifts are a manifestation of the life of the spirit. A spiritual life can be constructed as a narrative, a story of one's interior processes as they developed over time. This story should include the obstacles and challenges that a person faced and the inner resources that helped him or her to surmount these difficulties. Tracing the pivotal events and beliefs in story form can be conceived as presenting a person's spiritual stepping stones. (See the writings of Ira Progoff [1992] in *At a Journal Workshop* concerning spiritual stepping stones.) These stepping stones can include both interior and exterior events that have shaped a person's spiritual destiny such as a first communion, a bar or bat mitzvah, and a marriage or life separation that provoked great spiritual understanding and growth in one's life.

Usually, the individual begins to see certain patterns emerge as he or she identifies these spiritual stepping stones. The steps can be reenacted in some form through ritual as a way to memorialize them as a spiritual legacy. It is also possible to record the ritual for future generations so that others can have a visual record of an elder's spiritual journey through life.

SPIRITUAL LEGACIES AND CODAS

Residents in nursing facilities need to be assisted in completing their life process. Bringing life to fullness and completion should become part of what is truly a sacred mission of long-term care staff. Each resident has certain unresolved issues in his or her life. Although some unresolved issues need the expertise of clergy or a psychologist, others may only need a supportive community for expression and resolution. Residents need to find ways to explore their life history to know what issues in their life are the most meaningful. Usually, the resident will express his or her life history most easily with a supportive individual or in a group setting. Residents who do not receive regular visitors often need additional help to facilitate a process that meets their needs. The families of those who come to visit can be a rich source of anecdotes about their loved one and can help their loved one discover the areas of his or her life that need completion.

JEAN

After several weeks in a local hospital, Jean Grudzen could no longer eat solid foods and was limited to liquids such as peach juice, which she loved to sip. Rather than put her in a nursing facility, the family members arranged to have her return to her daughter's home, where she had lived for several years after selling her own home. She was taken by ambulance from the hospital to her daughter's home. All of her children and grandchildren were waiting for her at the home. When she arrived, she was taken upstairs to her bedroom. As the attendants placed her in her bed, she passed quietly from this earthly abode. It seemed that what Jean needed in order to complete her life was to feel completely "at home" and to share this moment with her family. She was apparently waiting to die and her family was able to help her find the closure she sought.

Residents in nursing facilities can also have unresolved spiritual questions or issues that need professional attention. Some older adults may feel a sense of guilt or shame about some earlier experience or failure in their lives such as a marriage that ended in divorce, the loss of a child, or the loss of a loved one through death. Any one of these factors can be a major issue for an older adult as he or she reaches the final chapter of his or her life story. The nursing facility staff can be very helpful in discovering these issues and making them known to the clergy or a social worker that facilitates individual and group counseling in the facility.

Each resident needs to have someone who will listen to his or her story and find avenues for him or her to feel a sense of life fulfillment. Sometimes, the best way to help a resident find life fulfillment is to talk about all of the positive contributions he or she has made in his or her life and to help that resident find some way to express his or her gifts in a tangible manner (e.g., storytelling, drawing, painting, poetry, writing a fairy tale).

Mirroring back to a person the spiritual gifts that have anchored his or her life is another way of capturing a spiritual legacy. When the third author's mother-in-law, Jean, was terminally ill, her younger daughter, Simone, wrote Jean a letter that recounted the spiritual gifts that she saw in her (see Figure 1). Jean posted this letter at her bedside for her friends and family to read. It enabled her to realize that her gifts had been recognized and would live on in her children and grandchildren. She could see the ultimate meaning of her life documented in this letter, and it brought her peace; it allowed her to let go. She died a week after receiving it.

Dear Grandma,   June 28, 1994

When I heard from my Mom that your condition was getting more and more serious, I began to hurt more and more. At first, I was angry, and then confused, and then numb, but now I don't feel any of these things, because all I can feel is you now, your presence.

However unaware you are of it, each and every one of your grandchildren has been forever loved and influenced by you. And although I've spent most of my life missing you and distanced from you, you have always been, and always will be with me.

You have instilled in me the kind of strength that will endure my struggle, as it did yours. And where it is that you're going I will also be someday. Everything that you have taught me guides me. I know that you knew pain in your life, but I also know that you knew joy, and I hope you are letting go of the pain.

I want more than anything to be by your side now, but fate has it that I am not. But please realize that your face is in my thoughts every waking moment, reminding me that I can, as you do, live with both dignity and compassion. I respect and love you more than I can ever say. As I said, you are with me now, as always.

Please know that you live through us. Grandma, you are the most beautiful woman I will ever know. I have always lived in awe of you. I miss you and I hope that you will visit me in my dreams and watch me from the HEAVENS.

          I LOVE you GRANDMA.

                    Simone

Figure 1. Letter from Simone to her grandmother, Jean Grudzen.

Even though the granddaughter wrote the message, it represents a living spiritual legacy for her grandmother. Very often, the children or grandchildren of elders are the ones who actually write their loved one's legacy and pass it on to the next generation. A spiritual legacy can be a powerful experience for everyone who is touched by the process.

A spiritual legacy need not be limited to written form. It can include certain objects that were once part of an elder's profession or household life. These objects are imbued with years of commitment and a certain kind of devotion. A doctor might want to hand down his or her favorite medical instrument to a younger doctor; a factory worker might hand over his or her tools to a son or daughter or a younger worker. A person who has cooked all of his or her life might want to hand down his or her favorite recipes.

The father of the author's husband worked as a tool and die maker, and his tools were precious to him. At the end of his life, he handed over many of these tools to his two sons. Similarly, the author learned to bake bread from the hands of a woman who became her spiritual mentor. The woman taught not only the skill of bread making but also conveyed the keys to her spiritual legacy. She put all of her love and energy into her role as a bakery chef for her religious community for more than 50 years. Bread making was an essential part of that dedication to her community and her friends. Eating her bread was like taking communion.

Another way elders can manifest a spiritual legacy is through rituals. A ritual can be as simple as a gathering of family and friends to share the final days.

ANTHONY

When Anthony was terminally ill, his family and friends staged a procession that included many of the elements that had been part of his life as a priest, teacher, and community leader. This procession symbolized the movement of his life through different transitions that he had made. It graphically enacted the drama of his life as a kind of contemporary Gospel narrative. Down through the ages, the Judeo-Christian tradition has interpreted the passage of time as a history of God's action in the lives of his people. For some, it can recapture the sense of God's immanence in their lives.

Anthony had been a pastor in the Mexican-American community of San José, and he established a small faith community called the Communidad de Ministerio Christiano, or Community of Christian Ministry. Many members of the Communidad had made outstanding contributions to the local community of San José, and they were able to express their sense of indebtedness to

Anthony for the example he had set for them through his life of service.

Anthony also had been founder and chairman of a major job-training agency in San José called the Center for Employment Training (CET). This program has grown into one of the model training programs for the western United States and has grown far beyond the local area to a national job-training model for the whole country. Many of the staff and board members of CET were able to visit Anthony in his final days, and he was able to share with them his own sense of spiritual identity and the vocation they shared in serving the thousands of people trained by CET for successful employment. Anthony was a man whose legacy lived on in his basic Christian community, the Communidad, and in the service that CET provided for the wider community. In one of his final acts of solidarity, he was able to give the sermon at a final liturgy held in his home and attended by his family and friends. He had to be brought out in a wheelchair, as he was very weak. The strength of his spirit shone through in his final words as he shared his hopes and dreams for his community of faith and his community of service.

DISCUSSION

1. In what ways would you like to be remembered by your family and friends? Would you feel comfortable with some kind of ritual that expressed a legacy you wished to convey to them?

2. Can you think of any particular ritual that is still very meaningful to you whether you experienced it in the past or present?

3. Do you have any favorite readings that express something important to you and could become part of your legacy?

4. Do you have someone in mind to be the custodian of your legacy?

CULTURAL RITUALS

Among many cultures of the world, the lives of loved ones continue to influence their survivors even after their deaths. The Mexican celebration of the Day of the Dead is one example of this kind of celebration. The deceased members of one's family continue to be part of the spiritual tradition through a memorial, which usually includes a meal. In many cultures, the meal actually occurs at the gravesite to indicate that the spiritual legacy of the loved one continues in that family. In Belize, the Garifuna people celebrate their connection with the deceased in the construction of a ritual "temple" or "tent" in which they sing, dance, and talk about their family members for a period of 1 week. This annual celebration is the central religious celebration of their culture. It ends with a ritual meal that evokes the presence of the deceased, and it includes the placing of the remaining food in a boat that is sent out to sea, symbolizing the journey through life that everyone takes toward a final destination in the world beyond the present temporal domain.

In today's fast-paced, youth-oriented culture, it is important to encourage greater respect for the spiritual legacy of elders. In many cultures, elders are the central figures who embody the wisdom tradition of their specific culture. With encouragement, these wisdom traditions can again become part of an honored and respected spiritual legacy. Renewing these traditions requires encouraging a variety of practices that express the spiritual legacies of today's elders, such as oral and written histories, ritualistic expressions of a person's life story, the handing over of physical symbols, and the celebration of a ritual meal or journey. A community must exist to create these events, and the nursing facility can provide such a community. The rituals can be wonderfully bonding experiences for all who participate.

In the nursing facility environment, staff members become part of the residents' extended families. The staff often provides the kind of support and encouragement that gives meaning to the resident's life experience. Staff members can contribute to future generations as well as to the life of individual elders by helping each resident to express the meaning of his or her life through oral or written form or through rituals that include the resident's family and friends. Staff members will undoubtedly discover higher levels of satisfaction in their work if they are able to assist residents in communicating their spiritual legacies.

Many forms of spiritual legacy, as well as ways to bring it into focus and explore, honor, and communicate it, have been discussed in this chapter. Individual case- and culture-specific examples have been described. What form spiritual legacies and codas take is often less important than the act of giving and receiving them, of having them recognized in some way and carried on. Many elders have very vivid imaginations and they can readily recall important, meaningful events and people who have become a part of their lives. It is possible to nurture these memories and celebrate them in many ways, particularly while the resident is still alive and able to appreciate the honor that he or she is receiving from a celebration of this legacy. Many of an elder's memories can enrich the lives of his or her family, friends, and the staff of the nursing home. One of the purposes of this book is to help staff members develop programs that encourage residents to express their memories in the form of a spiritual legacy. As was stated earlier in this chapter, the key to helping uncover a person's spiritual legacy often takes little more than asking about his or her life experiences—then listening and acknowledging their significance for the elder.

ACTION STEPS

1. Help your facility develop a program for remembering residents after their deaths.

2. Discover how elders in different cultures are honored by their families after they die.

3. What suggestions can staff members give to residents' families regarding ways to honor the resident either before or after his or her death?

4. Develop suggestions for rituals that staff members can develop for residents' families that will bring them comfort if they are not present for the death of their loved one.

5. Discuss ways the staff can begin to work more closely with clergy who service the nursing facility to develop services that involve the staff in storytelling and sharing about the lives of residents who have died unexpectedly.

REFERENCES

Achterberg, J. (1985). *Imagery in healing: Shamanism and modern medicine.* Boston: New Science Library.

Baines, B.K. (2002). *Ethical wills: Putting your values on paper.* Cambridge, MA: Perseus.

Frankl, V. (1992). *Man's search for ultimate meaning: An introduction to logotherapy* (4th ed.). Boston: Beacon Press.

Progoff, J. (1992). *At a journal workshop: Writing to access the power of the unconscious and evoke creative ability.* Los Angeles: J.P. Tarcher.

Singer, J. (1994). *Boundaries of the soul: The practice of Jung's psychology. Revised and updated.* New York: Anchor Books.

Spence, L. (1997). *Legacy: A step-by-step guide to writing personal history.* Athens: Ohio University Press/Swallow Press.

RECOMMENDED READING

At a journal workshop: The basic text and guide for using the Intensive Journal process by Ira Progoff (Dialogue House Library)

Elder wisdom: Crafting your own elderhood by Eugene C. Bianchi (Crossroad)

Ethical wills: Putting your values on paper by Barry K. Baines, M.D. (Perseus)

From age-ing to sage-ing: A profound new vision of growing older by Zalman Schachter-Shalomi and Ronald S. Miller (Warner Books)

Generativity and the gift of meaning by John Kotre in *Generations, 23*(4), 65–70

Religious views on legacy and intergenerational transfers by Stephen Sapp in *Generations* 20(3), 31–36

The clash of meanings: Medical narrative and biographical story at life's end by Sharon R. Kaufman in *Generations, 23*(4), 77–82

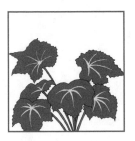

Afterword

You have just read 14 chapters that promote health and wholeness for residents and for staff of long-term care facilities. The chapters have dealt with vital connections that everyone needs in their relationship with others, themselves, and a higher being. These connections are spiritual and may include a religious faith, but essentially, these spiritual connections are at the core of people's existence and give meaning to life.

The authors have said that nursing facilities are *sacred places,* and the service that is performed there is *sacred work.* In addressing the spiritual needs of residents and ourselves, staff members realize that if they are not whole and healthy, the residents will not be whole and healthy, even when residents experience good clinical care.

Now that you have completed one cycle of exploring the spiritual dimensions of care, you may choose to start this workbook again. Another option is to explore spiritual well-being from other aspects of care. You will be surprised at the new depth of learning and practice these vital connections will create in your lives and in the lives of residents. Changing the way you think, act, feel, and perform services takes a lot of effort and practice, so the authors encourage you to find a friend, relative, or fellow worker to continue to discuss what you have learned and how you are putting what you have learned into practice. You will grow and learn from and through each other's encouragement. The possibilities for nourishment and renewal are unlimited.

Index

Page numbers followed by *f* indicate figures; those followed by *t* indicate tables.

Beyond the Law
Crime in Complex Organizations

Beyond the Law
Crime in Complex Organizations

Edited by
Michael Tonry and
Albert J. Reiss, Jr.

Crime and Justice
A Review of Research
Edited by Michael Tonry
with the Support of The National Institute of Justice

VOLUME 18

The University of Chicago Press, Chicago and London

This volume was prepared under Grant Number 90-IJ-CX-0016 awarded to the Castine Research Corporation by the National Institute of Justice, U.S. Department of Justice, under the Omnibus Crime Control and Safe Streets Act of 1968 as amended. Points of view or opinions expressed in this volume are those of the editors or authors and do not necessarily represent the official position or policies of the U.S. Department of Justice.

The University of Chicago Press, Chicago 60637
The University of Chicago Press, Ltd., London

ISSN: 0192-3234

ISBN: 0-226-80821-1 (cloth)
98 97 96 95 94 93   5 4 3 2 1

ISBN: 0-226-80823-8 (paper)
98 97 96 95 94 93   5 4 3 2 1

LCN: 80-642217

Library of Congress Cataloging-in-Publication Data

Beyond the law: Crime in complex organizations / edited by Michael Tonry and Albert J. Reiss, Jr.
     p.   cm.—(Crime and justice, ISSN 0192-3234 ; v. 18)
   Includes bibliographical references.
   ISBN 0-226-80821-1 (cl.: alk. paper).—ISBN 0-226-80823-8
   (paper: alk.   paper)
     1. Corporations—Corrupt practices—United States.   2. Commercial crimes—United States.   3. White-collar crimes—United States.
   I. Tonry, Michael H.   II. Reiss, Albert J.,   III. Series: Crime and justice
   (Chicago, Ill.): v. 18.
   HV6769.B49   1993
   364.1′68′0973—dc20   93-37641
                                                                   CIP

Contents

Preface

Beyond the Law—Crime in Complex Organizations is the sixth thematic volume in the *Crime and Justice* series and, like the first, *Communities and Crime*, of which Albert J. Reiss, Jr., was also coeditor, insists on looking at crimes and criminality as more than a matter of individual variation and individuals' decisions. *Communities and Crime* focused on community crime careers and their effects on individual crime careers. This volume focuses on organizations rather than individuals as violators of law. The essays in *Beyond the Law* examine illegal behaviors by, against, within, and among organizations in specific legal, administrative, regulatory, social, and economic contexts.

The essays describe business organizations as violators of law. Yet government and not-for-profit organizations also are violators of law. Businesses are major violators of environmental pollution laws. So are the U.S. Department of Defense and other federal, state, and local government agencies. Moreover, government organizations engage in behaviors that corrupt their authority as Watergate and investigations of police corruption and misuse of authority make abundantly clear. Scandals likewise involve not-for-profit organizations, particularly in the solicitation and stewardship of voluntary contributions. Rather than choose one or two examples from each of these types of organizational violators, we decided to focus on different types of business organizations to illuminate a range of structural and organizational issues in organizational law violations.

The focus on organizational crime, even the title of this book, reflects dissatisfaction with the much more widely used term, white-collar crime. Although the classic work *White Collar Crime* by Edwin Sutherland was a study of the criminality, reflected in official case records, of corporate organizations, white-collar crime is a plastic phrase that means many things in many contexts. White-collar crime is used to refer to behaviors as different as income tax evasion (in which the common denominator is income, not the colors of collars of shirts), financial crimes including embezzlement (of which the typical offense is embezzlement of small sums by bank tellers and bookkeepers), environmental offenses (which can range from sustained multiyear industrial toxic dumping to a lawn-service operator pouring used oil in a ditch), commercial frauds (which can range from sale by a street vendor of a counterfeit Rolex to multimillion-dollar securities scams), and violations of statutes and regulations affecting the finance and securities industries. Because white-collar crime can encompass those types of crimes, and many others, we narrowed our scope to particular kinds of crimes in which existing organizations were an essential component and in which changes in those organizations, or in the environments in which they operate, can change incentives and disincentives to unlawful behavior.

Thus, this volume focuses on organizational crime, broadly defined to range from relatively small, but long-term, waste management organizations in New York and New Jersey through nursing homes to multibillion dollar savings and loans, securities firms, and industrial corporations.

Throughout the essays, one aim is to obtain a better understanding of the motives and sanctions, the incentives and disincentives, and the structural influences that shape organizational crime. Another aim is to illuminate the diverse effects of self-regulation, industry regulation, administrative regulation, and criminal law approaches to eliciting compliance with applicable laws and regulations, discouraging illegality, and discovering wrongdoing.

This volume was supported by a grant from the National Institute of Justice. We are most grateful to then-director James K. Stewart, assistant director Paul Cascarano, Mary Graham, who oversees all *Crime and Justice* undertakings supported by the National Institute of Justice, and Lois Mock, the institute's specialist on white-collar crime in all of its manifestations and particularly crime within, by, and against organizations.

Michael Tonry
Albert J. Reiss, Jr.

Albert J. Reiss, Jr., and Michael Tonry

Organizational Crime

Perhaps the most striking revolution of the twentieth century was the rapid expansion of the population of organizations. As the century draws to a close, the population of profit, not-for-profit, and governmental organizations in the United States rivals in number the population of individuals.

Both organizations and individuals may be regarded as behaving under the law. Many organizations, created by the acts of individuals, of corporate organizations, or of governments, are given a legal identity. Under the law, organizations are accorded distinct properties, such as a corporate form, a domicile, and recognition as a not-for-profit, a profit-making, or a governmental entity. Organizations can be held accountable for their behavior under the law, without any of the individuals who took actions on behalf of the organization being held legally accountable. Capital and not-for-profit organizations, for example, can be fined for violations of law—even to the point of bankruptcy. They can be placed on probation for violations of laws and be required to meet special conditions or perform community service, much as is the case for sanctioned individuals.

This volume consists of case studies of organizational violations of law. Each is limited to patterned violations of civil and criminal law and patterned evasions of administrative regulations by organizations in an organizational network. The focus is on the behavior of organizations in that network, rather than on specific individuals who commit those violations. For example, in essays on savings and loan organizations, the central focus is not on any particular organization, such as the Lincoln Savings and Loan Association, but on understanding the widespread violations within the S&L industry. We are less interested in how and why individuals committed violations than in why so many individuals in particular roles in savings and loan organizations did

1

so. Hence, our interest in people working within organizations is in understanding their conduct in the pursuit of organizational purposes or in understanding how employees in the pursuit of personal goals victimize organizations by using their resources.

Violations by and within organizations are facilitated by the behavior of other organizations in their or other networks. For example, enforcers or regulators of organizational behavior in various ways may account for the pattern of violations by organizations in the network.

To return to the S&L example, in planning this volume we were not interested specifically in Charles Keating or in, say, the five U.S. senators who became known as the "Keating Five" but in how people in a class of organizations—the savings and loan industry—came to behave as they did, and how the Keatings, the regulators, and the congressmen came to behave as they did and do. Savings and loan violations are embedded within larger environments and exchange systems, such as the structures of savings and lending, of regulation, and even of congressional campaign financing, all of which are relevant to understanding how a particular industry becomes involved in violations and how a regulatory system is compromised.

A caveat is in order, lest readers be misled into thinking that we are not interested in specific cases such as the Lincoln Savings and Loan Association debacle. We most certainly are to the degree that specific cases enliven the exposition as examples. Writers were asked to seek out telling and colorful examples.

We are interested in common-law crimes such as fraud and theft only to the degree that they are part of the patterning of violations in an organization. To return again to the S&L example, employees and contractors of many specific S&L associations appear to have committed fraud in assessing the value of property for investment and may personally have gained from doing so. We are interested in that employee behavior and its sanctioning only to the degree that it helps us to understand how the industrial and organizational structure and the structure of regulation gave rise to such behavior throughout much of the S&L system. Many of the violations, for example, may be generic common-law crimes of employee theft and fraud, but this is not another book on how white-collar persons commit such crimes.

From an organizational perspective, however, violations by a particular class of individuals—for example, the affluent or those at the top of an industry, or of the less affluent who often become involved in the commission of violations—are less important than how persons of any class may become enmeshed in the patterned violations and hence be open to individual prosecution under the criminal law, to tort liability and litigation, or to regulatory sanctions like fines, loss of licenses, or registrations.

About a decade ago Lawrence W. Sherman (1978) published a book, entitled *Scandal and Reform: Controlling Police Corruption*, that illustrates an organizational approach to unlawful behavior within organizations. His central focus was on explaining how police organizations are corrupted and why the reforms that follow are often ineffective. Although scandals in cities such as New York and Oakland, California, are used as illustrations, the central argument focuses on the fairly widespread phenomenon of department corruption. Although in the corruption scandal a substantial number of officers and employees at different levels of police departments and organized criminal activity may be processed as violators, the core of the explanation is on how and why departments become corrupted and why there are repeated failures in controlling the conduct that leads to organizational corruption.

I. Four Features of the Legal Control of Organizations

Most theories and conceptions of law violation and of victimization center on persons rather than on organizations. Most criminological theories, including subcultural, social learning, and structural opportunity theories, focus on individuals and attempt to explain their behaviors. Causal theories in criminology center on individuals making rational choices to offend or offending because of the influence of a plethora of individual or situationally induced motives. Any examination of different kinds of law violations, however, makes it clear that an emphasis solely or preponderantly on individuals can provide only an incomplete and impoverished account of crime in America.

Once the search for improved understanding of the causes of crime is widened to include organizations, four implications stand out. One is that organizations are central offenders in many violations of law. Most major violations of environmental pollution laws, for example, are committed by public and private organizations rather than by private individuals. It is organizations that must be controlled in the public interest (Yeager, in this volume). Likewise, fraudulent record keeping and billing is endemic in the American nursing home industry. To remain financially solvent, many operators bill Medicaid for services that are not rendered. Similarly, institutional neglect of the well-being of nursing home residents is more of a problem for nursing home regulation than is employee abuse of residents (Braithwaite, in this volume).

Second, organizations and collectivities of individuals (such as taxpayers, or residents of a town or neighborhood, or members of an association) are a major class of victims of crimes by individual offenders and by organizations. Vandals who destroy public property, such as parks and schools and public transportation equipment and facilities, directly victimize a corporate entity and indirectly victimize collectivities of taxpayers and users. Organizations that collude in fixing the prices of commodities or services may target organizations as well as individuals as their victims. Reuter, in this volume, shows how collusion in the cartage industry in the New York metropolitan area has for many years significantly raised the price of garbage collection for commercial establishments. Two essays on the savings and loan crisis in this volume (Pontell and Calavita; Zimring and Hawkins) focus on both the victimization of particular S&L organizations that became insolvent and on the short- and long-run victimization of American taxpayers who must absorb losses that would otherwise have fallen to individual depositors and shareholders.

Third, many individual violations of law and almost all organizational violations involve use of an organization's position of significant power, influence, or trust to commit the violation (Biderman and Reiss 1968). The insider trader who uses a position of access to information that will affect the market price of shares is an example, as is the use of appraisal, loan officer, corporate officer, and directors' positions in the savings and loan crisis.

Finally, it is evident that many violations of law are committed neither by individuals nor by organizations acting separately. Much organizational lawbreaking involves the use of the organizational power created by a network of organizations or the coercive power of a syndicated network. Recent notorious examples include allegations of price-fixing in bidding on public construction projects in many cities, allegations of nationwide collusive bidding for military and public school supply contracts by dairy products companies, and allegations of price-fixing by domestic airlines. Reuter, in this volume, shows how the coercive power of the Mafia, the network power of trade unions, and ethnic and kinship networks were fundamental to creating and maintaining segmented local markets in the early years of the cartage industry in New York, New Jersey, and elsewhere. Later those combined powers and influences were replaced by racketeering organizations that maintain discipline among the conspirators and inhibit customer complaints. Reichman's account of insider trading in this volume depicts it as enmeshed in a web of deal-making roles and relationships and describes how insider trades can be unlawfully brokered through networks of even remotely connected participants. Those who unlawfully take advantage of trading information may be far removed organizationally from its source, as when the printer of financial documents relating to an impending stock split trades on that information.

II. Five Limitations of the White-Collar Crime Literature on Organizational Wrongdoing

Since Sutherland (1945), the empirical criminological literature on white-collar crime has abounded with examples of organizations as violators. Critiques of that literature have drawn attention to five limitations that the essays in this volume seek to address through intensive case studies of industrywide violations of statutes and administrative regulations.

The first, only partly addressed, is the general neglect of organizations as victims of law violations. This subject is only partly addressed because we have not included cases of substantial victimization of organizations by common crimes—how, for example, public transportation systems bear substantial losses of revenue from fare cheating or incur substantial costs owing to vandalism. There are many other examples of how minor crimes, such as employee theft, are more costly to organizations than are felonies; a retailer that suffers "shrinkage" of 2, 4, or 10 percent of its inventory bears far greater financial burdens from shoplifting and employee theft than from store robberies. The essays in this volume focus far more on organizations as violators than as victims and on individuals as indirect victims of organizational violations rather than on organizations as direct victims. The essays on the S&L crisis are a notable exception, focusing on the victimization of S&L organizations and its consequences for depositors and taxpayers.

A second major limitation of the white-collar crime literature is the tendency to focus solely or preponderantly on large profit-making organizations and on the behavior of corporate officers and managers as major offenders; many violations by and against organizations are committed by people in lower-ranking white-collar and blue-collar positions. The corruption of authority endemic in large public police organizations in the United States, for example, normally involves the rank and file and line supervisors rather than the top command. Reuter's description of collusion in the cartage industry demonstrates how organizational offending is grounded in the behavior of many small-scale entrepreneurs in one of the most demeaned occupations—garbage and trash collection.

A third limitation has been the tendency to focus on particular named organizations and the violations of their white-collar employees rather than on how industrial and commercial organization creates and sustains particular patterns of violation. The focus should be on opportunities the legal, economic, and regulatory structure of an industry provide for patterned law-breaking by organizations. For example, an examination of the highway construction industry might concentrate on major changes in the structure of competition in the industry, in the public bidding process and its regulations, and in supervision of performance contracts awarded.

By focusing on industrial systems and the environments they create, such as the savings and loan industry, or on market organization, such as that of garbage and trash collection or stock transactions, one can better understand how particular organizations and their employees become violators as a consequence of system organization and change. The two essays on the savings and loan industry and their lending and investment practices illustrate how organizational practices come to be regarded as law violations in a turbulent business environment. In the essay on insider trading, Reichman argues that the new forms of insider trading sought to corrupt the market itself—to change its dynamic features. To understand insider trading, she locates it within the changing structures of finance. Similarly, the essays on the S&L crisis locate it within the conjunction of deregulation and the dynamic forces affecting commercial real estate and the production and marketing of commodities such as oil.

This limitation is closely related to a fourth. Typically, the control of organizational law violations is investigated by studying the behavior of enforcement or regulatory agencies and their agents and only rarely by focusing on how enforcement or regulation interacts with an environment. Braithwaite's account of nursing home regulation in this volume shows how comparative societal studies of nursing homes and their regulation enhance our understanding not only of different regulatory processes but of the ways that organizations sometimes adapt to their regulatory environments in ways that can undermine efforts to attain their own goals. He demonstrates how the U.S. regulatory inspection of nursing homes, which emphasizes maintenance of paper records of staff and organizational compliance with rules and regulations, leads to organizations that are more concerned with ritualistic bureaucratic compliance than with the quality of the care they provide. In contrast, the more goal-directed regulatory regime in Australia generates small nursing homes focused on giving personal rather than institutional centered care. He concludes, moreover, that empowerment of staff and residents through local accountability and advocacy provides more humane care than does the more bureaucratized American approach. Such studies accordingly approach the problem of controlling organizational behavior in conformity with law as one of mutual adaptations of regulators and regulated.

Finally, there is a tendency to treat violations of administrative law as violations of criminal law. Although individual contributors to this volume have not always maintained a distinction between the two, in part because willful, persistent, or extreme violations of administrative regulations can constitute criminal offenses, many violations of law involve administrative regulations and are subject to administrative rather than criminal law proceedings. The failure to distinguish these two bodies of public law usually carries over into treating all organizational violators as white-collar criminals and all organizational violations as white-collar crimes.

This conflation of criminal and administrative law has some major consequences for consideration of strategies of social control over organizational behavior (Reiss 1984). Regulatory agencies are primarily intent on inducing *compliance* with the law—to prevent the violation of law. Criminal law systems, by contrast, are organized on *deterrence* principles—the detection of violations and punishment of violators to deter future violations. Because compliance systems are oriented toward prevention, they are *premonitory*. They attend to conditions that increase the risk of violation and seek to have the organization alter those conditions so as to increase the likelihood of conformity with the law. Because law enforcement systems seek to prevent future violations by punishing violators, they are oriented toward detecting violations, apprehending and charging violators, and imposing penalties that will deter the violators or others from violating. While each system seeks to prevent violations, they do so by quite different means.

Although penalties can be invoked in either compliance or deterrence systems, they are integral only to deterrence systems. Deterrence systems assume that penalties have a causal effect in preventing future violations. In compliance systems, the emphasis is on rewarding compliance or withholding the potential imposition of penalties to induce compliance. In compliance systems, penalties are principally used as threats rather than as sanctions. Typically, sanctions are suspended or withdrawn when acceptable compliance is demonstrated.

Some of the essays in this volume illuminate these contrasts between the two systems. Braithwaite's essay on nursing home regulation shows how inspections can be used to induce compliance rather than to punish violators. Yeager's essay on water pollution likewise demonstrates that compliance is a *process* rather than an end state and details the gradual evolution of a compliance system to control water pollution.

III. Controlling the Behavior of Organizations

A central problem of modern societies is to control the behavior of organizations in the public interest. There are several principal ways of doing so.

One is to rely on governments to make laws and rules governing the behavior of organizations and to establish techniques for their enforcement or compliance with them. Our civil, criminal, and administrative law systems are the foundation of legal control of organizational behavior. Public prosecution, civil litigation, and regulatory actions are their hallmarks.

Another is to trust that market mechanisms can control organizational behavior. Markets usually operate in conjunction with some form of formal or informal regulatory system. A presumption of formal deregulation is that an open or free market controls behavior in the public interest. The two essays on the crisis in the saving and loan industry examine from different perspectives the ways in which deregulation contributed to that crisis. Pontell and Calavita attribute the S&L crisis to the conjunction of thrift deregulation with federal insurance on deposits, which created a "criminogenic environment" that provided extensive opportunities for fraud at minimal risk to managers and attracted dishonest entrepreneurs to the industry. Zimring and Hawkins, by contrast, advance a more structuralist explanation. The structure of incentives produced by deregulation was a major explanation for the behavior that resulted in record losses. The symbolic politics of deregulation rather than technical market economics drove the deregulation of thrift institutions to their debacle.

Market mechanisms of control are more or less indifferent to the legality of commodities or services, however, and competition may be restricted by illegal means such as coercive violence, as well as by legal means. What is commonly called "organized crime" is a form of control imposed on the marketing of illegal commodities or services or the use of illegal means to control transactions in legal commodities. The essay on garbage collection by Reuter documents how the marketing of a legal commodity—garbage—in the New York metropolitan area has been dominated by a private cartage industry that operates in restraint of trade through customer allocation agreements that treat customers as assets. He shows that both law enforcement and regulation have failed to eliminate these agreements and, indeed, that they have achieved a more legal form, thereby enhancing the power of racketeers.

A third way to control the behavior of organizations in the public interest is to depend on aggrieved parties—typically private organizations or individuals—to exercise control over organizations through civil suits for compensatory or punitive damages. This form of control is limited, however, by the extent to which liabilities are insured as well as by the extent and liquidity of organizational assets. Federal insurance on thrift deposits effectively obviated the need for civil litigation for recovery of deposits in S&L institutions and may even have encouraged imprudent lending, as Pontell and Calavita argue. Severe declines in the market value of housing, offices, and retail buildings, moreover, limited the government's potential recovery of loss as an insurer.

Braithwaite points to other private alternatives—the use of advocacy groups to represent client interests in nursing homes, the empowerment of staff vis-à-vis the power exercised by management, and self-regulation. Self-regulation exists when collectivities of self-interested organizations develop or adopt norms of behavior and ways to get members to conform with them. It often is adjunctive to control exercised by regulatory agencies. Reichman in her essay on insider trading points out that the National Association of Securities Dealers (NASD) provides adjunctive support to Securities and Exchange Commission (SEC) rules governing conflicts of interest in multiservice securities firms. The erection of so-called Chinese Walls within a firm— invisible procedural barriers that separate conflicts of interest within the firm—is a recommended procedure by both NASD and the SEC. Braithwaite's essay on nursing homes emphasizes that the homes with the lowest rates of violations have a participatory regulatory structure rather than a strictly hierarchical management structure.

The thematic volumes in the *Crime and Justice* series are testament to the need and the difficulties for multidisciplinary research and theory that transcends the balkanizing partitions that divide academic disciplines. Too often, scholars and policy analysts from different specialties look at different aspects of a large and complex problem. The cumulative result too often resembles the portrayal of an elephant as a horse built by a committee. Criminologists interested in organizational crime have tended to adhere to the white-collar-crime emphases described earlier and too seldom have learned from sociologists of organization and bureaucracy, from economists and organizational theorists, and from legal and regulatory literatures. Each of these in turn generally fails to benefit from each others' learning and from the criminologists. In commissioning the essays in this volume, we asked writers to reach beyond their disciplinary grasps, and all have done so.

We hope these essays demonstrate that the understanding of organizational law violations is enhanced by bringing an organizational and social system analysis to the study of the behavior of organizations rather than relying principally on the traditional criminological analyses of white-collar and organized crimes and criminals. That understanding is enhanced also by expanding the horizons beyond the scope of the criminal law and criminal justice to include administrative law and legal regulation. These shifts in emphasis may open the way to better control of law violations through both organizational compliance and deterrence strategies.

REFERENCES

Biderman, Albert D., and Albert J. Reiss, Jr. 1968. "On Exploring the 'Dark Figure' of Crime." *Annals of the American Academy of Political and Social Science* 374:1–15.

Reiss, Albert J., Jr. 1984. "Selecting Strategies of Social Control over Organizational Life." In *Enforcing Regulation*, edited by K. Hawkins and J. M. Thomas. Boston: Kluwer-Nijhoff.

Sherman, Lawrence W. 1978. *Scandal and Reform: Controlling Police Corruption*. Berkeley: University of California Press.

Sutherland, Edwin H. 1945. "Is 'White-Collar Crime' Crime?" *American Sociological Review* 10:132–39.

John Braithwaite

The Nursing Home Industry

ABSTRACT

Nursing home regulation in most U.S. states is oriented more to
compliance than to deterrent strategies. Voluntary compliance is
surprisingly high. The major problem is not resistance to state commands
but what Merton called ritualism—going along with institutionalized
means for achieving regulatory goals while not attaining the goals
themselves. The nature of state regulation has driven the American
industry away from informal, intimate caring toward institutionalized care
in larger nursing homes and toward the ascendancy of large corporate
chains. These trends lead to the extraordinary disciplinary quality of U.S.
nursing homes. Practices are regimented and documented from
above—the federal government disciplines the states, state supervisors
discipline inspectors, inspectors discipline nursing home operators,
operators discipline nursing home staff, and staff discipline residents.
Achieving quality of life and quality of care for residents requires
substantial abandonment of this hierarchy of discipline in favor of local
debate about outcomes in which residents and their advocates are
empowered.

This essay is based on data from an international comparative study
of nursing home regulation in the United States, England, Japan, and
Australia. At the time of writing, only the U.S. fieldwork is complete
and analyzed. Hence, the situation in the United States is dealt with

John Braithwaite is professor at the Australian National University, Research School
of Social Sciences. This project has been supported by the Australian Department of
Housing, Health and Community Services, the Australian Research Council, the American Bar Foundation, and the Australian National University. I am indebted to my
colleagues Valerie Braithwaite, David Ermann, Diane Gibson, Miriam Landau, and
Toni Makkai for their support.

11

systematically, though frequent comparisons are made to the situations in other nations.

In investigating regulation of the nursing home industry in the United States, my colleagues and I in Australia first worked to understand the enforcement and regulatory system, which is largely a state government responsibility. Then we pursued greater depth of understanding in one locale—the city of Chicago. To accomplish a general understanding of the system, we sought to interview the key regulatory players in half the states and to observe at least one nursing home inspection in each state. Only one state government, Pennsylvania, refused to cooperate with the study. A letter of introduction from the Australian minister for aged care was effective in securing cooperation from the others.

In all twenty-four states where cooperation was secured, we observed at least one nursing home inspection, totaling forty-four inspections overall. Unstructured interviews were conducted at all levels of the state regulatory agency or agencies—inspectors, middle management, and senior management. In all states, at least some of the specialist staff were also interviewed—complaints officers, ombudsmen, lawyers, or criminal investigators. In addition to observing meetings of inspectors at the nursing homes, we sat in on some tactics meetings with more senior staff in head offices and some meetings that decide or review the imposition of penalties on nursing homes. In most states, we interviewed representatives of industry associations and consumer organizations. At the national level, we met with the influential industry, professional, and consumer groups in Washington and with the Health Care Financing Administration (HCFA) in Baltimore. Most of the key regulatory players nationally and in the twenty-four states were included among more than three hundred people whom we interviewed for the study. I conducted most of the U.S. fieldwork, the remainder being undertaken by my colleagues Valerie Braithwaite, David Ermann, and Diane Gibson, whose assistance I gratefully acknowledge. Fieldwork was conducted during six visits to the United States, which totaled fifteen months between 1987 and 1991.

The states were selected purposively rather than randomly. First, the twenty states with the largest numbers of nursing home beds were selected. These accounted for three-quarters of the nursing home beds in the country. Second, five smaller states were selected because these were states where we were advised that distinctive regulatory strategies were being adopted. For example, Rhode Island was selected because it had the most frequent nursing home inspections (state law mandates at least six inspections per year). The states visited were California, Washington, Arizona, Colorado, Oklahoma, Missouri, Indiana, Illinois, Wisconsin, Michigan, Ohio, Massachusetts, Rhode Island, Connecticut, New York, New Jersey, Maryland, Virginia, North Carolina, Florida, Texas, Tennessee, Georgia, and Louisiana.

In Chicago, it was possible to range more widely in choosing what kinds of actors to interview (e.g., to interview private attorneys who represent nursing homes, to observe ombudsmen and inspectors from other agencies doing their job) and more systematically to observe the regulatory process. All but one of the twenty-two state nursing home inspectors working in the city of Chicago (in 1988) were observed doing their job, most of them many times during the eighteen inspections that were observed. These were all the inspections that occurred in the city during a three-week period in 1988, a one-week period in 1989, and a one-week period in 1990.[1] Because we returned to Chicago for each of our six fieldwork visits, we were able to interview the same actors many times during the five years of fieldwork. In Chicago, we also spent a lot of time observing self-regulatory processes in nursing homes—staff meetings where regulatory issues were discussed, care planning conferences, and meetings of quality assurance committees.

Here is how this essay is organized. Section I describes the nature of law violations in the nursing home industry. How the industry came to acquire its present structure and the regulatory framework is discussed in Sections II and III. Sections IV and V, respectively, examine governmental and self-regulatory strategies used to secure compliance. Section VI gives an account of the structure and culture of nursing homes that sees them as profoundly shaped by regulatory structure and culture.

I. The Nature of Law Violations in the Nursing Home Industry

The focus in this section is on violations of regulatory standards by nursing homes—including building and fire safety standards, but mostly quality-of-care standards. Financial fraud is also a major prob-

---

[1] This meant they were not inspections that were especially selected for us, which was the case with some of the inspections we attended in the other states. But even with our visits to most states, there was little choice involved, as we generally attended whatever inspection happened to be on at the time within reasonable proximity to where we were doing our interviews.

lem in the nursing home industry. The Medicaid program is an easy target for unscrupulous nursing home operators, many of whom get most of their income from these programs (Vladeck 1980, pp. 174–91). Claims are frequently made for the care of residents who have been discharged permanently or temporarily to the care of relatives. Claims are made in higher categories of dependency than apply to the resident concerned. Claims are made for ghost staff. Since our fieldwork involved quality-of-care rather than financial inspectors, fraud is not a major focus in this essay. It is worth pointing out, however, that some of the homes we saw that were infamous for poor quality care were also infamous for welfare fraud. One reason for this is that similar types of rationalizations or techniques of neutralization are used to justify both types of offending. As the deputy director of one state department of social services put it, "They say 'The reason we can't meet the standards is that you're not giving us enough money.'" Because of the professional acceptability of fraud that is seen as necessary to "stand by [their] patients," many in the industry were surprisingly open about admitting it. Even the head of one state nursing home regulatory agency said, "When I worked in the industry I tried to keep reimbursement up by keeping records of people being on services they didn't need."

Some nursing homes owned by organized crime are regarded by regulators as less than exemplary on both quality of care and fraud. This, however, could be a stereotypical reaction fostered by disconcerting practices such as putting a gun on the table for the duration of the regulatory negotiation at an exit conference.

Nursing homes also sometimes conspire with residents to conceal assets so that they satisfy the eligibility threshold for Medicaid benefits. Fraud against Medicaid by residents and their families shuffling assets is pandemic in the United States. The temptation is huge because even well-to-do middle class people are sure to be rendered indigent by an extended period of nursing home care. In this sense, the United States does not have a social security system; it has a social insecurity system. For anyone concerned that infirmity or accident will cause a need for long-term care (as opposed to acute care, which is covered by Medicare), there are only two paths to social security in the United States: being wealthy or being dishonest.[2] As the nation ages, this simple

---

[2] If you are very wealthy, you can afford to pay thousands of dollars for every month you spend in a nursing home. If you are moderately wealthy, you can afford expensive long-term care insurance to cover you against such a catastrophe.

structural reality of public policy is making the United States more and more a nation of crooks. In nations like Australia that have universal nursing home benefit systems, this type of fraud does not exist at all.

There is also fraud connected with quality-of-care regulation. We observed the detection of falsification of medical and other records at many nursing homes. In one case, for example, the falsification of minutes of an "infection control committee" (required by law) was detected by reference in the minutes to a man who had died a year before the meeting supposedly took place. This type of fraud is never, in our experience, punished under the criminal law of fraud. In the case just described, the nursing home was cited for failing to convene a meeting of the infection control committee, and no action was taken against the nurse manager who committed the fraud. One experienced criminal investigator with a state regulatory agency saw the connection between criminal neglect of residents and fraud as an iron law: "If it's a neglect case that rises to the standard of criminality under American law that crosses that line, you will find falsified records."

Besides fraud, the other problem that is clearly worse in the United States than in Australia (and other countries as well, we suspect) is abuse. We cannot prove this with systematic, comparable statistics on abuse, nor can we report that we have directly observed much violence against residents during our American fieldwork (apart from many shocking cases of physical and chemical restraint). Even so, we believe that there is a sharp contrast to report here.

The basis for our claim of a huge difference between Australia and the United States is our interviews with inspectors and complaints coordinators. Ask the complaints coordinator in an Australian state to tell you the worst abuse case they have known in the past year and most tell a story of a nasty shoving or bruising incident. To the follow-up question: "Haven't you had a worse case than that? What about someone punching or slapping a resident?" some answer "No we haven't had a complaint like that since I started in the job." Ask the same question of people in a comparable position in the United States, and they often tell a story of the murder of a nursing home resident by a staff member. In one state, the story was even of the murder of five residents by two staff members in a single nursing home. Moreover, the details of the American stories are comparatively horrific. They will tell of a male resident having his penis severed with a razor blade (a story that actually recurred in two different times and places).

They will tell a story of rape of an elderly woman or of stuffing a washcloth with feces on it in the mouth of a ninety-year-old woman on two separate occasions.[3] In the United States there seems to be more of a problem of pathological individuals moving from job to job in the nursing home industry so they can prey on vulnerable people. Ask the complaints coordinator of an American state nursing home regulatory agency how many confirmed abusers she knows of, and in a number of states the answer is that she has a list of more than fifty people, or even over a hundred, who are on her blacklist of abusers. Most or all of these will have been referred for criminal investigation to a local or state prosecution office. Most Australian counterparts have no cases that have been referred for criminal investigation and only a few cases "that I have concerns about" where informal warnings have been given to nursing homes contemplating employment of these people. Partly, we think that this difference is because Australian authorities are much less vigilant and systematic in their attention to the problem of nursing home abuse than they should be. Equally, we think it is because the problem of abuse is much less in Australia than in the United States. In the United States, 197 individuals were convicted criminally in 1989 for abuse of nursing home residents; there have been no such criminal cases in Australia during the five years of our study.

Physical restraint of residents is a form of abuse that can be shown statistically to be much worse in the United States than in other nations. Judging by the number of residents we observed with symptoms of long-term psychotropic drug use (e.g., repeated blinking or facial movements and protruding tongue), we suspect the same is true of chemical restraint, but there is no credible, systematic way of confirming that this impression is correct because of the lack of credible surveys in Australia.[4] Only in the last few years has widespread use of restraint ceased being a professionally and legally sanctioned way to deal with management problems in American nursing homes. In 1988, 41 percent of nursing home residents were subject to daily physical restraint—mostly tie restraints around the lap.[5] Unknown numbers of

[3] The latter case was the subject of a criminal conviction in Jefferson County Court, New York, on October 28, 1987. See the National Association of Attorneys General (1987), p. 23.

[4] Also see n. 15 below.

[5] Figures are supplied by the Health Care Financing Administration from annual surveys (see also United States Senate, Special Committee on Aging 1990, p. III: "an estimated 50 percent of all nursing home residents are restrained in some form").

further residents were subject to chemical restraint and lesser forms of physical restraint such as the routine use of bedrails to restrict freedom of movement at night. In Australia, too, there is excessive use of restraint, but in no Australian nursing home have we seen a level of physical restraint approaching the average level for U.S. nursing homes (and we have visited one-third of the 1,400 nursing homes in Australia during the course of our study).

The contrast with Britain is even more striking. In the fifty homes we visited during our English fieldwork, we did not notice a single tie restraint. An English inspector who has twenty or thirty nursing homes on her beat can often name the one or two residents who are physically restrained in her nursing homes, so rare is physical restraint. Caring for the frail elderly is no simple challenge; fragility and proneness to broken bones cannot be dismissed. But the evidence of British restraint practices and the growing number of restraint-free homes in the United States are powerful testimony that for every problem there is almost always a better way to solve it than tying people down.

The foregoing comments should not be interpreted as an attempt to show that in all ways American nursing homes are worse places than nursing homes in other countries. American nursing homes have higher fire safety standards than Australian nursing homes, better food and nutrition standards than English nursing homes, better trained administrators, better care planning, and more varied activities programs than in both these other nations. Nor should my comments later on the deficiencies of the U.S. regulatory process be read to mean that the U.S. process is necessarily inferior: in some important respects it is superior to those in England and Australia. My purpose here, however, is not to give a balanced international comparison of nursing home standards, it is to identify law-breaking and regulatory problems that are particularly acute in U.S. nursing homes.

In all countries, including the United States, the most serious problems of law-breaking in nursing homes are neither fraud nor abuse, but neglect. The suffering of residents left in their own feces, sometimes with massive bedsores, sometimes with bodies infested with maggots, is suffering hard to imagine for those who have not seen it, hard to forget for those who have. The nonphysical suffering of bedfast or chairfast residents who spend years in one spot without adequate mental or physical stimulation is also terrible and is getting worse as lives are further extended in a medicalized care system. That it is against the law for residents to be denied the opportunity for the stimulation, activities, and conversation they need to be human does not change the reality of widespread denial of such opportunities.

Those of us lucky enough to live into our eighties will likely have a direct personal interest in ensuring that these regulatory challenges are met. By the end of this essay, I hope to cast some light on how this might be achieved. First, however, I set the scene by briefly telling the story of how the nursing home industry came to be the way it is.

II. The Structure of the Industry

The nursing home industry is a twentieth-century phenomenon. The predominantly private nursing home industry that we see in the United States today is a late twentieth-century phenomenon. The industry is a product of increased life expectancy. However, it is also a result of increasing geographical mobility, the changing nature of the extended family, and changing patterns of care. In the nineteenth century, the aged infirm were cared for at home, though poor laws introduced throughout the Western world saw expanded opportunities for institutional care for the indigent aged without family. Nineteenth-century poorhouses accommodated the aged infirm together with a motley collection of younger persons requiring institutional support, a situation that continued through the 1930s. The expansion of mental hospitals also increasingly picked up the aged infirm. By 1930, there were more people over sixty-five in mental hospitals than in almshouses and private nursing homes combined (Vladeck 1980, p. 35).

The first half of the twentieth century saw considerable growth in specialist charitable (mainly church) and governmental institutions for the aged. These dominated the nursing home scene until after World War II, when a rapid proliferation of private nursing homes occurred. The turning point was the Johnson administration's introduction of Medicare and Medicaid in 1965, which provided government benefits for those who needed nursing home care and could not afford it. In 1954, there were fewer than 250,000 nursing home beds in the United States, but around 1970 it passed the one million mark (Vladeck 1980, p. 103). For elderly people who do not require continuous nursing care, there has also been an expanding continuum of care—from home nursing to retirement villages to board and care homes that approach the level of care in nursing homes.

Medicaid is not the only way in which the state shaped the structure of the industry. Other essays in this volume have many interesting things to say about the way the structure of an industry shapes the nature of law enforcement and law violation within it. The more interesting phenomenon with the nursing home industry is the way that law enforcement has shaped the structure of the industry. Today in the United States, the conventional economic wisdom of the industry is that a nursing home with fewer than eighty beds is of suboptimal size; the result is that most nursing home residents live in institutions of more than one hundred beds. In Australia, the median number of beds for nongovernment nursing homes is thirty-eight; in England and many European countries, smaller still. The reason a thirty-bed nursing home is economically viable in Australia but not in the United States is to be found in the nature of the regulatory system.

The structure of the industry in the United States once was rather more like that in Australia or England. In upstate New York, for example, the average number of beds in private nursing homes in 1949 was fourteen, increasing to twenty-four by 1958 and thirty-four by 1964 (Thomas 1969, p. 157). Data supplied to us by the Rhode Island Department of Human Services shows how this trend continued—with the average size of nursing homes increasing from thirty-two beds in 1972 to seventy-three by 1978. We get a clue to how this happened by noticing that the number of nursing homes in Rhode Island dropped during the same period from 180 to 110. Continuing a trend that started earlier, how much earlier varying from state to state, a combination of tougher regulatory standards and economies of scale began to close down the smallest nursing homes. Fire safety standards were preeminently important here. The trend started in 1971 in Rhode Island when eighteen homes that failed to meet the "life safety code" were closed. The "mom-and-pop" nursing home run by a family in a large converted house that had been the backbone of the industry during the 1950s rarely survived the 1970s. Larger purpose-built homes were the way to meet tougher fire safety standards. This development was not without paradox. More than anything, what fire safety standards do is ensure design principles that will contain fires within limited sections of large buildings. This way, say, only twenty beds will be exposed to fire instead of the 140 beds in an entire facility—an ironic accomplishment since a major effect of modern fire safety standards has been the abandonment of stand-alone twenty-bed facilities.

While fire safety standards were the most important regulatory factor in rendering the "mom-and-pop" nursing home uneconomic, they were not the only one. The United States has higher regulatory standards than other countries requiring access of nursing home residents to specialist professionals such as social workers, physical therapists, consultant pharmacists, and dieticians. Small nursing homes are not required to have a full-time dietician, but they must at least have a part-time dietary consultant working with the cook.[6] Specialist overheads such as these are more easily borne by nursing homes with a large income base than by smaller homes that pay the same overhead from a smaller income. Australian nursing homes, because they are not required to have these specialist overheads, can be cost-efficient with fewer beds than in the United States. American law imposes much more detailed documentation requirements for residents than does Australian law: again there are economies of scale in setting up the information systems required by the regulators.

Regulation is even more directly implicated in the smaller average size of nursing homes in England. Most English health authorities believe that smaller nursing homes provide better quality care than do larger, more institutional facilities. Consequently, they are extremely reluctant to issue a licence to any facility that approaches the size of the average American nursing home. They almost certainly have no legal authority to refuse licences to larger nursing homes, but they do it anyhow.

American regulation created conditions in which approved beds (for which the state had issued a certificate of need) were available for sale by the "mom-and-pop" nursing home to large corporate owners that built chains of nursing homes with standard designs of economically optimal size. By the mid-1980s there were some fifteen thousand nursing homes in the United States, a thousand of them owned by the largest chain, Beverly Enterprises.

But as the chains were built on the ashes of an old industry razed by a new regulatory order, so some of the chains have been threatened by a second wave of regulatory change that has been under way for the past five years. This is particularly true of the largest, Beverly Enterprises. Nursing homes owned by some of the largest chains became dispiriting places—regimented, standardized, institutionalized, relying heavily on restraint to maintain order, and devoid of a warm, homelike atmosphere. They were often excellent at getting the standardized inputs mandated in the law right—the fire rating of building materials, the minimum number of grams of protein required in the diet for each resident each day, and the charts recording the time each

---

[6] According to Vladeck (1980, p. 154), "Consultants receive exorbitant fees at public expense, essentially for filling out forms."

resident was toileted. Even on these standardized inputs, which are the forte of the chains, however, problems emerged as the chains got bigger and management control became increasingly remote from actual care giving. The largest chains had such a large span of control as to make flexible response to ever-changing care needs difficult. The chains drew on the same labor force as the fast food chains to deliver the hands-on care (often paying even less to nurses aides than McDonalds did to counter workers). But the nursing home chains found that it is easier for massive organizations to sustain high quality with hamburgers than with people who have radically different and constantly changing care needs.

The advocacy groups and regulators increasingly reached the conclusion that the chains—particularly Beverly Enterprises, which came to symbolize the new corporate care in the eyes of the critics—delivered cold and unresponsive care. Beverly was vilified by consumer groups, subjected to major law-enforcement actions in a number of states, had many of its homes closed as a result of these actions, and in some states was forbidden from operating altogether. As a result of this regulatory and consumer onslaught, Beverly suffered substantial losses in 1987, 1988, and 1989. It sold off many of its nursing homes, reduced its work force to 92,000, rethought a decentralized management system for the smaller organization, increased investment in quality assurance, and returned a modest profit in 1990.

Like the nuclear and pharmaceutical industries, regulation is so important in the nursing home industry that it has shaped the fundamental structure of the industry.

III. The Regulatory Framework

Health-care programming in the United States, including regulation, was dominated by state governments until Medicaid and Medicare emerged as federal programs in 1965. Medicaid and Medicare shifted the center of decision making about funding and standard setting to the federal government, but responsibility for program delivery and regulatory implementation remained with the states. Today, the U.S. Congress enacts the most important nursing home regulatory laws and these are fleshed out into regulations by the HCFA. The standards cover health-care quality, activities, resident rights to privacy, information, personal possessions and control of patients' financial affairs, dietary standards, pharmaceutical services, physical environment, infection control, and disaster preparedness, among other issues of vital concern to the quality of life of institutionalized people. These standards are then monitored and enforced primarily by state governments. The HCFA runs "look-behind" inspections to check that the state governments are doing their jobs and takes its own enforcement actions on problems it discovers.

In addition to enforcing federal laws that are conditions of participation in Medicaid and Medicare, state governments have their own additional standards that are conditions of state licensure. The latter are the only standards that apply to facilities that choose not to participate in Medicare and Medicaid (i.e., nursing homes catering exclusively for better-off private pay residents). State surveyors (inspectors) have the awesome task of assessing compliance with some five hundred federal standards, plus in some cases hundreds of additional state regulations. Some cities and counties also have nursing home inspectors, as does the federal Veterans Administration. During our fieldwork there were many occasions when, on entering a nursing home with one agency, we encountered an inspector from another government agency in the facility.

For all this, the main game is the work of the state Medicaid and licensure surveyors, and it is on their work that I concentrate, contrasting them with other government inspectorates where appropriate. Federal law requires annual surveys for nursing homes participating in Medicaid. Some state laws require more frequent visitation. Unlike the situation in many regulatory settings in which an inspection policy of annual visits is rarely achieved, in practice the annual visitation cycle in the United States is virtually universally achieved. This is a consequence of the regulation of the state regulators by the HCFA, which cuts off funds for nursing homes that are not certified in time, with the state government in effect then having to find those funds.

Not only is the consistent frequency of inspection much more impressive than in other areas of regulation, the intensity of the scrutiny is far more fine-grained than for occupational health and safety, environmental, food, or pharmaceuticals inspectors in any country we know. Typically, a team of at least three and often five or six inspectors will spend three days or more at a facility. A 1990 HCFA survey found that the average inspector-hours on site was 156, but to this must be added time paid for by the state to survey additional state requirements. Where there have been serious problems in large facilities, we are aware of cases where as many as ten inspectors have been camped in the nursing home for two weeks.

The inspection (or survey as the federal government calls it) begins with an initial tour of the facility and then selection of a sample of residents who are interviewed and whose charts are audited for evidence of compliance with the standards. Most surveyor time is spent on the checking of charts. But in addition, there is a physical inspection of the building, observation of treatments, calculation of an error rate for the administration of medications, observation of the cooking, distribution and eating of meals, interviewing of staff, checking nursing home policies, and a meeting with the residents' council. At the conclusion of the survey, an exit conference is held at which nursing home management, and often a representative of the residents' council, are informed of the results of the survey. Some preliminary discussion of what sort of plan of correction will be required may occur at the exit conference.

In all states, over 90 percent of failures to meet standards are dealt with by lodging a satisfactory plan of correction without any law-enforcement action being taken. Formal enforcement action occurs only where there is a very serious initial offense or where there is repeated failure to correct a violation. In the situation of a serious initial offense, administrative penalties have become an increasingly popular sanction. For example, an error rate for the administration of medications over 5 percent in some states results in an immediate administrative penalty of some hundreds of dollars. Most states have had administrative penalties available as a sanction for some years, and recent amendments to federal law have given all state regulators access to them. In 1989, almost all states actually imposed administrative penalties on fewer than a hundred occasions, though California imposed 1,800 and Texas 1,700 administrative penalties (Gardiner and Malec 1989, pp. 7–8). Some of the states that make heavy use of administrative penalties—such as California and Wisconsin—did not use the next most popular sanction, suspending new admissions (Gardiner and Malec 1989, pp. 8–9). Almost all states have this sanction available in their law, and most of them use it. It is a sanction that is generally more damaging to nursing homes than relatively low administrative penalties. In addition to the greater financial cost of reduced income, there is the adverse publicity from having to advise residents that they cannot be admitted to empty beds in the facility because of an enforcement action. New Jersey used this sanction on more than 130 occasions in 1989, Texas on 218 occasions (Gardiner and Malec 1989, pp. 8–9). Most states have had for some years the capacity to appoint a receiver to run a noncompliant nursing home or designate a monitor paid for by the nursing home to report back to the regulators on progress. Few states that use these remedies do so more than once or twice a year, with the notable exceptions of comparatively frequent use of monitors in Illinois and Indiana.

The ultimate sanction in all states is license revocation—corporate capital punishment. In most years in most states it is never used for fear of what will become of residents after a home is closed. Only thirteen states used the sanction in 1989 (with three states also suspending licenses rather than revoking them). Georgia revoked ten licenses, with Kansas, New Jersey, and Illinois each revoking eight (Gardiner and Malec 1989, pp. 11–12). For most nursing homes, Medicaid decertification is as clearly a death sentence as license revocation since most nursing homes cannot survive without the majority of their residents being supported by Medicaid. There were twenty-five Medicaid decertifications in Massachusetts in 1989, thirty-seven in Texas, and fourteen in Oregon. Overall, fifty-three nursing homes in the United States had their licenses revoked in 1989, but 130 were decertified for receiving Medicaid benefits (Gardiner and Malec 1989, p. 15). It is extremely rare in all states for criminal penalties to be imposed on nursing home organizations for breaches of quality-of-care standards, and in most states organizational criminal penalties are never used. Celebrated homicide prosecutions for neglect of residents in nursing homes have failed in the courts (Schudson, Onellion, and Hochstedler 1984; Pray 1986; Long 1987). Almost all states, however, refer charges against individuals who abuse residents for criminal investigation by state prosecutors.

Some states initiate large numbers of enforcement actions that they never formally implement because they reach settlement agreements with the nursing home. States that do this routinely, such as Massachusetts at the time of our fieldwork in 1988, appear on paper to have a worse enforcement record than in fact they have. Consent agreements sometimes contain onerous provisions, such as California's 1986 agreement that Beverly Enterprises pay a fine of $800,000 and set up a substantial quality control program.

An extensive critical literature exists attacking the weakness of American nursing home enforcement (Brown 1975; Butler 1979; Blum and Wadleigh 1983; Johnson 1985; Institute of Medicine 1986; General Accounting Office 1987; Long 1987). Yet the United States has tougher nursing home enforcement than any country we know; stronger than in

Australia, and much stronger than in England or Japan. The literature attacking regulators for enforcement weakness may be one of the factors that has caused American regulation to get tougher and that continues to keep the pressure on regulators to persist with toughness. Yet armchair scholarly commentators read these critical literatures as evidence that enforcement is weak. The truth of the matter is that it is precisely in regulatory domains that lack such critical literatures (e.g., nursing home regulation in the United States during the twenty years after World War II or nursing home regulation in Japan) that we are most likely to find weak enforcement. Armchair commentators on an industry who seek truth in the weight of popular critiques, rather than through systematic empirical comparison, may obscure the truth. Yet at the same time they may play a significant role in reinforcing social constructions of an industry that lead to change. The social construction, "American nursing home enforcement is weak," is shown to have a rather limited truth claim when one asks, "Weaker than what?" It turns out that it is tougher than at any other point in American history, tougher than nursing home regulation in the rest of the world, and much tougher than most other domains of business regulation in America. Yet scholarly acceptance of the social construction reinforces it, even legitimates it to the point where opinion leaders in the community, some regulators themselves, and many legislators come to accept this social construction as fact. When this happens, the widespread perception of regulatory weakness will cause a response that is likely to deliver tougher regulation.

Unfortunately then, criminological constructions of enforcement weakness that are not grounded in fieldwork with the industry risk subscribing to the received wisdom of popular critique in a way that conceals more truth than it reveals. Indeed the scholarly construction may be subservient to a transformative political campaign that causes the scholarly construction to become just the opposite of the truth. In the worst (yet perhaps common) case, criminologists read the popular critiques of enforcement failure as the raw data for their own construction of the world *after* those critiques have already done their work in changing the world (see fig. 1).

In the most implausible of political contexts, such as the period of the deregulation-oriented Reagan administration, one can find evidence of popular critiques of regulatory failure effecting change. The scholarly construction of the Reagan era as a period of deregulation is also false. It was certainly a period of deregulatory rhetoric by the govern-

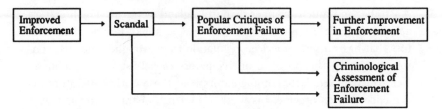

FIG. 1.—Lagged criminological assessments

ing administration, combined with denunciation of the seeming fact of deregulation by critics of the administration. In practice, it was a period of regulatory flux during which substantial shifts in both deregulatory and proregulatory directions occurred (Ayres and Braithwaite 1992, pp. 7–12). One reason why this turned out not to be an era of deregulation is that the denunciation of the social construction of the "era of deregulation" produced a lot of regulatory growth.

That this occurred with the backlash against the first Reagan administration's environmental policies is now fairly widely accepted. Nursing home regulation is a less well-known case study. When Reagan first came to power, there was a failed attempt to replace government inspection of nursing homes with a self-regulatory scheme administered by the Joint Commission on the Accreditation of Hospitals (Jost 1983, 1988). When political opposition foiled this reform, there were substantial cuts to federally funded health facility inspection personnel (mostly nursing home inspectors) from 2,400 to 1,800 in 1982. In this latter sense, there was a factual basis initially in conceiving of this as a period of deregulation. However, the reaction against it was sustained and effective by consumer groups, by the courts and members of Congress who supported consumer groups, and by supporters of strong regulation within the health care professions and state and federal bureaucracies.[7] While the turnaround in nursing home regulation by the end of the Reagan administration was not as visible as enforcement growth on Wall Street, where handcuffs were being slapped on the rich and famous, it was perhaps more fundamental in its implications for regulatory strategy. In terms of regulatory resources, the bottom

[7] In the courts, the most important case was *Smith v. Heckler*, 747 F.2d 583 (10th Cir. 1984), while the preeminently important legislative extension to nursing home regulation was the Omnibus Budget Reconciliation Act of 1987, Pub. L. No. 100–203, paras. 4203–13. An authoritative document by the Institute of Medicine (1986) was the most important watershed where regulatory bureaucrats, consumer advocates, and, most important, health care professionals came together to urge stronger regulations and tougher enforcement.

line of the Reagan administration was a period of unparalleled regulatory growth. The cut of federally funded health facility inspectors from 2,400 to 1,800 in 1982 was more than erased by the end of the Reagan administration, by which time there were over 4,000. There was substantial further growth under President Bush, with a 40 percent increase in inspection resources promised in the early nineties to implement reforms passed in the 1987 Omnibus Budget Reconciliation Act (OBRA). More fundamentally, during the Reagan era, the federal policy of support for a "consultative" approach to nursing home regulation was sharply reversed and replaced with a law enforcement policy.

The next section, however, shows that policy and practice are not exactly the same thing. While inspection practice has shifted from consultation toward enforcement, consultation remains a major part of the practical reality of regulation.

IV. Regulatory Strategies

Day and Klein (1987) conducted an exploratory study of nursing home regulation in New York, Virginia, and their own country, England. They concluded that, in terms of Reiss's (1984) dichotomy, New York was a case of deterrence regulation, England and Virginia of compliance regulation. Our own fieldwork generally confirms their conclusions, though we would want to advance even more strongly the qualifications they concede to the categorization of New York state as a deterrence regulator. Day and Klein (1987, p. 333) found New York program administrators to be strongly animated by the desire to prevent field staff from playing a consultancy role: "We have continuously to remind them that they shouldn't be consultants." We found this, too. But in New York and in other states that rejected the consultancy philosophy (most states were more like New York than Virginia in this regard), we found a great deal of consultancy going on in defiance of official policy.

These agencies are "street-level bureaucracies" (Lipsky 1980) where the real work is done by surveyors out in nursing homes remote from their supervisors. As noted earlier, in all states over 90 percent of detected violations are dealt with by means other than formal enforcement action (in some states over 99 percent). It is simply not an option to launch enforcement actions for a majority of detected violations. Comparatively well resourced as American nursing home inspectorates are (compared to, say, the Occupational Safety and Health Administration or foreign nursing home inspectorates), there are not, and never can be, sufficient resources to impose deterrent sanctions against a majority of infractions. So when New York is described as a deterrence regulator, something of comparative force has been said, but we are still describing a regulatory agency that gets most of its compliance by means other than deterrence.[8] Moreover, even in New York, inspectors see cooperative compliance strategies as a good way of working the cross-cutting allegiances within regulated organizations to get staff to volunteer information that might later be used in a formal enforcement action. A New York inspector commented, "How do you get staff to give you incriminating evidence? You don't get it by going in as a poker-faced regulator."[9]

The street-level bureaucrats, even in New York, tend to regard it as their job to get compliance even though deterrence will not be an option for more than 90 percent of the violations they detect. In a sense, this overstates the problem, however. Voluntary compliance, even in the comparatively adversarial, litigious New York described by Day and Klein (1987), is high. Without exception, in the forty-five jurisdictions in four countries where we did fieldwork, overwhelmingly, the most common industry response to a detected violation was to accept it and agree on a plan of correction without any threats being issued. Making threats about enforcement action is almost as rare as enforcement action itself. At the same time, making threats is hardly necessary in jurisdictions like New York that do have a demonstrated capacity to take tough enforcement action. The record speaks for itself: if the nursing home "plays the game" (an expression that recurred cross-nationally during our fieldwork) and agrees to fix the problem, the regulator is most unlikely to take enforcement action, even if the initial problem is quite serious; if the nursing home refuses to play the voluntary compliance game, it will not shake the regulator off its back so easily, and if it persists with resistance on a matter of some seriousness, enforcement action becomes likely.

[8] Even when voluntary compliance breaks down and the state of New York proceeds with a formal enforcement action, most of these are resolved at a settlement conference before the proposed penalty even goes to an administrative hearing, let alone the courts. New York is a comparatively litigious jurisdiction, but even in New York, going to court is a rare event. A number of informants also argued that there is a big difference between New York City and Upstate: "It's not for the most part a problem in getting compliance Upstate, even without regulations to cover it. They will take notice if we suggest something. But it's a different story in New York City" (Upstate New York supervisor).

[9] Australian inspectors proffer the same advice: "I try to call them [the staff] by name always to encourage familiarity. Then by the second day it's all 'Hello Mary,' and they are at ease with me and will start to tell me things about the place."

In jurisdictions that, unlike New York, lack a credible will to enforcement (e.g., Louisiana, most English health authorities) the process is still very similar in this fundamental way: most of the action is voluntary compliance without threat. Whereas in New York resistance triggers a regulatory attention cycle that may well lead to enforcement, in Louisiana or England resistance triggers a regulatory attention cycle that gives the *appearance* that it may well lead to enforcement, without the fact of enforcement. Hawkins (1984) calls the latter process "bargain and bluff." But note that "bargain and bluff" is not the standard approach of toothless nursing home regulators; the standard approach is to eschew all suggestion of threat; "bargain and bluff" only comes into play in the unusual cases where there is resistance.

Yet, in a way it is wrong to say that 90 percent of the time compliance is achieved without an invocation of deterrent threats; in these cases deterrence is either implicit and real (New York) or implicit and imaginary—based on bluff (England).[10] This is not to say that at the moment of voluntary compliance, it is fear of implied sanctions that mostly motivates the compliance. The empirical evidence suggests that this is not the main story (e.g., see Braithwaite and Makkai 1991). The capacity for deterrence is part of what lends authority to the state when it requests compliance with the law (or the doing of things that will make life better for nursing home residents even if that is not strictly required by the law). Or perhaps Durkheim (1961, p. 10) was closer to the truth on this question: "Punishment does not give discipline its authority, but it prevents discipline from losing its authority." Nursing home compliance arises more from a desire to go along with authoritative requests to comply with the law or authoritative suggestions to act in a professionally responsible way than from any rational weighing of the costs and benefits of compliance. This is why bargain and bluff, while it sometimes fails, works better than would be predicted by a rational actor model. Voluntary compliance is underwritten by deterrence, but not in a way that often leads the nursing home operator to calculate about the actual levels and probabilities of deterrent threats. Because of this, even when these actual levels and probabilities are zero, orchestration of an appearance that they are nonzero will often be enough to do the job: "This is the government talking. And ultimately they have the authority to make their demands stick

[10] Actually, in many English health authorities, bluff is replaced by a creative use of alternatives to formal punishment—like the power of adverse comment in relevant professional circles or threatening the license of a nurse to practice her profession.

when you are acting outside the law." Needless to say, however, such state authority is a fragile accomplishment and therefore hardly a basis for sound regulatory policy.

In this respect, it is New York that has the more robust and principled policy settings. The following statement by a New York inspector could never be made by an inspector from a typical English health authority: "You can maintain the same demeanor when confronted with tension and stress, when the facility gets aggressive and unpleasant. You can be friendly if they don't correct. You just pass it on. You never have to be anything but assured and friendly. The enforcement system will take on the battle. . . . The team leader just tells them [the nursing home] what the repercussions are if you don't correct. You just let the system take over. That's all you have to do. A good team leader is confident, friendly, and explains consequences. She never uses a standover approach."

This assurance and composure in New York is underwritten by the capacity to "pass the case on" to the agency lawyers. It enables accomplished New York inspectors to project a demeanor of inevitability about compliance, an inexorability about enforcement escalation when confronted with resistance, a capacity to communicate the (slightly misleading) implication that "if you want to go off and fight with the lawyers about this, that's fine and that's your right. It won't be my problem; it will be your problem and the lawyers' problem." When inspectors have productivity targets to meet and another inspection to start tomorrow, they really don't mind handing over a recalcitrant noncomplier to the enforcement system.

The foregoing discussion might be read as suggesting that the major problem with nursing home regulation is the resister to regulatory commands. This is not so: determined resistance to regulatory commands by nursing homes is quite rare, even in comparatively adversarial and litigious New York.[11] The politics of rebellion against regulatory commands is much more common at the level of industry association resistance than at the individual nursing home level. At the nursing home level, what Merton (1968, p. 194) calls "ritualism" is the greater problem than what he calls "rebellion." Merton identifies the

---

[11] The following statement of a surveyor from a southern state is typical: "In most cases—95 percent—the plan of correction is acceptable. We write back to the 5 percent saying it's not an acceptable plan of correction. Mostly it's unacceptable dates—beyond ninety days. Then the vast majority come back with an acceptable plan. Much of it is sorted out on the telephone."

TABLE 1

Merton's Typology of Modes of Adaptation

Modes of Adaptation	Goals	Institutional Means
I. Conformity	+	+
II. Innovation	+	−
III. Ritualism	−	+
IV. Retreatism	−	−
V. Rebellion	±	±

Source.—Merton (1968), p. 194.
Note.—See text for explanation of symbols.

five types of adaptation to a normative order in table 1, where +
signifies "acceptance," − signifies "rejection," and ± signifies "rejection of prevailing values and substitution of new values." Here we
apply Merton's model, with only a little distortion, to acceptance and
rejection of regulatory goals (outcomes) and means to achieving those
goals institutionalized in regulatory specifications (inputs).

Ritualism is a more effective means of resistance to regulation than
rebellion because it is less confrontational and more subtle. Rather
than resist the objective of reducing chemical restraint that management does not really accept, the services of a captive physician can be
retained to complete medication orders required by the law whenever
management requests them. It is generally regarded as imprudent in
the nursing home industry to force a confrontation with the state by
openly refusing to comply. Typically the legal costs of such a confrontation will exceed the expected penalties one is seeking to avoid and
the costs of compliance, which are usually not high (Braithwaite et al.
1990, p. 94). Moreover, nursing home regulatory agencies in most of
the jurisdictions we have studied, even in New York, have a good track
record at winning their infrequent legal battles. As a result, rebellion is
often motivated by reasons such as professional pride rather than rational economic calculation, as in the anger of a nursing home client
reported by one American defense attorney: "I didn't do this. I want
to fight it whatever it takes." Exceptions where legal resistance occasionally becomes economically rational arise in U.S. states—like Illinois and California—that provide for automatic severe consequences
of repeat violations. But generally the "check's always in the mail"
strategy, as some regulators refer to it, is the more effective one for
those who wish to cut corners on compliance. First, all regulatory

agencies have less than perfect mechanisms for confirming that checks are actually paid or that plans of correction are implemented. Second, it is often possible to write a plan of correction that follows institutionalized means for securing regulatory goals but that in practice can be implemented in a perfunctory fashion, as the following exchange illustrates:

> *Administrator for chain:* "You can win the battle and lose the war. There's the fear of retaliation next time round. When we disagree, sometimes the best policy is to lie down and play dead. Just put in a plan of correction that will make them happy."
> *Interviewer:* "And then what? Do you mean you have only perfunctory compliance with the plan of correction, enough to get them off your backs?"
> *Administrator:* "Yes."

The nursing home can agree to write a new policy—a piece of paper that changes little in terms of how things are actually done—or it can agree to run an "in-service" program to train staff in how to avoid noncompliance in future. Such plans of correction can be hard to reject as unsatisfactory and can readily be shown to have been implemented. But organizations that opt for such ritualism are likely to become what the regulators call "roller-coaster" nursing homes—that make a few changes to come into compliance only to be found out of compliance again at the next survey because of their fundamental lack of commitment to regulatory goals. Some large American nursing home chains are like this. They respond to a finding of noncompliance in one nursing home with a plan of correction to put extra staff onto the problem. The extra staff are simply shifted from another nursing home in the chain and once the first nursing home has been certified as back in compliance the extra staff may drift back to the second home, which meantime has been out of compliance in some other area because of the staff shortage. If this violation is detected by another survey team, staff may be temporarily shifted from a third facility to plug this gap. In this way a ritualistic corporation can have roller-coaster compliance in all its facilities. Chains that claim to be "playing the game" can actually be taking the regulators for a ride.

Industry informants in both Australia and the United States were often quite open about their commitment to ritualism: "I wrote it [the plan of correction] to pacify them [the regulators]." Our favorite example of ritualism is of an Australian director of nursing who did not want to oppose an inspection team who "made a big heap out of ethnic diet" under an Australian standard that requires sensitivity to cultural preferences for different types of food: "So we bought ethnic diet books—a ragout, goulash is a stew—give it a foreign name and they'll be happy." In many American states the virtues of ritualism are a deeply ingrained part of the received wisdom of the industry: it is repeatedly pointed out to you that the facilities with the highest levels of compliance are not the best facilities: "They are the best facilities at keeping the paperwork on the particular things required," said one Chicago nursing home administrator. Ritualism can also be a source of profound injustice. With more serious matters, the administrator will sometimes fire the director of nursing in a plan of correction as a ritualistic sacrifice because, said a Midwestern inspector, "It's his butt or hers when actually it's him who is the problem and she's doing a reasonable job."

That ritualism, rather than rebellion, is the main problem with nursing home regulation, takes us back to the claim that inspectors cannot rely on deterrence to deliver compliance most of the time. Unless they can coax and caress nursing home management into a commitment to regulatory goals, they will confront endemic roller-coaster compliance from organizations that correct some institutionalized means without tackling the underlying causes of chronic noncompliance. Effectiveness therefore crucially depends on embracing both compliance and deterrence strategies. Compliance without deterrence regulation puts inspectors at risk of having their bluff called; deterrence without compliance regulation puts inspectors at risk of accepting ritualism rather than conformity with regulatory goals. American street-level bureaucrats who are perceptive enough to realize the truth of the latter claim (actually, quite a large proportion of them) defy federal and state policies that forbid the evil practice of "consultancy." They usually do not recommend institutionalized means that the nursing home must follow to secure compliance. This really would be an evil of consultancy since commitment to regulatory goals is most likely when nursing home staff own the solutions designed to meet regulatory goals. The goal is more often to be a catalyst, to get the administrator to analyze and remedy the root causes of failure to attain regulatory goals, as is explained by one experienced New York inspector: "The feds say: 'Do not survey for root causes.' New York State has always surveyed for underlying causes [a statement that would horrify those in head office in Albany

who espouse the official line]. We talk with the administrator prior to
the exit: 'Gee, there's a lot of problems here [in this area]—X, Y, and
Z. What do you think about the competence of the department head?'
Or, 'Why do you think these systems aren't working?'"

Sophisticated street-level bureaucrats first seek to persuade management that regulatory goals really are desirable if evidence of this management commitment is lacking. Then they will help the nursing home
do their own diagnosis of the problems of their organization that must
be solved if compliance is to be sustained (see Bardach and Kagan
1982, pp. 148–49; Braithwaite 1985, pp. 101–3). Unfortunately, however, the regulatory process in most American states does not readily
accommodate the coaxing of compliance at these two levels. Consider
the following example of a citation of a Southern nursing home:

> Each resident did not receive care necessary to prevent skin
> breakdown as evidenced by three decubiti that developed in the
> facility.
> *Plan of Correction Written by Nursing Home:* The medical director
> examined the residents in which the alleged decubiti were found.
> He did not feel that two of the three residents had evidence of
> decubiti. However, all three residents were placed on treatment
> schedule to prevent further skin breakdown.

Legally, it is hard to reject such a plan of correction as unsatisfactory. Yet its acceptance succumbed to two regulatory failures. First,
there was a failure to persuade the nursing home that they had a serious
problem (or if not that failure, a failure of the inspection team to admit
they were wrong and that there was no problem).[12] Dialogue is needed
to persuade the nursing home that skin breakdowns representing even
the early stages of decubiti on three separate residents is a problem of
a seriousness that should not be tolerated by responsible management.
Second, there was a regulatory failure to persuade the nursing home
to rethink their whole prevention program with regard to skin breakdowns instead of just offering to patch up the three detected cases.
Dialogue is needed to diagnose the deficiencies in prevention programs

[12] Sometimes these failures of persuasion are even more explicitly portrayed in plans
of correction, as in the following (admittedly unusual) submission by a Chicago nursing
home: "These 'plans of correction' are being submitted only because they are asserted
to be required by law. In submitting these plans, the facility does not intend to admit
to any of the allegations in this statement or elsewhere, or to the violation of any
regulation or law, nor does it intend to waive or limit in any way its right to contest
any alleged violation or other action of any governmental authority or person."

and to catalyze the serious redesign of policies and procedures required. What happened instead was the triumph of ritualism with the acceptance of the proffered plan of correction. The U.S. process leaves little space for the required dialogue: "Anything that's the least bit acceptable will be approved because we have to turn these around in 45 days. Unless it's right out of left field, we'll accept it," said a Midwestern inspector.

The deadlines that deliver the impressively reliable annual inspection cycle in the United States, combined with the official policies against "consultation," make the dialogue difficult. Yet we have seen some rays of hope, of change. One reason for the oppressively high levels of restraint in American nursing homes has been a failure to engage in regulatory dialogue with nursing homes that respond ritualistically to concerns raised about high levels of restraint. Repeatedly during 1988 and 1989 we observed regulatory inertia in the face of nursing homes that inspectors knew, or should have known, had unacceptable levels of restraint. As soon as management could produce signed physicians' orders for all residents who were restrained, that was the end of the story. The right piece of paper would keep them out of trouble even if it were signed by a medical automaton who rarely saw the residents, who was a captive of nursing home management (for a suitable fee), and who signed everything that the nursing home put in front of him. In 1990, in the aftermath of the brilliant "untie the elderly" campaign run by a coalition of consumer groups, nursing home professionals and progressive state regulators were required to put their stamp on the interpretation of nursing home reform laws implemented that year, and we observed regulatory practices becoming more dialogic on the restraint issue. Even where the nursing home could produce physicians' orders for all restraints, inspectors persisted with questioning. "But why is the restraint needed? Don't you think you need a more detailed assessment than this? What about an assessment by a psychiatrist? What are your procedures for reviewing restraints? Aren't you worried about litigation for the improper use of restraints? Have you thought about why you have so many more restrained residents than other facilities in our region? Did you know that X [an industry opinion leader] has halved the number of physically restrained residents in her facility in the past six months, and she says that it's the best thing she's ever done for the residents and for the staff?" The aides rose to the challenge.

Levels of restraint in American nursing homes are falling dramatically; some states having already halved the percentages of their residents who are physically restrained. Deterrence has not produced this change; deterrence may even have decreased in this area during 1990 and 1991. It is the combination of the processes of regulatory dialogue described above driven by the communitywide clamor for reform of the "untie the elderly" campaign and the 1987 OBRA regulatory reforms that is delivering dramatic change. So often scholars of regulation lose sight of the possibility that the year-by-year regulatory failures they see during long periods of regulatory inertia ought to be qualified by noticing that there are periods of history when dramatic regulatory accomplishments are secured in a relatively short space of time. Sometimes these are later reversed. But often they are not. I predict that the regulatory progress on nursing home restraint will not be reversed, but will be cumulative; twenty-first century Americans may look on twentieth century practices of tying up the infirm elderly as incomprehensible barbarism to which it would be unthinkable to return.

While regulatory dialogue over the restraint issue manifests some mellowing of the official U.S. doctrine that inspectors are law enforcers whose job is simply to rate the nursing home for compliance with the standards, and not "consultants," the dialogue remains limited. Moreover, U.S. inspectors receive training, consistent with the official policy, which is unsuitable for preparing them for a dialogic role. At least until 1990, HCFA training of state inspectors emphasized the need for inspectors to be in control during exit conferences, not to be distracted by questions raised by nursing home staff, to stick to the facts of the deficiencies that require a written plan of correction. Occasionally, we have seen surveyors take this training depressingly seriously, as by refusing to answer questions from nursing home management as to whether, in spite of their deficiencies, they had improved since the last survey. This particular survey team was strongly of the view that there had been great improvement at this nursing home, but they declined to express this view at the exit lest it compromise their demeanor as "law enforcers" whose function does not extend beyond dispassionate monitoring and reporting of compliance with the law. Here, as Albert J. Reiss, Jr., pointed out in commenting on an earlier draft of this essay, it is the inspectors who are being ritualistic by shying away from positive feedback that might help sustain regulatory goals. Fortunately, such an extremist interpretation of law enforcement ritualism is not typical among the street-level bureaucrats who make the regulation work.

In terms of Merton's typology, I have so far discussed conformity, rebellion, and ritualism. Retreatism, where there is a disengagement of commitment to both regulatory goals and institutionalized means for attaining them, does occur from time to time, particularly when the chief executive of the organization is "burnt out" by the pressures of running a health care institution (see Braithwaite et al. 1992, app. E). Indeed, it is when "burnout" happens that some of the more draconian regulatory interventions occur, such as putting in a government-appointed administrator to run the facility. Some of the disengaged nursing home managers we have seen have been alcoholics, one of Merton's classic types of retreatists. While it is a less common occurrence in the United States than ritualism, when retreatism does occur, the consequences for everyone concerned can be serious.

Innovation—achieving regulatory goals but by other than the institutionally approved means—has been substantially destroyed by decades of input-oriented regulation. As the head of one large state industry association put it, "You manage facilities according to the standards written rather than according to what's best for patient care. You quickly learn how to play the game, to give them what's required to meet the standards." This is today widely recognized—by scholarly commentators, governments, industry, and professional and consumer groups—to have been a bad thing. American nursing home regulatory policy today claims that it is undoing this regulatory stultification of innovation by shifting strategy from input- to outcome-oriented regulation. The theory is that the law should specify quality of life and quality of care outcomes for nursing home residents, allowing nursing homes to achieve them through whatever means they see fit. In my view, the shifts in U.S. policy toward more outcome-oriented nursing home regulation have been very marginal. Australian government policy has matched the rhetoric with more genuinely outcome-oriented regulatory practices than one sees in the United States, even though input regulation still has an important place on the Australian scene. To illustrate the difference, if an Australian nursing home achieves good outcomes for residents with staffing levels that are below the industry average, or with professionally unqualified staff, regulators might applaud this as cost-efficient accomplishment of the outcomes. Notwithstanding the rhetoric of outcome-orientation, regulatory practice in the United States will punish nursing homes that skimp on staffing inputs or that fail to use staff with mandated professional qualifications, regardless of resident outcomes.

In summary, then, American nursing home regulation achieves a surprising degree of voluntary conformity, a great deal of ritualism, and occasional retreatism and rebellion, and it tends to systematic destruction of innovation. While American nursing home regulation uses deterrence much more than in other countries, it still relies heavily on compliance strategies, though not heavily enough to grapple with widespread regulatory resistance through ritualism.

V. Self-regulation

Our fieldwork was attentive to self-regulation as well as government regulation. We interviewed people at industry associations who claimed to run self-regulation schemes; we visited the Joint Commission on Accreditation of Healthcare Organizations and interviewed both surveyors and nursing homes that had been through, or were preparing for, their accreditation process in different parts of the country; we attended a meeting of the Accreditation Committee of the American College of Health Care Administrators; we sat in on thirty-six care planning conferences in nursing homes and eight meetings of facility quality assurance committees.

In its short history, the U.S. nursing home industry moved quickly from being totally unregulated to heavy government regulation. There has never been an era when self-regulation was the primary control strategy. The Reagan administration, as I have noted, tried unsuccessfully to change this situation in 1981. There has long been the Joint Commission on Accreditation of Hospitals (JCAH), which changed its name to the Joint Commission on the Accreditation of Healthcare Organizations (JCAHO) in the 1980s, with an eye to the nursing home business in particular. In Texas, JCAHO accreditation is deemed to satisfy state licensure, but not federal certification, which requires a government inspection. The penetration of the commission's voluntary accreditation has always been weak, as the vice president for quality assurance with one nursing home chain explained: "The Joint Commission accredits only three percent of the nursing homes in the country and it's decreasing. Forget it, we're up to here [signifies her neck] in inspection." Most of the industry is not remotely interested in applying for accreditation and is totally unaffected by this self-regulation process.

The 1981 proposal to waive federally mandated inspection for nursing homes accredited by the JCAHO was resisted on a number of grounds (Jost 1983, 1988). First, the JCAH had no enforcement powers. Second, its reports were treated as confidential quality assurance feedback to management that was not available to consumers. Third, its standard accreditation cycle is three years instead of the one-year government cycle. Fourth, it was rightly criticized for an extremely input-oriented (ritualistic) approach to self-regulation. The JCAH has been as bad as government regulation in the United States in stultifying innovation to deliver better health care outcomes. Accepting some truth in the latter criticism, the JCAHO has sought to move to a somewhat more outcome-oriented approach in the last few years, but as with U.S. government regulation, outcome-orientation at JCAHO remains more a matter of rhetoric than reality.

Over the years, some state industry associations have developed self-regulatory schemes to ensure that their members had satisfactory quality assurance programs as a condition of membership. The most ambitious of these was the Washington Health Care Association's (1990) Quality Validation Program conducted in cooperation with the JCAHO. At the time of our visit to Seattle in 1990, this seemed about to fold, effectively removing industry associations from any substantial involvement with self-regulation, though some state associations (e.g., Virginia) run low-key voluntary peer review programs for administrators. Professional associations continue to play important roles in accrediting health care professionals. Of particular interest in the nursing home industry is the American College of Health Care Administrators, which accredits 6,500 administrators. Some of the professional development plans developed with nursing home administrators during their accreditation process amount to quality assurance programs for the facilities they run (American College of Health Care Administrators 1987). Doctors are subject to peer review organizations (Jost 1988). This may be important in hospitals where doctors exercise great power, but in nursing homes where doctors are generally part-timers with minimal involvement in organizational decision making, this form of self-regulation has a small impact. In any case, in the entire American health care sector up to September 1987, only fifty-four health care providers had been excluded from Medicare, with another twenty-five being subjected to monetary penalties, as a result of peer-review organization deliberations (Jost 1988, p. 591).

The self-regulatory action that counts most is at the level of particular nursing home organizations themselves rather than at the level of national or state associations. For years, many nursing home chains have had quality assurance programs, often headed by a vice president for quality assurance. Some of these have impressive manuals. Our observation is, however, that most corporate quality assurance programs demand no more than is required by government regulation. This contrasts with quality assurance programs in the pharmaceutical industry that often demand much higher standards than those imposed by the law (Braithwaite 1984). The function of the vice president for quality assurance in a nursing home chain tends to be to get her facilities up to speed when a government inspection is due. The objective, in other words, is not so much to improve quality as to minimize deficiencies detected by the regulators. This reality is reflected in the incentive systems of the chains, which pay bonuses to administrators who obtain low numbers of deficiencies in government inspections rather than to administrators who are rated by corporate quality assurance systems as delivering good quality outcomes. At worst, corporate quality assurance personnel train staff in the art of ritualism. But this is not always the case. For example, the national quality assurance program mandated by a 1986 Californian consent agreement with Beverly Enterprises—a past master of ritualism and roller-coaster compliance—according to several knowledgeable informants and our own limited observation of the Beverly quality assurance program in operation, is seriously oriented to improving the quality of care and has probably done so.

The Beverly consent agreement was a pioneering example of government-mandated self-regulation in this industry. This has been taken a big step further with the implementation of OBRA in 1990.[13] Under OBRA, each nursing home is required to have a quality assurance program coordinated by a quality assurance committee. The nursing home is allowed a lot of discretion in choosing whatever quality assurance objectives seem most needed to the nursing home in each area of its operation. This seems a paradigm shift away from command and control regulation and toward fostering self-regulation, and in impor-

---

[13] See n. 7 above. This was legislated in 1987 after a stunning campaign in which the National Citizens Coalition for Nursing Home Reform effectively persuaded the nursing home industry and professional associations to support the reform, even though it involved measures such as tougher enforcement. Regulations and a new inspection protocol to give effect to the law did not come into force until October 1990.

tant ways it is. However, the culture of an industry inured to government command and control, indeed, to government discipline, as I argue in the next section, pervades the quality assurance process. Ritualism is endemic. The question that holds center stage during quality assurance meetings is not, "What is the best way to design this program to deliver maximum improvement in quality of care?" It is, "What is it that they [the regulators] want of us here? What is the minimum we have to do to satisfy the requirement of having a quality assurance program?" We could illustrate this with some shameless instances of ritualism during quality assurance meetings. The following interaction is a more subtle case that is closer to the modal reality of quality assurance ritualism:

> *Director of nursing:* "Are you looking for 100 percent [with your outcome evaluation]? What are you going to do about it if it's 95 percent?"
> *Dietician:* "An in-service."
> *Quality assurance coordinator:* "Shoot for 100 percent and put 90 percent [on the written evaluation plan]. Don't hesitate to change the design to make it more realistic. They [the state] don't mind that. You don't get penalized for not meeting your quality assurance objectives. You'll get penalized for failing to take action on the problems you find. Do we all agree? Ninety percent."

Here the parameters of the quality assurance program are being set so as to avert the need for any follow-up action to improve quality. In the most blatant cases of ritualism, the very selection of quality assurance evaluation is driven by a search for nonproblems that will guarantee a near-100 percent result. Ritualism cannot therefore be simply fixed by changing the structure of the law away from command and control. Ritualism is a deeper problem of regulatory culture. It is also a problem of infinite regress. This was illustrated in one quality assurance committee meeting when linking quality assurance data to employee evaluations was discussed: "In my area, if we specify clearly their employee evaluation criteria, they won't do anything else." Ritualism is such a deeply embedded, multilayered problem in the American nursing home industry that nothing short of a cultural revolution in the industry and its regulation may be needed to conquer it. I turn to this question in the next section.

VI. The Structure and Culture of Nursing Homes

Nowhere, not even in prisons, do I get so powerful a sense as in American nursing homes that there may be some merit in the social theory of Michel Foucault (1977). American nursing homes (like Japanese nursing homes, though less so with English and Australian homes) are disciplinary societies. Many of them have explicitly panoptic designs—nurses' stations are hubs from which radiate wings of rooms. The corridors of each wing and the front rooms of each—usually public areas such as activities rooms, TV and dining rooms—can be subjected to surveillance from the nurses' station in such homes. Residents whom it is thought unwise to leave unsupervised in their room are put into, often tied into, a wheelchair and positioned adjacent to the nurses station. Often a dozen or more silent, sullen, slumped subjects are congregated around the nurses' station. Occasionally, homes that are architecturally ill-suited to surveillance compensate with closed-circuit television surveillance. In these nursing homes, television monitors adorn the nurses station. I am not saying that panoptic design or television surveillance characterizes a majority of American nursing homes. What is remarkable from the perspective of another culture is that they exist at all and exist in significant numbers; they would, for example, be in clear breach of Australian "homelike environment" and "privacy and dignity" standards. In more subtle ways, almost all American nursing homes are designed as surveillance institutions.[14] My hypothesis about this is much stronger than simply a failure of American regulation to prevent this; it is that American regulation was centrally involved in causing it.

My argument in this final section is that: the organizational structure of the American nursing home industry has been driven by the regulatory structure (the conclusion I reached in Sec. II); the disciplinary nature of American nursing homes is connected to their comparatively large size, distant management, and institutional structure; the disciplinary nature of American nursing homes is connected to the disciplinary nature of American nursing home regulation; the disciplinary nature of both American nursing homes and American nursing home regulation makes ritualism an inevitable pathology; and therefore, the key point of intervention to deal with the dual problems of ritualism

[14] Albert J. Reiss, Jr., has pointed out to me that this is a more general American medical institutional model: many hospitals also have panoptic designs: in the recovery room with all its monitors the surveillance institution reaches its highest form, with almost total abandonment of privacy as a value.

and disciplinary oppression is a radical transformation of the regulatory framework.

The disciplinary nature of American nursing homes is most apparent in the physical surveillance described above, which, as oppressive of privacy and dignity as are its effects, is nevertheless motivated by a well-meaning desire to protect residents from harm and to protect the nursing home from legal allegations of negligence. Similarly with the other most visible sign of the disciplinary order of the American nursing home—the shocking level of physical restraint.[15]

Consider this deficiency citation for a Beverly Enterprises home: "Resident #13 was found . . . with her right hand restrained to the bedrail with mitt in place. The hand and lower arm were swollen and cyanotic. Indentation marks from the strings were noted where tied. . . . The resident has no mitt restraint order."

Question staff and they will say (usually both mistakenly and sincerely) that restraint is necessary to protect the residents by preventing falls and to protect the nursing home from lawsuits and regulatory sanctioning.[16] Less commonly, they will concede it represents a policy of the corporation to save staff time on the management of difficult residents. These most visible manifestations of the disciplinary society are complimented by an infinity of smaller less visible disciplines. In many parts of the United States, nursing home residents do not have what we might call a "right to be fat." Mrs. Smith, who has enjoyed eating to excess and put up with being fat for eighty long years is forced to diet when she enters a nursing home. Why? Because the nursing home dietician is concerned at what might happen when the

---

[15] Chemical restraint may be even more pernicious, though it is less visible. Some surveys have found as many as 50 percent of nursing home residents on antipsychotic or sedative/hypnotic drugs when only 10 percent of the sample had clearly documented mental illness (Sherman 1989). National Nursing Home Survey data analyzed by the National Institute of Mental Health found 62 percent of residents to be on psychiatric drugs, though only 5 percent of them had psychiatric diagnoses (United States Senate, Special Committee on Aging 1990, p. 40). As one state inspector who was a qualified pharmacist put it, in many nursing homes "drugs can be causing more confusion than psychosis."

[16] In truth, there have been more successful lawsuits in the United States about residents strangling on restraints than about residents who fell for want of a restraint. Indeed, it is likely that there have been very few successful lawsuits of the latter type (see United States Senate, Special Committee on Aging 1990, p. 33, and elsewhere; see also Evans and Strumpf 1989). While it is true that American health care professionals are more vulnerable to lawsuits than their peers in other countries, this observation has less force in the nursing home industry because the frail aged everywhere are disinclined to sue. Also families are very reluctant to push their loved ones into a lawsuit during the last of their time on this earth.

inspectors see in Mrs. Smith's chart that she is so overweight and that the nursing home has failed to protect her health by putting her on a diet. This might get the dietary department a deficiency (and therefore cost the dietician a bonus for a deficiency-free inspection). Even if in fact the nursing home is likely to get enlightened inspectors who would not count Mrs. Smith's not being on a diet as a strike against the home, the disciplinary order of nursing home employment requires the dietician to play it safe ("Who ever got a deficiency for putting a fat person on a diet?").

A good illustration of protective discipline being applied arose during an inspection on the East Coast of the United States in a nursing home specializing in the needs of Asian residents. The inspectors observed many of the residents, as would be customary in their own homes, to remain all day in house-coats like bathrobes. Following a cultural pattern, they did not wear underwear, and old people being as they are, this resulted in various incidents of exposure of private parts observed by the inspectors. The inspectors said they did not want to discourage the residents from customary modes of dress, but they wanted staff to be more sensitive to the privacy and dignity issues involved, and in any case they could not ignore the standard. So they wrote the following citation: "Privacy and dignity was not always maintained: i.e., four patients were observed with their personal parts exposed and they lacked underwear." The following plan of correction came back from the nursing home: "Staff to be inserviced further on patient dignity and the need to maintain the privacy of all patients. Underwear to be purchased for patients who lack them; underwear to be worn."

One is reminded of Foucault's (1977, p. 222) aphorism that "the 'Enlightenment' which discovered the liberties, also invented the disciplines." Indeed, one is tempted to extend it to the present by saying that the postwar United States, which claims some credit for spreading the liberties behind the iron curtain, imposed the disciplines on its own elderly and then sought to export the disciplines through the international expansion of its nursing home chains. Even in countries like Australia, which has experienced only very minor market penetration by American nursing home chains, there is still some percolation of the American model, mediated through textbooks, gerontology journals, marketing men with new surveillance technologies, industry associations that see more of a future in corporatized caring than in a cottage industry, and visiting gurus. There is even a group which manages thirteen Australian nursing homes called Conforme Management. A South Australian director of nursing captured well the concern some feel about the direction of change: "It's no longer a cottage industry. They are individual people with needs to us. In the new factory industry, they are units. That's why we now need complaints systems and the rest."

This is an interesting quote, I think, because by making the connection with the "factory," this director of nursing, doubtless without having read Foucault, is tapping into Foucault's key idea of the carceral archipelago: "Is it surprising that prisons resemble factories, schools, barracks, hospitals, which all resemble prisons?" (Foucault 1977, p. 228).

The large American nursing home chains cannot help but spread the disciplines. They operate in an industry that poses large regulatory risks, as the near bankruptcy of Beverly Enterprises in the late eighties illustrates. There is no choice for them, therefore, but to follow the logic of regulatory risk management. That means highly disciplined institutions in which risks (*read* people) are monitored, recorded, and subjected to preventive controls (or at least the appearance of preventive control, so that the organization can be seen not to have neglected the risks embodied in the five-hundred-plus standards). We have already seen how the large American chains owe their very existence to the imperatives of largeness and institutionalization that were products of regulatory choices made in the United States two decades ago, different regulatory choices from those made in other countries. The risk with large institutions is that people and problems can fall between the cracks. Size therefore motivates surveillance, record keeping, and control. This is the essence of Foucault's notion of power as discipline. Disciplinary power does not grow out of the barrel of a gun, not from the edicts of a monarch or a judge, not from the control of capital, as do other forms of power. Disciplinary power works through the construction of routine; it can be seen in its most developed form when a total institutional environment is designed as a technostructure of control. Bauman (1982, p. 40) summarizes well the change Foucault sees in the way power is exercised with the growth in discipline:

Power moved from the distant horizon into the very center of daily life. Its object, previously the goods possessed or produced by the subject, was now the subject himself, his daily rhythm, his time, his bodily actions, his mode of life. . . . It wanted to impose one ubiquitous pattern of normality and eliminate everything and everybody which the pattern could not fit. Unlike the sovereign power which required only a ceremonial reminder of the timeless limits to autonomy, the emergent power could be maintained only by a dense web of interlocking authorities in constant communication with the subject and in a physical proximity to the subject which permitted a perpetual surveillance of, possibly, the totality of his life process.

The crucial theoretical limitation of the Foucauldian perspective for the present problem is that it assumes that disciplinary power is used for "normalization," by which Foucault means bringing under control, back to "normal," the slightest irregularity of conduct. Foucault sees the clinical sciences as instruments of normalization. Yet the clinical sciences and regulation can be instruments of individualization rather than normalization.[17] Ironically, there is a literature on "normalization" in gerontology. The author of the term, Wolfensberger (1972, 1985), a gerontologist, means exactly the opposite to the meaning Foucault gives the term.[18] For Wolfensberger and the many health care professionals influenced by the idea, normalization means shifting power back from institutional routine to individual residents—allowing them to live in a nursing home as free, choosing individuals, just as they do in the "normal" outside community. Put another way, these health care professionals have the agenda of normalizing the institution instead of normalizing the subject of the institution.

Garland (1990, p. 174) has made the point in his critique of Foucault that there is no inevitability that regulation destroys freedom; regulation, equally, can constitute freedom. Cases in point are the Australian standards that require nursing homes to guarantee "privacy and dignity," a variety of specific "freedoms," including the wonderful legal mischief of the "right to take risks" (Commonwealth/State Working Party on Nursing Homes Standards 1987, p. 49). A useful way of comprehending what is happening within the nursing home industry in the modern world is as a battle between the two normalizations. Health care professionals are warriors on both sides of this battle;

---

[17] Garland (1991) has made a similar critical point about Foucault's view of the relationship between criminology and discipline.
[18] See Wolfensberger (1972). In the 1980s, Wolfensberger reformulated his normalization concept somewhat as "social role valorization" (Wolfensberger 1985).

regulation is a weapon used on both sides of the barricades, though the modalities of regulation favored by the two sides are very different.[19]

Furthermore, we must not forget that it is specific regulatory choices that created the conditions for a factory industry. Smallness dissolves many of the disciplinary imperatives of the chains of large institutions. Tiny English nursing homes can be justifiably criticized for sloppy record keeping and abysmal care planning. Yet, in their defense, they do not need such discipline as do American institutions managed by a remote corporate headquarters on the other side of the country. When there are only eighteen residents in the nursing home, the director of nursing knows the problems of all of them personally and intimately. She does not need a systematic information system to ensure that problems do not fall through the cracks. She does not have to worry so much about shuffling staff from A wing, where they know the residents, to F wing, where they do not, because there is only one wing. She does not need a pervasive surveillance system to cover the nursing home because she herself gets into every part of the nursing home many times every day. The more intimate knowledge of every resident's needs that can be accomplished when all staff get to know all the residents means that particularized solutions can be found to problems that more bureaucratized institutions feel they can only handle with a form of control such as restraint.

The structural imperatives of scale and bureaucratization therefore combine with a disciplinary regulatory system (that is forgiving so long as the appearance of remedial inputs is documented) to create disciplinary institutions for the elderly. A little more should be said on how the disciplinary regulatory system is created, though my colleagues and I will have a great deal more to say about this when we write a book on the subject. What we are describing is a disciplinary regress. Mrs. Smith is disciplined by the dietician onto a diet. The dietician has been in turn disciplined to do this by the existence of a state inspector, who is unlikely to understand the details of Mrs. Smith's preferences as well as the dietician and who therefore may react to the appearance of poor health care when overweight residents

---

[19] The battle is joined on one side by the majority in the corporatized caring sector who want to be "given the rules of the game so we can play by them" and the rulebook regulators. On the other side are the bulk of the consumer movement and the outcome-oriented regulators who are interested in a regulatory process that includes dialogue about resident rights and freedoms.

overeat. The state inspector, in turn, is disciplined by the existence of supervisors and HCFA look-behind inspectors, who are even less likely to get close to a nuanced understanding of Mrs. Smith's case but who can readily pick up a failure of an inspector to notice an unclosed loop in documentary records the inspector should have checked. A regulatory system has been created where everyone is regulated by someone else in a culture of distrust in which all are ground through the disciplinary mincer. Demands for regulatory accountability are met with ever more layers of regulation, usually heavily documented to vindicate the new discipline.

Structurally, this situation conduces to ritualism. Getting the documentation right is the way to protect yourself. The way to persuade the disciplinary actor above you is to show her that you are a credible agent for her discipline, passing it on to those below in a way that can be documented to those above. It is the documents and the disciplinary practices that are your defense, not any imaginative or dedicated things you might have done to improve the quality of life of nursing home residents. That is, ritualism is your defense—devoting your energies to institutionalized means rather than to a goal like reducing pain. The contrast is palpable at every layer of the regulatory apparatus, between the United States and England or Australia, in the proportion of the time people spend working on documentary defense rather than hands-on problem solving. Nurses in the United States spend very little of their time giving care to residents; that must be left to untrained nurses' aides because practically all of the registered nurse's time must be dedicated to the more important task of keeping documents in order.[20] Inspectors in the United States spend most of their time alone in a room poring over resident charts, whereas English and Australian inspectors spend most of their time out in the nursing home observing care and talking to staff, residents, and visitors about care. The theory of the recent OBRA reforms was that the inspection process would become more resident-centered and less document-centered. But our research team's observation is of no significant change because the new element of resident interviews has been balanced by extra documents for inspectors to check and extra pieces of paper for them to fill out.

[20] This, in turn, exacerbates the disciplinary quality of nursing homes because there is evidence that registered nurses are less "custodial" in their attitudes to residents than are licensed practical nurses and that licensed practical nurses are less custodial than nurses aides (Bagshaw and Adams 1986, p. 242). Nurses, with their more caring, patient-centered professional socialization, are sorely needed on the front line as role models of noncustodial care.

Enormous resources in the United States are dedicated to documentary accountability checks to ensure that inspectors have completed all their records in the right way; few resources are dedicated to evaluating whether they have done anything to improve quality of care or even to talking with them about how to better accomplish this.

At every level in this hierarchy of mistrust, actors have a more jaundiced view than they should of the competence and capacity for responsibility of those they wish to discipline. The social scientists who advise U.S. governments on the design of nursing home surveys, for example, almost uniformly have the view of nursing home inspectors as incompetents who are incapable of dialogic problem solving, who must be disciplined against deviating from "objective" survey protocols. These are registered nurses whom they view as incapable of the responsible exercise of discretion, some of whom have run much larger organizations than the departments in which the academics work. The social scientists typically have acquired this stereotype of the untrustworthy, incompetent inspector without ever seriously interacting with inspectors on the job about their reflections on how they achieve progress. Instead, they sit at their computer terminals designing protocols for inspectors-as-dopes, thereby increasing the prospects that inspectors will become dopes. Our truth is that it is the dopes at each level who create dopes at the next rung down on the disciplinary ladder. Hence, the inspector who does not trust nursing home management will insist on making "recommendations" that they expect to be followed instead of opening up a dialogue that encourages management to design their own solutions. At the next step down, good managers empower their staff: in the best nursing homes, one sees nurses' aides actively involved in decision making and rising to the challenge of exercising their discretion to better serve the residents who are their responsibility (Tellis-Nayak 1988). In the worst nursing homes, one finds care managers manifesting the jaundiced view of the competence and trustworthiness of aides of this Australian director of nursing: "A checklist was my way of getting it done. We have to accept that we are dealing with girls who are rote learners. So it's the way I get them to learn. It's not checked off so they say, 'Oh, I haven't done it.'"

Breaking out of the hierarchical culture of mistrust and ritualism requires advocacy of a new regulatory maturity, a radical break with the documentation-driven obsessions of the past. American social scientists and health care scholars who work in this field hold out limited hope because they are central communicators of the culture of mistrust.

They tend to view the industry as rapacious and untrustworthy, regulatory managers as captured and feckless, and inspectors as incompetent. Managers in the industry are the least capable actors of effecting a profound change in regulatory culture, notwithstanding the conventional incantations about the power of capital. This is because they are the most mistrusted in a culture of mistrust, because they have most to gain by being untrustworthy. The federal regulators—within the Health Care Financing Administration—are in a better position to lead than the industry, though they still suffer from considerable mistrust as "captured regulators" and they have a poor record of policy entrepreneurship, probably because of their structurally weak position within a spending agency driven by the imperative to keep costs down.

The greatest hope for policy leadership toward a radical shift in the culture of U.S. nursing home regulation resides with the group who have been the policy entrepreneurs during the past decade—the National Citizens Coalition for Nursing Home Reform (NCCNHR). This consumerist coalition has as outstanding a leadership in Elma Holder and Barbara Frank as one can find in a consumer movement anywhere in the world. They enjoy a surprising degree of grudging respect from their adversaries in industry and the state. They are in touch with the grass roots of their constituency—the nursing home residents. This gives them a good grasp of the failures of U.S. nursing home regulation from a resident-centered perspective. It is this grasp that led them to campaign so vigorously and effectively for reform in the use of restraints—reform, as we have seen, that has challenged the ritualism of regulation that accepted a pile of physicians' orders as sufficient justification for restraint.

At the same time, advocacy of a radical renegotiation of the ground rules of U.S. nursing home regulation poses risks and threats to an organization like the NCCNHR. First, there is the risk that major accomplishments of their social movement would be lost in a radically redesigned regulatory order. One of these, for example, is that the United States was perhaps the only country in the world with a demonstrated capacity during the 1980s, even if an underused capacity in many states, to take tough enforcement action against nursing homes with deplorable standards. Second, there is the threat involved in conceding that the consumer movement shares with the industry, the lawyers, the regulators, and the social scientists a significant part of the blame for the disciplinary, ritualistic quality of American nursing home regulation. The consumer movement does share in this blame because it has been at the forefront of demanding new layers of discipline, the filling out of more pieces of paper to ensure that residents are protected. The consumer movement position has not been without paradox in this regard. While it has been an advocate of more and more specific new regulations that require new pieces of paper, in the broad it has been an advocate of a more resident-centered process that is less oriented to checking documentation. The policy it has advocated as a matter of broad regulatory strategy has been at cross-purposes with the aggregation of its piecemeal advocacy of an extra bit of discipline here and there. In this, the consumer movement is no less guilty than the industry associations that call for regulatory simplification as a matter of broad regulatory strategy and scream for tighter specification (ergo, multiplication) of regulations as soon as their members complain of inconsistent application of a broader rule.

As politically difficult as it would be for them, it is perhaps only the NCCNHR who have the political respect to initiate a cooperative process with the other industry players of fundamentally rethinking the culture of American nursing home regulation. Early success with the "untie the elderly" campaign is a taste for them of what can be accomplished down this path for the people they represent. Moreover, they already have succeeded with some path-breaking reforms in the direction of an alternative accountability model to more and more layers of discipline. These involve increased empowerment of advocacy groups outside nursing homes and of residents' councils within them. Examples are the recent OBRA reforms empowering representatives of residents' councils and advocates to participate in exit conferences at the conclusion of inspections and earlier reforms to give discussions with residents' councils an important role during the inspection process and to give residents more effective access to inspection reports.

VII. Conclusion

My view would be that dialogic, local accountability based on broad outcome-oriented standards and well-resourced local advocacy is a more hopeful strategy than national accountability based on demands for detailed documentation and a myriad of inputs (see Handler 1986). This, indeed, is the path that nursing home regulation is heading down in Australia, with reasonably broad, if fragile, support from industry, the consumer movement, and the state. Out of the energetic process of nursing home reform proceeding in the United States, a somewhat different model of nursing home regulation better suited to American realities may be developing. The American consumer movement has successfully lobbied for a new accountability model based on dialogue with consumers and advocates, though this has been allowed to grow alongside the oppressive old accountability model based on ritualized inputs and paper warfare. So there are grounds for both hope and despair about the future. A next step might be to open up a dialogue about a coherent program to effect the demise of this old accountability model. While it is hard to break out of cycles of mistrust, it should be possible to persuade consumers, workers, owners, and bureaucrats that a less disciplining industry culture would allow them all more rewarding lives. How such a process might unfold is better left for others to consider. Outsiders with comparative knowledge can occasionally glimpse a little clarity of perception in observing regulatory rituals that are taken for granted by locals. But they lack the appreciation of cultural and procedural subtleties to advise on ways of reforming local institutions. Americans must seize their own history. In the meantime, history may prove us to have also followed the wrong path in Australia.

REFERENCES

American College of Health Care Administrators. 1987. *The Professional Certification Program for Nursing Home Administrators.* Bethesda, Md.: American College of Health Care Administrators.

Ayres, Ian, and John Braithwaite. 1992. *Responsive Regulation: Transcending the Deregulation Debate.* New York and Oxford: Oxford University Press.

Bagshaw, Margaret, and Mary Adams. 1986. "Nursing Home Nurses' Attitudes, Empathy, and Ideologic Orientation." *International Journal on Aging and Human Development* 22(3):235–46.

Bardach, Eugene, and Robert A. Kagan. 1982. *Going by the Book: The Problem of Regulatory Unreasonableness.* Philadelphia: Temple University Press.

Bauman, Zygmunt. 1982. *Memories of Class: The Pre-history and After-life of Class.* London: Routledge & Kegan Paul.

Blum, Stephen R., and Elizabeth Wadleigh. 1983. *The Bureaucracy of Care: Continuing Policy Issues for Nursing Home Services and Regulation.* Sacramento, Calif.: Report of the Commission on California State Government Organization and Economy.

Braithwaite, John. 1984. *Corporate Crime in the Pharmaceutical Industry.* London: Routledge & Kegan Paul.

———. 1985. *To Punish or Persuade: Enforcement of Coal Mine Safety.* Albany, N.Y.: State University of New York Press.

Braithwaite, John, and Toni Makkai. 1991. "Testing an Expected Utility Model of Corporate Deterrence." *Law and Society Review* 28:7–40.

Braithwaite, John, Toni Makkai, Valerie Braithwaite, and Diane Gibson. 1992. *Raising the Standard: Resident Centred Nursing Home Regulation in Australia.* Canberra: Department of Health, Housing, and Community Services.

Braithwaite, John, Toni Makkai, Valerie Braithwaite, Diane Gibson, and David Ermann. 1990. *The Contribution of the Standards Monitoring Process to the Quality of Nursing Home Life: A Preliminary Report.* Canberra: Department of Community Services and Health.

Brown, Robert N. 1975. "An Appraisal of the Nursing Home Enforcement Process." *Arizona Law Review* 17:304–56.

Butler, Patricia A. 1979. "Assuring the Quality of Care and Life in Nursing Homes: The Dilemma of Enforcement." *North Carolina Law Review* 57:1317–82.

Commonwealth/State Working Party on Nursing Home Standards. 1987. *Living in a Nursing Home: Outcome Standards for Australian Nursing Homes.* Canberra: Australian Government Publishing Service.

Day, Patricia, and Rudolf Klein. 1987. "The Regulation of Nursing Homes: A Comparative Perspective." *Milbank Quarterly* 65(3):303–47.

Durkheim, E. 1961. *Moral Education: A Study in the Theory and Application of the Sociology of Education,* translated by E. K. Wilson and H. Schnurer. New York: Free Press.

Evans, Lois K., and Neville E. Strumpf. 1989. "Tying Down the Elderly: A Review of the Literature on Physical Restraint." *Journal of the American Geriatrics Society* 37:65–74.

Foucault, Michel. 1977. *Discipline and Punish: The Birth of the Prison,* translated by A. Sheridan. London: Allen Lane.

Gardiner, John A., and Kathryn L. Malec. 1989. *Enforcement of Nursing Home Regulations: OBRA Plus Two.* A Report to the U.S. Senate Special Committee on Aging. Chicago: University of Illinois at Chicago, Office of Social Science Research.

Garland, David. 1990. *Punishment and Modern Society.* Chicago: University of Chicago Press.

———. 1991. "Criminological Knowledge and Its Relation to Power." Paper presented at the British Society of Criminology Conference, York, August.

General Accounting Office. 1987. *Medicare and Medicaid—Stronger Enforcement of Nursing Home Requirements Needed: Report to the Ranking Minority Member, Special Committee on Aging, U.S. Senate.* Washington, D.C.: United States General Accounting Office.

Handler, Joel F. 1986. *The Conditions of Discretion: Autonomy, Community Bureaucracy.* New York: Russell Sage Foundation.

Hawkins, Keith. 1984. *Environment and Enforcement: Regulation and the Social Definition of Pollution.* Oxford: Clarendon.

Institute of Medicine. 1986. *Improving the Quality of Care in Nursing Homes.* Washington D.C.: National Academy Press.

54   John Braithwaite

Johnson, Sandra H. 1985. "State Regulation of Long Term Care: A Decade of Experience with Intermediate Sanctions." *Law, Medicine and Health Care* 13(September):173–87.

Jost, Timothy Stoltzfus. 1983. "The Joint Commission on Accreditation of Hospitals, Private Regulation of Health Care and the Public Interest." *Boston College Law Review* 24:835–923.

———. 1988. "The Necessary and Proper Role of Regulation to Assure the Quality of Health Care." *Houston Law Review* 25:525–98.

Lipsky, Michael. 1980. *Street-Level Bureaucracy: Dilemma of the Individual in Public Services.* New York: Russell Sage Foundation.

Long, Steven. 1987. *Death without Dignity: The Story of the First Nursing Home Corporation Indicted for Murder.* Austin: Texas Monthly Press.

Merton, Robert K. 1968. *Social Theory and Social Structure.* New York: Free Press.

National Association of Attorneys General. 1987. *Medicaid Fraud Report.* Washington, D.C.: National Association of Attorneys General, December.

Pray, John. 1986. "State v. Serebin—Causation and the Criminal Liability of Nursing Home Administration." *Wisconsin Law Review* 1986:339–66.

Reiss, Albert J., Jr. 1984. "Selecting Strategies of Social Control over Organizational Life." In *Enforcing Regulation,* edited by K. Hawkins and J. M. Thomas. Boston: Kluwer-Nijhoff.

Schudson, C. B., A. P. Onellion, and E. Hochstedler. 1984. "Nailing an Omelet to the Wall: Prosecuting Nursing Home Homicide." In *Corporations as Criminals,* edited by E. Hochstedler. Beverly Hills, Calif.: Sage.

Sherman, David E. 1989. "Psychoactive Drug Use in Long Term Care: Some Contributing Factors." *Long-Term Care Review* (Spring), pp. 8–14.

Tellis-Nayak, V. 1988. *Nursing Home Exemplars of Quality.* Springfield, Mass.: Charles C. Thomas.

Thomas, William C., Jr. 1969. *Nursing Homes and Public Policy.* Ithaca, N.Y.: Cornell University Press.

United States Senate, Special Committee on Aging. 1990. *Untie the Elderly: Quality Care without Restraints.* Serial no. 101-H. Washington, D.C.: U.S. Government Printing Office.

Vladeck, Bruce C. 1980. *Unloving Care: The Nursing Home Tragedy.* New York: Basic Books.

Washington Health Care Association. 1990. *We've Taken a Pledge to Provide Quality Care: Quality Validation Management Guide.* Olympia: Washington Health Care Association.

Wolfensberger, W. 1972. *The Principle of Normalization in Human Services.* Toronto: National Institute on Mental Retardation.

———. 1985. "Social Role Valorization: A New Insight, and a New Term, for Normalization." *Australian Association for the Mentally Retarded Journal* 9(1):4–11.

Nancy Reichman

Insider Trading

ABSTRACT

Insider trading involves the unlawful use of material, nonpublic
information. Regulation and the push to innovate in the securities
industry create new information demands and changing webs of
entitlement and obligation that place many different roles and
relationships at risk of abuse and corruption. Transactions are pushed to
the limits of norms of practice by combinations of information-driven
commodities; complicated networks of transaction-oriented exchanges with
conflicts of interest; and organizational cultures, including legal and moral
ambiguity about insider trading rules. Social controls, where they exist,
are not well suited for managing the dynamic of the market.

Insider trading is known to the public as *the* white-collar crime of the
1980s (Coffee 1988; Szockyj 1990). The Boesky and Milken "scandals"
that erupted in the middle of that decade recast the popular conceptions
of insider trading from a technical issue of "investor protection" to an
issue of "cultural significance . . . a manifestation of undue greed
among the already well-to-do" that led Congress to pass the Insider
Trading and Securities Fraud Enforcement Act of 1988 (Langevoort
1991, p. 1).

But the scandals did much more than expose the greed of Wall
Street. The elaborate networks of unlawful tips and transactions exposed by the Levine, Boesky, and Milken scandals revealed for the
first time the organizational dimensions of what had traditionally been
understood only as individual trust violations. We began to see the

Nancy Reichman is associate professor of sociology at the University of Denver. She
is indebted to Susan Shapiro for her scholarship and collegiality. Charlie Gwirtsman
and Albert J. Reiss, Jr., made helpful comments on earlier drafts.

organizational value of insider information and how its abuse could be used to enhance market positions and create market momentum that served particular clients. Indeed, a critical reading of the insider trading scandals exposes an industry at risk of participating in its own corruption.

The vast majority of research on insider trading has been conducted by legal scholars who track the changing technical requirements of securities law and by economists who debate whether insider trading is efficient for the market. Few sociologists examine the behavioral dimensions of insider trading or its regulation. Most scholarly business journals bypass the topic.

This essay analyzes the securities industry and its structural and cultural vulnerabilities to the unlawful use of inside information by traders and securities organizations.[1] Although insider trading has been typically understood as occupational crime, this essay shows how individual violations both reflect and construct organizational misconduct, misfeasance, and malfeasance. Insider trading as practiced in the 1980s is a form of crime that combines elements of the traditional categories of organizational and occupational crime. It represented a departure from the traditional forms of intracorporate self-dealing and market pilfering. These new forms of insider trading sought to corrupt the market itself, to change its very dynamic. None of this would have been possible without changes in the conditions of the market. Thus, to understand insider trading we must locate it within the changing structures of finance.

Section I describes insider trading and its organizational bases. The typical violations and violators are respectively examined in Sections II and III. Section IV describes the organizational context of insider trading. A model of market vulnerability is described in Section V. Trading conditions, organizational structures, and organizational cultures are examined. Section VI discusses the governmental response to insider trading and relates the response to the interorganizational dimensions of contemporary insider trading activity.

[1] This essay is based on disparate sources. Legal treatises, specialized seminar papers, lists of cases compiled by former SEC enforcement staff, the SEC Docket, and government reports provide data on behavior and responses to it. Histories of the securities industry (e.g., Mayer 1955; Carosso 1970) and contemporary accounts, both scholarly and popular (Wolfson 1980; Hayes, Spence, and Marks 1983; Auerbach and Hayes 1986; Auletta 1986; Eccles and Crane 1988; Stone 1990; Levine 1991), provide insight into the structural and cultural factors that shape and perpetuate insider trading.

I. Insider Trading and the Law

Trading rules prohibit individuals with access to privileged information about securities from trading in them or tipping others to trade in them without first disclosing to the other side of the transaction their possession of material, price-sensitive information that might affect that transaction. Prohibitions to abstain from trading are not statutorily defined. They are grounded, instead, in more sweeping securities fraud regulations such as Securities and Exchange Commission (SEC) Rule 10b-5, which prohibits individuals from engaging in any act, practice, or course of business that would operate as a fraud or deceit on any person in connection with the purchase or sale of a securities product. Securities and Exchange Commission Rule 14e-3, adopted in 1980, makes it illegal for *anyone* with inside information about a takeover to trade the target company's stock. An investor violates this rule even if he or she did not get the information directly from the insider but simply "knows or has reason to know" that the information came from an insider (Herlihy 1987).

Insider trading rules buttress beliefs that markets are fair arenas for transacting stock trades. By prohibiting individuals who have material, price-sensitive information from trading, insider trading restrictions attempt to neutralize the advantage of being an "insider" and, thus, invite participation by outsiders who would not trade if they thought the market was rigged against them. Insider trading rules convey an impression that parties to transactions have equal standing and that market information is neutral, or at least available, to all who wish to trade. Some commentators argue that the practice of trading on insider information promotes efficiency in the markets and oppose insider trading rules on those grounds. (See the debate in Beck-Dudley and Stephens [1989], and, for a classic statement, see Manne [1966].) Others view the laws "as crucial to the capital formation process that depends on investor confidence in the fairness and integrity of our securities market" (U.S. House of Representatives 1988, p. 8; and see Tomasic and Pentony [1989] for a discussion of the Australian markets).

While intentionally avoiding defining insider trading, Congress enacted two pieces of legislation in 1984 that clearly situate the behavior as a public wrong worthy of government intervention. The Insider Trading Sanctions Act of 1984 (ITSA) stipulates that persons found guilty of insider trading violations may face civil penalties up to three times the profits made (or losses avoided) as a result of the unlawful trading. Previously, offenders faced only the possibility of injunctions and disgorgement of actual profits.

Reacting to the scandals of the mid-1980s that exposed complex insider trading activity, Congress passed the Insider Trading and Securities Fraud Enforcement Act of 1988 (ITSFA) to augment the enforcement provisions of ITSA. ITSFA authorizes the establishment of a bounty program to enhance detection of insider trading abuses, expands the potential penalties for those found to have violated insider trading rules, broadens private rights of action, and imposes a possible jail term of five years for those who violate insider trading rules. Most important for our understanding of insider trading as organizational crime, ITSFA expanded the scope of the rules to include "controlling persons" who fail to take adequate steps to prevent abuse. Broker-dealers and investment advisors are now required to "establish, maintain, and enforce written policies 'reasonably designed' to prevent misuse of material, nonpublic information by the firm or any of its employees or associated persons" (U.S. House of Representatives 1988, p. 7). This rule establishes that securities-related organizations have a legal responsibility to recognize the potential for insider trading within their organizations and are obligated to take steps to prevent its occurrence.

A. Violations of Trust

Insider trader prohibitions apply only to *unlawful* trading on material, nonpublic information. They do not cover mere possession of inside information or *lawful* trading when in such possession. "There are numerous instances where persons who possess material nonpublic information can trade lawfully" (Langevoort 1991, p. 6). The legal conclusion that insider trading is unlawful is based on a breach in the fiduciary relationship of the involved parties.

The legal reference to a breach in fiduciary relationships underscores the important trust dimensions of insider trading. When trading on material, nonpublic information violates normative understandings and expectations of securities roles and relationships, it is a transgression of organizational trust (Shapiro 1987), a violation of the fiduciary relationships agents have with their principals and employers with their employees.

Two principal theories of liability have been applied to insider trading cases; their use depends on the type of fiduciary relationship contaminated by the leak of information (Langevoort 1991). The "abstain or disclose theory" holds that corporate employees have a fiduciary duty to their shareholders, and, thus, they must abstain from trading on material, nonpublic information if they have not disclosed that they are in possession of such information. It is applied to cases where corporate executives with access to material information trade for themselves on the basis of that nonpublic information. In *Dirks v. SEC*, 463 U.S. 646 (1986), the Supreme Court recognized that fiduciary obligations with respect to material, nonpublic information could include knowing "confederates" or "quasi insiders": "The majority opinion in *Dirks* recognized that under certain circumstances, such as where inside information is revealed to an underwriter, accountant, lawyer, or consultant working for the corporation, with the expectation that the disclosed information will remain confidential and in the context of a relationship at least implying a duty of confidentiality, such agents of the corporation should be treated as 'quasi-insiders,' with a fiduciary duty to refrain from trading on such information [*Dirks*, 463 U.S. 655, n. 14]" (Ferrara and Dozier 1988, p. 11).[2]

The "misappropriation theory" of liability for insider trading applies to cases where a person trades on material, nonpublic information about Company ABC when that information comes from a source other than Company ABC. The fiduciary obligation is not to the shareholders of Company ABC but to employers who can expect that their employees will refrain from profiting on confidential information entrusted to them in the course of their employment. The SEC, for example, charged Anthony R. Tavani with unlawful trading on the basis of inside information he gathered in the course of his employment with an insurance brokerage firm hired to review the insurance programs of a potential corporate takeover target (Securities and Exchange Commission 1991*a*).

Just how far securities regulation based on theories of misappropriation can extend beyond individuals directly involved in the purchase and sale of securities products was tested in the case against Foster Winans, a reporter for the *Wall Street Journal* (Winans 1986; Parsons

---

[2] But note that in Chiarella v. United States (445 U.S. 222 [1980]) the Supreme Court reversed the conviction of a financial printer who had obtained the identity of takeover targets from the bidder's financial tender offer materials and purchased the stock of the target before the tender offer was public. The justices argued that the printer had no fiduciary or agency relationship with the target and, therefore, was not bound by the abstain or disclose rule.

1987). Winans's "Heard on the Street" column was a daily "gossip" column that focused on stock price movements and prospects. In October 1983 Winans struck a deal with Peter Brant, a Kidder Peabody stockbroker, to supply him with the subject matter for the column. Knowing that Winans would write a story that included the information he supplied, Brant traded on the basis of what he expected would happen to the stocks once the column hit the streets. Brant and Winans split the profits. Winans's agreement with Brant was clearly a violation of the *Journal*'s conflict of interest policy. *Journal* employees are prohibited from disclosing the subjects or schedules of forthcoming articles and prohibited from trading in stocks about which they are writing or know that an article is about to appear. Once the scheme was exposed, Brant pled guilty to two counts of securities fraud and became the government's star witness against Winans and two co-conspirators: Kenneth Felis, another Kidder Peabody stockbroker, and David Carpenter, Winans's roommate. The men were convicted of mail and wire fraud and securities fraud. The case was appealed to the U.S. Supreme Court, which was asked, among other things, to rule on whether the securities law applied in this case. The government argued that, since the column in the *Journal* was a central feature of the market, the actors were operating a *fraud in connection with the purchase or sale of securities*, and thus Rule 10b-5 applied. The defendants argued that the *Journal* was not a direct market participant, and therefore the deception was not material to an investor. The justices divided evenly on the question of whether the action violated securities law. Although the Winans conviction was technically affirmed, the decision leaves open how far securities law extends (*U.S. v. Winans*, 612 F. Supp. 827 [SDNY 1985]; 791 F.2d 1024 [2d Cir.], cert. granted, 107 U.S. 666 [1986]).

B. The Problem with Rules

Even the most cursory review of the legal treatises on the subject of insider trading discloses a legal structure that is technically complex at the same time that it is uncertain or imprecise in terms of its meaning, intent, and reach. Rule uncertainty or imprecision adds to the vulnerability of the securities industry to insider trading in several ways. First, the lack of a clear definition of violative conduct generates a great deal of confusion at the operational level of securities transactions. Tidwell and Aziz (1988) studied stockbroker understandings of insider trading law. They asked stockbrokers whether descriptions of hypothetical situations violated securities rules. In all factual situations presented, brokers had trouble applying judicial definitions. The degree of difficulty depended on the facts of the case. Tidwell and Aziz conclude that the lack of a statutory definition creates confusion among practitioners in distinguishing lawful from unlawful conduct.

Second, the possibility that multiple interpretations may be applied to rules creates a kind of legal risk for regulators should official legal action be invoked (see also Hawkins and Thomas 1989). In theory, legal ambiguity opens up the possibility that both the prosecution and the defense can fit the facts and mold the rules in ways favorable to their interests; in practice, that advantage often falls to the defense attorneys, who as a rule have more resources to construct a substantive defense. Kenneth Mann's (1985) portrait of white-collar defense attorneys provides many examples in which defense attorneys who enter a case early are able to establish an evidentiary setting favorable to their clients. The case of *U.S. v. Chestman*, 947 F.2d 551 (2d Cir. 1991), is illustrative. In this case a stockbroker received a tip about a takeover from a relative of an insider and traded on the basis of that information. His attorney successfully maintained that the existence of family relationships does not necessarily give rise to a fiduciary duty. The appeals court dismissed the insider trading charges brought under Rule 10b-5. Although the Rule 14e-3 conviction was affirmed, the ruling offers a direct challenge to the regulatory program.

Third, ambiguity gives offenders moral justification for insider trading. In systematic study of white-collar offenders, Benson (1985) concluded that white-collar offenders used many of the techniques of neutralization that delinquents use to "excuse" their delinquent conduct (Sykes and Matza 1957). Tax violators and antitrust violators relied on the complexity of the law and historical traditions of moral ambiguity about "technical" violations to deny guilt. Normative ambiguity about the effect of insider trading, fueled by economists' assertions of its market efficiency, similarly may allow some offenders to deny that their actions are wrong.

Finally, imprecision can create structural pressures to test the limits of law. As discussed below, individuals and organizations in the securities business compete on the basis of information that they can provide for their clients. The success of securities firms and the career paths of their employees depend in large measure on their abilities to channel information in profitable directions. In the face of normative ambiguities about the role that valuable information *ought* to play in capital markets, competitive pressures on securities professionals will tend to push them to the margins of norms of practice.

II. Typical Patterned Violations

The insider trading violation is itself deceptively simple. A person obtains material, nonpublic information and trades securities on the basis of that information without disclosing to the opposite side of the transaction that he or she has that information. The complexity of the violation is associated with the circuitous route information might travel before it is exploited, from the mix of individual and organizational gains that might accrue, and from the cover-ups that might be involved.

The material, nonpublic information that has been the traditional focus of SEC enforcement includes information about a company's operations, assets, and liabilities that when made public may affect the price of a publicly traded stock. The landmark U.S. Supreme Court decision affirming the illegality of insider trading involved executives of Texas Gulf Sulphur Company who purchased significant quantities of their own stock before they made public their discovery of huge mineral deposits (*SEC v. Texas Gulf Sulphur Co.*, 107 U.S. 666 [1969]), material information that once disclosed could be expected positively to affect the company's assets and general financial health. Indeed, once the discovery was made public, the value of the stock shot up, and the executives made handsome profits. In some cases, self-dealing piggybacks other violations of the securities law such as falsifying financial records in an initial public offering and trading in the stock while in possession of material, nonpublic information.

The information chain that can be unlawfully exploited can be quite long and far removed from the corporate suites. In early 1991, the SEC filed a complaint against Robert H. Willis, the psychiatrist of Joan Weill, wife of Sanford Weill, the former chief executive officer of Shearson Loeb Rhodes. On two separate occasions, Willis apparently traded and tipped others to trade securities on the basis of information obtained from his patient (Securities and Exchange Commission 1991*b*).

In the 1980s, insider trading enforcement began to focus on material information regarding plans to merge or acquire companies. When a takeover bid is announced, the stock price of the targeted company often rises. This is because those who want to take over the company are generally willing to pay more than the market price for the stock to insure that they will obtain controlling interest. Advance information of a takeover permits a potential investor to buy the stock at a lower price before the takeover attempt is announced. Once the announcement is made, if the stock price rises, the stock can be resold for substantial profit.

The web of interorganizational relationships woven around deals to merge and acquire offers many possibilities for self-dealing insider information. The celebrated exchanges between investment bankers and Ivan Boesky, one of the "street's" most savvy arbitragers, are illustrative. Investment banker Dennis Levine traded inside information with arbitragers in exchange for intelligence about future clients and deals. According to some analysts, Levine passed tips about impending takeovers gratis to Boesky in hopes of obtaining another source for his information network (Stewart and Hertzberg 1986). Others have suggested that Levine was in awe of Boesky's wealth and wanted to be in his favor (Stevens 1987). Whatever the motivations, the flow of information between the two was allegedly extensive, one report suggesting as many as twenty contacts per day (Stewart and Hertzberg 1986). Boesky allegedly used this information to purchase large blocks of stock before the takeover attempt was made public and then sold the stock when the tender offer was announced. Boesky's unlawful trades were covered up by illegally "parking" the transaction with yet another brokerage firm. (Parking stock occurs when an investor, in this case the brokerage firm, buys stocks for another, in this case Boesky, who did not want to be identified as the owner.)

Less often, but perhaps more significant, insider trading has direct organizational dimensions; that is, it is committed with the implicit, if not explicit, support of the organization or is intended to advance the goals of an organization as well as its participants. In its simplest form, confidential information gleaned from clients is used unlawfully to bolster organizational profits. This was the case when Martin Siegel used inside information obtained from his activities as a takeover specialist to buttress Kidder Peabody's arbitrage profits. His unlawful actions "turned Kidder Peabody's arbitrage unit, virtually overnight, into one of the firm's principal profit centers" (Stewart and Hertzberg 1987, p. 1).

In other cases, organizational gains are achieved by exploiting the complex transactional environment of securities trading. When investment bankers leak confidential information to arbitragers in order to create strategic market swings for their clients they engage in this kind of interorganizational dealing. Just before Martin Marietta announced a counterbid against a takeover by Bendix Corporation, Martin Siegel, the investment banker leading Martin Marietta's defense, leaked the information to Boesky who purchased the Bendix stock (and subsequently sold it for a $120,000 profit). Boesky's purchase stoked demand for the Bendix stock, causing its price to rise and fueling a rumor that a raider was after the company. Faced with the possibility that it might itself be a takeover target, Bendix withdrew from its attack on Martin Marietta—a success for Siegel and his firm, Kidder Peabody. The SEC's case against Drexel Burnham Lambert, Inc., and Michael Milken further illustrates the general pattern. The core charges in the indictment were, in Milken's words, "reciprocal accommodations" he made with Boesky. Among other things, Milken was willing to pass along insider information to Boesky in order to put Drexel clients into "play." Drexel (Milken) and Boesky agreed to split any illegal profits that might accrue from the use of that information. Milken subsequently pled guilty to six felonies including conspiracy, stock parking, fraud, and the filing of a false document. He was sentenced to ten years in prison and ordered to pay a $600 million fine. (For more detailed accounts of these cases, see Stewart 1992.)

According to the U.S. Government Accounting Office (1988), 50 percent of the SEC's successful enforcement actions during the fiscal years of 1985 and 1986 involved unlawful trading prior to a tender offer. Review of litigation releases about insider trading from January 1, 1989, through September 30, 1991, suggests that this general trend continued through the end of the decade. There are some indicators, however, that trading insider information in advance of a takeover is declining. William R. McLucas, director of enforcement for the SEC, commented in 1992 that he saw more selling on bad news than buying in advance of a merger (*Securities Regulation Law Report* 1992). Research by Seyhun (1992) supports that position. He found that insider trading volume and profitability continued to increase during the 1980s, despite the increased regulatory focus. During that decade, however, insiders became less likely to trade before earnings announcements and announcements of corporate takeovers. He concludes that insider trading continues unabated but that insiders trade with information that is not currently restricted by case law.

III. Kinds of Violators

To get a better sense of what kinds of insiders have been identified as violators of insider trading rules, I reviewed the LEXIS data base for all SEC litigation releases between January 1, 1989, and October 15, 1991, that involved issues of insider trading. The litigation releases cover a wide range of SEC actions—for example, the filing of civil complaints, criminal actions, administrative hearings—and yet, because they cover only the most formal of SEC actions, may miss a great deal.

There appear to be three distinct types of insiders in the sample. The first type includes those who have direct access to inside information and take advantage of that special relationship. Traditionally, this group includes corporate insiders who owe a duty to their investors. But it also includes journalists and other service providers who have a special relationship to the market as a whole. The second type of insiders includes individuals who are related to the source of inside information and who take advantage of that special connection. This type is best represented by the family member who obtains information from an insider and breaks that confidence to trade for his or her own account. The psychiatrist who traded on information obtained from his patient fits within this category of offender as well. What is striking about the list of known violators is that people who are only remotely connected to the securities business can be so easily embroiled in its violation. The third type of offender includes individuals or organizations who broker information across the market. These individuals and organizations are the conduits of capital, responsible for generating market momentum. In the 1980s financial professionals involved in mergers and acquisitions were often at the forefront of the capital formation process and were well positioned to obtain and broker inside information that could be easily exploited. As noted above, the financial transactions that dominate the 1990s are likely to generate new sources of inside information and new networks for trading.

What separates those with access to that information who engage in unlawful trading from those who do not? What motivates people with money to steal so much more? Dennis Levine, in perhaps a self-serving account of his own motivation, describes his behavior in terms of the quest for action, a motivation not unlike the stickup men described by Jack Katz in *The Seductions of Crime* (1988). Levine describes his participation in insider trading as intoxicating: "Something deep inside me forced me to try to catch up to the pack of wheeler-dealers who always raced in front of me. . . . It was only in time that I came to view myself as an insider trading junkie. I was addicted to the excitement, the sense of victory. Some spouses use drugs, others have extramarital affairs, I secretly traded stocks" (Levine 1991 p. 390). Members of Michael Milken's investment community attribute similar motivation to his actions. He reportedly enjoyed the game, "got joy from the adrenaline, from the action" (Stone 1990, p. 45).

IV. The Context of Insider Trading: Deal-making Roles and Relationships

This section focuses on deal making in the securities business, the backdrop for most of the interorganizational forms of insider trading. "Deals" are the financial arrangements constructed to raise or restructure capital. They include a company's public offerings of stock, private placements (the sale of stocks, bonds, or other investments to institutional investors), mergers and acquisitions, and the sale of corporate debt. The investment banker whose job it is to mediate the flow of assets between those who want to sell and those who want to buy is at the center of all these transactions. Complex networks of relationships and information exchanges are formed to get the job done (Eccles and Crane 1988).

Unlawful insider trading occurs when actors, by virtue of their position in a deal-making network, become aware of material, nonpublic information and unlawfully trade or tip others to trade on the basis of that information. Deal-making networks and organizations within those networks become susceptible to this kind of corruption when the inside information they trade has personal or organizational value beyond the deal itself. When the unlawful trade or tip generates something more than its intrinsic dollar value—for example, future information, new clients, new investors, or even market momentum—insider trading takes on a decidedly organizational cast.

To appreciate the complexity of deal making around plans to merge and acquire companies and to underscore the vulnerabilities that develop, the following section outlines the roles and relationships that are most at risk of abusing the confidential information that is legitimately and routinely exchanged. This is followed by a discussion of the industry and organizational factors that make the securities business particularly susceptible to the organizational dimensions of unlawful trading. The thesis is advanced that deal making in the securities industry is constitutionally vulnerable to insider trading by virtue of the abstract, information-driven commodities it "produces," the complicated networks of transaction-oriented exchanges that organize "production," the changes in information technology that promote the free flow of information across jurisdictional (regulated) space, and the competitive drive to be on the "leading edge" of financial innovation.

A. The Structure of the Market

The securities industry is best understood as a confederation of markets where stocks, bonds, and other financial instruments are traded. Each market consists of loosely connected, differentiated service functionaries and institutions organized around the production and distribution of corporate ownership (stocks) and financial debt (bonds, commercial paper, etc.). Stocks are representations of proportionate ownership of an organization and of the right to share in the net proceeds from corporate activities. They are a corporation's promise of a future "piece of the action," given in return for an investor's willingness to provide capital today (Sharpe 1985). Corporations issue stock to raise capital. Investors engage in subsequent stock trading, that is, purchases and sales beyond the initial transaction, in the hope that the price of the stocks tomorrow will be greater than their purchase price today, yielding a financial return on their initial investment. An alternative approach to raising capital is for a company to issue a debt instrument. In effect, this means that corporations take out loans from collections of investors. In theory, debt differs from equity (stock) financing in two ways. First, principal and interest payments are formally obligated. Second, interest payments are considered expenses and can be deducted from a corporation's taxable profit.

In recent decades, lines between equity and debt have been obscured. Preferred stock, like debt, promises a designated rate of return that has priority over payment of dividends on common stocks. "Futures" are traded that create a contractual right to buy or sell a security at a set price at a later date. Many debt instruments come with options that permit their conversion into stocks or warrants that permit purchase of stocks at set prices. Debt instruments can be traded in secondary markets when, for example, they are packaged and sold as a kind of security. These permutations are nearly limitless.

The production and distribution of these financial instruments is the core industry task performed by complex networks of service providers. Securities firms may specialize in one or another of the highly differentiated tasks necessary to affect securities transactions. Some firms, for example, specialize in deal making (i.e., they put together the financing structure for a takeover or the prospectus for a new stock offering). Other so-called multiservice firms provide a full range of services connected to the distribution of stocks and bonds. At the periphery of the market are services and service providers that support the construction of the products (accountants, lawyers, insurance agents, financial printers, and the like) and functionaries who affect the distribution of their products (journalists, investors, arbitragers, and regulators).

B. The Power of Information

The securities market is largely a market of information and speculation—"a transactional world based on tipsterism, rumor, gossip, and eavesdropping" (Shapiro 1984, p. 88; but see also Rose 1966; Smith 1981). Trades are based on social understandings and evaluations of the current financial conditions of firms, currencies, debt, and other general economic indicators (Adler and Adler 1984, p. 85). Information, particularly that not generally known on the street, is a valuable commodity. To individual investors, good, accurate information, particularly that which is not generally known, can be the difference between their success or failure in the market. To an organization, effective information networks can be critically important for maintaining market share (Hayes, Spence, and Marks 1983; Eccles and Crane 1988). The more complete the information available to a firm, the better able it will be to sell its services, price its products, and, in general, position itself in the market. Diversification and product innovation, two important competitive strategies for securities firms, depend on key information that can be lawfully and unlawfully exchanged.

Corporate insiders have the best access to material, nonpublic information that can be exploited in unlawful trading. Insider information networks expand, however, when a firm goes outside either to the public or to private investors to raise capital. It is in these financing arrangements that one sees the organizational dimension of the violation.

When a firm decides to raise money through a public offering of securities or through the sale of debt, teams of outside consultants are called in to assist in the construction of those instruments. Investment bankers and their teams of financial professionals are obliged to conduct a formal investigation into issuing companies. These reviews are conducted to insure that the issuing company has sufficient accounting and management procedures to meet the additional reporting requirements of a public company and to insure that information provided in a security offering is accurate.[3] Case law establishes an investor's right

[3] Because of their role as mediator between issuers and investors, bankers often stand in an uneasy relationship with their clients. As one investment banker told me, "Entrepreneurs expect to give up some control of their company to their public shareholders.

to sue should losses arise because bankers failed to perform this important duty. Similarly, according to SEC Rule 2(e), lawyers, accountants, and other professionals who perform inadequate "due diligence" investigations, fail to comply with generally accepted accounting standards and practices, or fail to uncover and disclose material facts about an issuer can be suspended from future practice before the SEC. During the course of these reviews, these professionals gain access to information about their clients that, if publicly disclosed, might affect the trading price of the stock.

Inside information networks also expand during plans to merge and acquire. To acquire a company means to buy up substantial shares of the company's stock in order to achieve a "majority" position. To "do" these deals, investment bankers and their teams of professionals put together the details of the tender offer, provide tactical and strategic advice regarding proxy fights and antitrust implications, arrange for financing, and help execute the plan of attack (Bloch 1986; Hirsch 1986). Once again, investment bankers must probe into the financial and operational details of prospective merger targets and are likely to uncover information that is material to stock price.

Mergers and acquisitions, recapitalizations, and leveraged buy outs also must be financed.[4] Securities products or bonds are created and sold to raise the necessary capital. And, once again, inside information networks expand to get the job done. The financing of takeover activity in the 1980s was fueled by a new twist in underwriting practice, the use of junk bonds.[5] The junk bond market was largely a creation of Michael Milken, who ran the High Yield and Convertible Bond Department at Drexel Burnham Lambert from his Beverly Hills office. According to one analyst, Milken built the junk bond market as a "one of a kind" proprietary network at the margins of traditional investment banking (Bianco 1986). To nourish the market, he apparently dissemi-

---

What they don't expect is that they also give up control to the brigade of legal, accounting, and financial experts who must approve every step they now take."

[4] Leveraged buy outs are transactions in which investors borrow all or most of the funds needed to acquire a company with the expectation of repaying the debt plus interest from the cash flow of the acquired company.

[5] Junk bonds are corporate debt instruments that have been given low (below investment grade) credit ratings because they are perceived to have a high probability of default. To compensate for the greater risk involved, the yield on junk bonds is relatively high compared to safer debt instruments such as federal government bonds or debt instruments issued by financially sound companies. (For more detail, see the analysis by Worthy [1987].) Because traditional financial arrangements were not available to the many corporate raiders in the 1980s, they turned to alternatives, notably the junk bond market, to finance their transactions.

nated confidential deal information and helped clients conceal ownership of large blocks of stock. In short, insider trading helped hold his
market together.

Finally, corporate takeovers require a kind of market momentum.
Raiders must be able quickly and quietly to accumulate majority stock
positions or coalitions. Arbitragers and off-exchange traders can create
the necessary market swings that promote accumulation.[6] Arbitragers
try to profit from the difference between the market price and the offer
price for the stocks of companies involved in mergers, acquisitions,
and restructuring. They purchase the stock of the suspected takeover
company and wait until the takeover is announced. When the public
announcement is made, the stock goes up, and the arbitrager sells at a
substantial profit. Enormous profits that arbitragers sometimes gain
are derived from their extraordinary techniques for ferreting out information before it is publicly known. As long as arbitragers' timely action
is based on rumor, analysis of public information, and the like, the
trading is perfectly legal. Trading on the basis of explicit tips from
insiders is expressly prohibited.

The importance of arbitragers to takeovers lies in their ability and
willingness to take large positions in the market. Since arbitragers often
hold substantial numbers of shares of an outstanding issue, they can
be important assets to both parties as they attempt to build majority
stock positions. Investment bankers report that they are often "com-
pelled" to "talk to the arbs."

The possibilities for insider trading mirror the information and trading patterns generally found in the markets. New mechanisms for
raising capital (e.g., junk bonds, the securitization of debt, and the
like) generate new information dynamics and patterns of exchange that
can be exploited. Thus, while insider trading cases might be expected
to decline with a decline in merger and acquisition activity and increased enforcement attention, it is also reasonable to expect an increase in insider trading in other product areas. Indeed, the attention
of regulators has shifted to problems in the area of debt securities and
the internationalization of securities transactions (McLucas, DeToe,
and Colachis 1991; *Securities Regulation Law Report* 1992).

---

[6] Arbitrage generally means the practice of trading like articles in different markets
to profit from price discrepancies between them. If a stock was selling for one dollar on
the New York Stock Exchange and fifty cents on the Toronto exchange, an arbitrager
would take a position that would enable him or her to profit from that difference (i.e.,
buying on the Toronto exchange and selling on the New York Stock Exchange).

V. The Road to Scandal

While norms of fiduciary responsibility and fair trading combine with formal regulatory restraints (e.g., insider trading rules) to discourage players from taking unfair advantage of the information routinely provided to them, under some conditions, the engines of the market drive market participants to the boundaries of fair play, and beyond. Insider trading rules try to neutralize the advantage of being an insider, but, as any number of popular books about stock investing suggest, market profit means having an "edge," generating new ways to capture and take advantage of stock pricing, and finding new arenas of "action" that can excite money into motion. Markets, if they are to survive, must balance the push to innovate, to find new structural arrangements for making a profit, with regulations both formal and informal that promote stability and fair trade (Moran 1984; Stenning, Shearing, and Addario 1986).

Models of crime in financial markets must locate the behavior within this dynamic of the marketplace. Pfeffer and Salancik (1978) and Clinard and Yeager (1980) argue that "corporate behavior generally and violations in particular are attempts to manage the industry environmental conditions that businesses face" (Clinard and Yeager 1980, p. 50). Organizational theorists have long recognized the environment as a contingency of organizational action (Thompson 1967, elaborated by Vaughan 1983, 1992). More recently, organization theorists have taken the view that organizations interact with their environments—shaping as well as being shaped by them. (See, e.g., the essays in Mizruichi and Schwartz 1987.) They recognize that organizations are governed by rules and simultaneously transformed from within as actors adapt and reconstruct the rules that govern their life. (See Burk's [1988] description of regulated financial markets.)

Insider trading can be usefully understood using this conceptualization of "enacted" organizations. While environmental conditions cannot predict which actors or organizations are most likely to engage in rule-breaking behaviors, they provide a sense of the structural vulnerabilities, changing opportunities, and adaptations that enable such crime. I believe that the introduction of new forms of insider trading represented by the shift away from pure self-dealing to more organizationally focused crime must be understood within the context of changing structural arrangements that changed the characteristics of the market, the incentives for misconduct, and the distribution of power among potential players. To elaborate this argument, the following subsections examine the institutionalization of the market, the pressures to innovate, and the structural and cultural responses. The focus then narrows to the investment banking world of mergers and acquisitions, the source of a good deal of the interorganizational forms of insider trading most significant to this essay.

A. *Changing Informational Dynamics*

By definition, patterns of information exchange are the core of insider trading violations. To understand the emergence of insider trading as a form of organizational crime one needs to consider how the structures of information processing have changed. Two changes are particularly salient to contemporary accounts of insider trading: the institutionalization of the market and changes in the technologies for processing that information.

1. *Changing Demographics.* More individuals with expertise in seeking out and analyzing information have joined the markets. Throughout the 1980s, the number of persons involved in securities-related work grew rapidly. The number of persons employed in "security, commodities brokers, services" increased from 227,000 in 1980 to 449,000 in 1988, nearly a 100 percent increase (U.S. Bureau of the Census 1990). The number of securities and commodities establishments increased from 11,279 in 1980 to 18,843 in 1985, a 60 percent rise (U.S. Bureau of the Census 1988, p. 446). Each increase has had the effect of multiplying the number of information networks circulating on "the Street" (see Carrington 1986).

The deals securities professionals can talk about proliferated as well. In 1980, the estimated gross proceeds from primary security offerings exceeded $78 billion. In 1988 that number had increased more than two and one-half times to more than $219 billion (Standard and Poor's 1990, p. 20). In 1990, 3,663 mergers were completed compared with only 2,328 in 1981, a 57 percent increase (*Mergers and Acquisitions* 1991).

Players and their information needs also became more sophisticated. Institutional investors increasingly dominate the market. They have both the savvy and the expertise to take advantage of inside information that is seldom available to small individual investors. In 1952, the volume of stock trading accounted for by institutional investors was 30.8 percent compared with 69.2 percent for individuals. By 1969, the relative share of public trading by these two investor types had shifted; 55.9 percent of the trading was conducted by institutional investors while 44.1 percent of the trading was undertaken by individuals. By

1980, institutional traders had captured 65 percent of the market (Burk 1988). Individuals did not leave the market altogether. Rather, they became indirect stock owners through participation in mutual funds, pension plans, and the like. Nearly half of the U.S. households who own stock do so through mutual funds (Russell 1986).

The growth of these institutional players has enhanced the field of play for information brokers of all kinds. The institutionalization of the market means that there are now more concentrated, powerful outlets for manipulating and exploiting the market. Certainly, the concentration of market positions that institutional players represent makes it easier technically, if not morally, for someone casually to drop information in a few select places and reasonably expect that the market will move in a direction favorable to his or her position.

2. *New Information Technologies.*   Computers transformed the securities business. They increased the efficiencies of the back offices, the clerical parts of the operations. Advances in telecommunications also created global markets that make it as easy to trade on the Tokyo Exchange as on the New York Stock Exchange. They have also made it easy to create satellites and regional offices, even renegade offices, within firms.

Computerization makes the technical analyses and processing of insider trading possible. Computers help hide illegal profits and market positions. They facilitate the easy transfer of money to offshore bank accounts. Computers also make it easier to park stock—to hide its ownership.

But computers did more than simply change the efficiency of the market or its abuse. They altered the meaning of market and investment. The faster pace and aggregation that computerization allow adds new dimensions to investment decisions about how and when to invest. Because computerization allows stock market participants to move quickly into and out of the market, timing has become an ever more important variable in investment calculation, so important that investment managers are often willing to compromise on the old market standard, price (Light and Perold 1987). Arbitrage, Ivan Boesky's game, seems hardly possible on a large scale without these advanced technologies.

Finally, computerization changed enforcement of securities laws. Computerized surveillance systems have been adopted by the Securities and Exchange Commission, the New York Stock Exchange, and the National Association of Securities Dealers. Among other things, these systems track the price, trading volumes, and ownership of stocks traded in the market. Unusual trading patterns that might suggest illegality are flagged for further analysis. Most significant, computers provide a tool for connecting trades, public events, and traders.

B. Competitive Pressure and the Push to Innovate

The competitive dynamics have changed as new coalitions of players developed. Competition is important for understanding organizational crime not just because of the motivational strain and pressures it creates. (For analysis of the criminogenic nature of organizational strain, see Staw and Szwajkowski 1975 and Vaughan 1983.) The instability of competition can be exploited and often reproduced by deviant actors seeking to cross the boundaries of normative practice. Three sources of competitive tension in the securities markets during the 1980s changed the securities markets: public ownership of securities firms, negotiated fee structures, and increased client mobility in the 1980s. Each relates to a corresponding change in the distribution of power in the market and to changes in the normative structure of "doing deals." Each creates a new incentive for breaking the rules.

1. *Public Ownership of Securities Firms.*   The capital needs and profit potential of members of the New York Stock Exchange, the elite of the industry, were drastically changed in the 1960s and 1970s by the large size of the institutional trades and the increased trading volume that was being generated by them (Keenan 1979; Burk 1988; Poser 1990). The basic constraint facing brokerage firms was capital; firms needed more money to finance the large trades and to upgrade their back office operations, the accounting and clerical processes that facilitate trading. Thus, in the early 1970s the New York Stock Exchange relaxed its rule that prohibited public ownership of member firms. Diversification was often achieved through the merger of theretofore functionally distinct firms.

The increased size and diversified composition of the new firms influenced how power was distributed across the industry. It also changed how normative cultures were made to fit within firms. When investment banking was the province of an elite community of financiers, informal controls based on reputation and loyalty worked fairly well (Mayer 1955; Carosso 1970). Power was concentrated among groups of men who shared a common understanding of how far the rules prohibiting insider trading could be stretched. As corporate structure diversified, the power within a firm became more dispersed and fluid. Personalized forms of control lost some of their saliency. In the newly consolidated firms, multiple normative understandings, including some deviant ones, were forced to coexist.

2. *Negotiated Brokerage Commissions.*   The introduction of negotiated brokerage commission rates on "May Day" 1975 is generally believed to have altered the "economics" of investment banking and the fostering of competition. Prior to 1975, commission rates for all transactions were fixed across firms. After May 1, 1975, firms had to negotiate the terms of their commission for each transaction, thus opening up competition between firms on the basis of the commissions they charged for their service. Faced with sinking profits, brokerage firms unbundled their products and sought out new kinds of business that would generate substantial fees. Mergers and acquisitions activity, arbitrage, and junk bonds were three "products/services" that were assumed to be able to provide huge new sources of capital for an industry that "judged capital to be the decisive weapon for competing effectively in the global marketplace of the future" (Metz 1987, p. 27). Advisory fees and returns from investing capital in takeover stocks were much sought after.

3. *Client Shopping.*   Also, in the 1980s, securities firms involved in raising capital found for virtually the first time that they had to compete for clients. Hayes, Spence, and Marks (1983) show that overall in the period 1970–78 traditional investment banking leaders maintained a hold on most of their client bases, but an overwhelming perception exists that in the 1980s clients shopped around (Auletta 1986). To attract clients successfully, firms developed new products that at the very least brought customers in to talk (Eccles and Crane 1988, pp. 40–41). New conduits of information exchange and new coalitions of actors were created.

The connection between new products and expanded information networks is well illustrated by Drexel Burnham Lambert's annual Institutional Research Conference, the brainchild of Michael Milken. The event was also known as the "High Yield Bond Conference" or the "Predators Ball." It was a four-day affair, held in Beverly Hills (Milken's base of operations), close to the Academy Awards ceremony. Information about new bond offerings was made available, but, more important, bond buyers were given an opportunity to mingle with bond issuers. Confidential information exchange was facilitated, if not directly encouraged. "High-roller" money managers, institutional investors, corporate raiders, and even entertainment personalities were invited to attend. An invitation to the Predators Ball was a sure sign that you had made it in the mergers and acquisitions world (Stone 1990).

C. Organizational Structure

Organizational responses to changes in market environments may exacerbate the opportunity, if not the motivation, for the formation of *maverick*, and unlawful, networks for brokering information. The focus in this section is on the investment banks that generated the mergers and acquisitions deals.

Organizational structures are reflective of their environments (Chandler 1962). As noted above, deal making involves a highly differentiated, loosely coupled network of agencies and actors focused around the production of a deal product. The structure of their operations reflects the myriad sets of interests that must be accommodated in deal making. Eccles and Crane (1988) studied the design structure of investment banks, the coordinators of deal making. There are several critical design features that provide clues as to how organized insider trading can develop within the context of legitimate business operations. First, investment banks, and by extension securities firms, tend to be self-designing organizations. This means that there is a high degree of autonomy for people to determine how to organize units and relationships among units (Eccles and Crane 1988, chap. 6). Second, securities organizations tend to have dispersed authority structures in which the decision-making authority itself is "ambiguous, loose, flexible, and constantly changing. [Indeed,] it is not so much a hierarchy of authority as a network of relations" (Eccles and Crane 1987, p. 184). Management specialists argue that such loosely coupled sets of complex "information-oriented" relationships make traditional hierarchical control structures obsolescent. Third, as a rule, investment bankers are rewarded for how they manage the external financial environment and the profit taking that follows from that management. The relative value of maintaining external relationships compared to internal ones is illustrated by the fact that "movement up the hierarchy indicates professional competence and external client responsibility, rather than more authority for internal management" (Eccles and Crane 1987, p. 183). Reward structures (bonuses) are based on one's capacity to bring resources (profits, clients, etc.) into the firm.

While providing necessary flexibility in arenas of rapid change, flexible, flat, network forms of organization create a number of control problems. "Management in investment banking, particularly in the largest firms, can be described as a massive differentiation and integration problem because of the large number of specialists and the many interdependencies that exist among them" (Eccles and Crane 1988, p. 126). These problems are particularly acute when investment banking is just one of the many financial services offered by a particular company. Two types of control problems are noteworthy for the analysis of insider trading: weak or diffused normative control systems and conflicts of interest.

1. *Emergence of Deviant Subcultures (Lack of Normative Controls).* The autonomy afforded to individuals and organizational units creates a number of coordination problems for firms. In a classic statement of this problem, Lawrence and Lorsch note that "organizations faced with the requirement for both a high degree of differentiation and tight integration must develop *supplemental* integrating devices, such as individual coordinators, cross-unit teams, and even whole departments of individuals whose basic contribution is achieving integration among other groups" (1969, p. 13). Eccles and Crane (1988) describe relationship managers whose jobs are to coordinate the internal ties within firms. Coordinators do not necessarily provide normative guidance, however. As Vaughan (1983, p. 74) notes: "Though directed toward integrating the separate parts of the organization, the potential for rules and procedures to achieve internal coordination and control varies considerably." One factor influencing the efficacy of coordination is the relative power of the coordinator to the unit. Power generally means the ability to bring resources (clients and profits) to the firm. Powerful, that is, profitable, subunits that continue to make money for the firm tend to operate autonomously.[7] Deviant normative structures, if recognized at all, may simply be ignored as long as the firm continues to profit. This was apparently the case with Michael Milken's high-yield bond operation in Beverly Hills. Coworkers on the East Coast were essentially denied access to the operations. Management, if aware of some shady dealings, seemed content to look away (Stone 1990).

Normative controls over powerful subunits within securities firms, should they exist, are often extraorganizational. Indeed, one's reputation in the financial community has been an important source of control in investment banking. The new transactional environment, however,

---

[7] Clinard and Yeager (1980) and Gross (1980) argue that authority structures that isolate decision making often lead to less conformity with the rules because decisions are less open to organizational scrutiny.

lowers the efficacy of some of these personal forms of controls. External contacts between investment bankers and their clients are often instrumental and consequently are not likely to produce the collective conscience that would form some kind of internal social control. Loyalties are often to deals rather than to clients of firms. Most important, the interorganizational character of many deal-making transactions means that self-regulatory strategies grounded in organizational practice may be less effective.

2. *Conflicts of Interest.* The second control problem follows from the conflicts of interest that are an intractable component of highly differentiated organizational designs (Lawrence and Lorsch 1969) such as those that organize deal making. Conflicts of interest are particularly acute when the primary deal makers (investment banks and their agents) are housed within multiservice securities firms. Conflicts of interest occur "when two or more interests are legitimately present and competing or conflicting. The individual (or firm) making a decision that will affect those interests may have a larger stake in one of them than in the other(s), but he is expected—in fact, obligated—to serve each as if it were his own, regardless of his own actual stake" (Schotland 1980, p. 4). Although multiservice firms owe many duties to their clients, those most frequently discussed in the context of insider trading include the following: duties to keep investment clients' confidences (Restatement [second] of Agency, sec. 3295 [1958]); duties to the investing public to disclose or abstain from trading or recommending to trade securities on the basis of confidential information (requirement of SEC Rule 10b-5); and duties to firm customers to disclose, to know the "merchandise" in which it deals, and to deal fairly.[8] Conflict develops out of the competing duties to channel material information in particular, often diametrically opposite, directions, for example, both to maintain confidences and adequately disclose. It is the *competing uses of information*, not the mere possession, that generates the conflict.

To attend to the inherent conflicts of interest in multiservice firms, securities organizations have erected "Chinese walls"—invisible works of procedural architecture—that, in theory, organizationally separate conflicts of interest within the firm (Lipton and Mazur 1975; Doty and Powers 1988). Chinese walls are policies and procedures, reasonable

[8] This duty is based on the "shingle" theory of agency adopted by the SEC in the 1930s, which states that brokers/dealers, by "hanging out their shingles," have made implied representations that they would act fairly with the public.

under the circumstances, to ensure that unpublished, price sensitive information is not passed between departments.

A classic illustration of the conflict for which Chinese walls are built is found in *Slade v. Shearson, Hammill & Co.* (517 F.2d 398 [2d Cir. 1974]). Shearson's brokerage customers filed suit against the firm alleging that the defendant, in its capacity as investment banker to Tidal Marine Company, received adverse information about that company and yet continued to promote the sale of Tidal Marine stock to its retail clients. Shearson pressed for a summary judgment arguing that as a matter of law it was precluded from using material, nonpublic information obtained in one context to prevent solicitation of the purchase of Tidal Marine stock in another. Moreover, the defendant argued, a Chinese wall was in place to insure that such confidences were not inadvertently breached. In the ruling favoring the plaintiff, the district court agreed that Shearson was not permitted to reveal inside information about its investment clients but disagreed that the firm was prohibited from preventing the brokerage organization from soliciting business on the basis of public information that it knew to be false. Citing the U.S. Court of Appeals landmark decision, *SEC v. Texas Gulf Sulphur*, 107 U.S. 666 (1969), the district court in *Slade v. Shearson, Hammill & Co.* argued that, if corporate confidences precluded disclosure of adverse information, a securities firm must abstain from trading or recommending the affected securities. Shearson appealed. The U.S. Court of Appeals referred the case back for further fact-finding arguing that the implications of the case were so considerable that solutions to the conflict ought to be found in extrajudicial bodies (Wolfson 1980). A judicial resolution of this issue was never reached.

Despite its uncertain status as a defense against liability, the Chinese wall has become, through legislative action, a centerpiece of regulatory compliance for multiservice financial firms. Securities Exchange Commission Rule 14e-3, adopted in 1980, is an antifraud rule specific to insider information obtained in the tender offer context. Section b of that rule offers a safe harbor exclusion to firms that have established Chinese walls. The adopting release issued by the SEC states that "it may be appropriate to advise customers of its use of the Chinese Wall, because the institution would not be using all information that it received to the benefit of a particular customer."[9]

[9] Tender Offers, Final Rule, Release nos. 33-6239, 34-1720, 45 Fed. Reg. 60,410 (September 12, 1980).

D. Organizational Culture

Robert Jackall argues that the condition of work shapes moral consciousness. "The hierarchical authority structure that is the linchpin of bureaucracy dominates the way managers think about their world and about themselves" (1988, p. 17), including the moral rules-in-use that guide their behavior. Similarly, the structural conditions of deal making, that is, the competition, loose authority relations, and the need to cultivate information networks generally, influence the cultural rules that guide the behavior of deal makers. Most significant, the structure of deal making allows for, supports, and, in some instances, facilitates the construction of meaning systems favorable to rule violation, or, at the very least, favorable to blatant disregard for the rules systems and their agents. Studies of the organizational culture most manifest within the securities industry are rare. Popular accounts of a renegade morality are everywhere. While perhaps academically suspect, they provide a glimpse into the world of insider trading.

1. *Game Metaphors.*   Paul Hirsch (1986) describes the cultural significance of game metaphors in the business world. He argues that linguistic framing is one important way that actors can make sense of and normalize disruptive social relations. After analyzing the language used to describe hostile takeovers, Hirsch concludes that "without concrete terms, metaphors, and contexts in which to describe and interpret new unexpected events, it is unlikely that they [hostile takeovers] can become conceptualized as normal, routine, and acceptable forms of behavior" (1986, p. 821). Game metaphors neutralize the blatant disregard for order that hostile takeovers represent. Game metaphors are also used to normalize deviant activities. According to Dennis Levine, "All too often the Street seemed to be a giant Monopoly board, and this game-like attitude was clearly evident in our terminology. When a company was identified as an acquisition target we declared that it was 'in play.' We designated the playing pieces and strategies in whimsical terms: white knight, target, shark repellent, the Pac-Man defense, poison pill, greenmail, the golden parachute. Keeping a scorecard was easy—the winner was the one who finalized the most deals and took home the most money" (Levine 1991, p. 19). Game terminology helps to mask or neutralize the moral significance of one's action.

2. *Culture of Competition.*   Coleman (1987) describes how the culture of competition may provide some of the motivation for white-collar crime. Obviously, this includes pressure to be the best, to jump the furthest, to have the biggest bonus. To be on the top in the investment

world is to be a "player." Money is important to have, but more important is control.

One critical but not as obvious component of the culture of competition—the drive to get ahead—is the "pervasive sense of insecurity that has always been a powerful undercurrent in the culture of industrial capitalism" (Coleman 1987, p. 416). The "fear of falling" that Weisburd et al. (1991) describe as motivating at least some white-collar offenders seems particularly acute in the fast-paced world of contemporary securities trading.

3. *Alienation.* Some Wall Street "players" describe the knack of being able to "compartmentalize" their thoughts and to disassociate the "deal" details from particular operational concerns or from personal relationships. "The harassed dealmaker must be able to put Carnation here, Union Carbide there, RCA somewhere else. He must strictly segregate his motives in dealing with different suitors for the same company. Thus, he acquires the ability to compartmentalize making money from the fact that he may be stealing from his firm's own customers by so doing" (Stein 1987, pp. 16–22).

The ability to compartmentalize or to disassociate your actions from the effect those actions might have on individuals or firms has been made easier by the transactional nature of many interactions. No longer trusted advisors, some investment bankers see themselves simply as distributors of another person's product (Auletta 1986; Bianco 1986). The transactional character of the relationships between investment bankers and their clients (both issuers and investors) creates a kind of moral alienation. In this kind of environment, many of the rationalizations identified by Sykes and Matza (1957) as important supports for otherwise law-abiding individuals to engage in unlawful conduct flourish: " 'You gotta do it,' Levine told Wilkis [part of Levine's insider trading ring]. 'Everybody else is. Insider trading is part of the business. It's no different from working in a department store. You get a discount on clothes you buy. You work at a deli. You take home pastrami every night for free. It's the same thing as information on Wall Street.' [When Wilkis continued to balk, Levine said,] 'I know you want to help your mother and provide for your family. This is the way to do it. Don't be a schmuck. Nobody gets hurt' " (Frantz 1987, p. 64).[10]

[10] Frantz (1987) reconstructed conversations from interviews with the participants in the insider trading ring. Although the conversations might not represent the exact words spoken by each participant, Frantz argues that he used standard journalistic techniques

4. *Marginality.* It is noteworthy that many of the key players in the insider trading scandals were associated with the firm Drexel Burnham Lambert, Inc. Drexel was an important player but arguably the "bad boy" firm on the playing field. Drexel employees were acutely aware of their negative reputation (Welles 1987). To some extent, the firm cultivated its outsider image. Drexel employees ran against the tide. They were the "hardmen," the "badasses" of Wall Street. Stone's (1990) description of life at Drexel suggests that the firm set out to buck the system, to question the authority of Wall Street. One wonders, however, whether in cultivating this image, the firm simply went too far. In their own way, they created a culture of action, chaos, and control that Katz (1988) describes as typical of street robbers and stickup men.

5. *Moral Ambiguity.* Legal and economic debates abound over the moral and practical value of insider trading prohibitions. These are not merely academic exercises. They reflect a great deal of uncertainty by those who practice the craft of deal making about the wrongfulness of insider trading. Stanley Sporkin, formerly head of enforcement for the SEC, notes that the Reagan administration's deregulation agenda and laissez-faire attitude with respect to mergers sent out mixed signals that may have encouraged the insider trading scandals (Taub 1989). Moral ambiguity creates room for the construction of vocabularies of evasion— ways to say that the rules do not apply or do not apply to you. Consider this from one investment banker in Milken's shop: "All the people who worked for Michael Milken believed him to be honest, they think that the laws are wrong" (Stone 1990, p. 119).

VI. Structure of Governance

Insider trading captured the public's attention in the 1980s as a kind of public morality tale about greed on Wall Street. But public scrutiny is far from a precise indicator of the extent of unlawful insider trading. There are few data on incidence. Occasional newspaper accounts claim that it is widespread. Studies of enforcement activity (a problematic, yet practical, measure of incidence) are few and structurally flawed. A 1988 study by the General Accounting Office shows that SEC records reveal only fifty-three insider trading enforcement actions from 1934 through 1979. Over three times that number of cases (a total of 177

---

to insure the most accurate representation possible. Indeed, he says that "in nearly every instance, the dialogue represents the best recollection of at least one participant in the conversation" (Frantz 1987, p. 354).

cases) were brought in the next eight years (1980–87). In a 1992 interview with the *Securities Regulation and Law Report*, SEC Director of Enforcement William McLucas said that his office had brought more than thirty-five insider trading cases in each of the last three years ("39, 38, and last year maybe 43 cases") (*Securities Regulation and Law Report* 1992, p. 699). Litigation by the SEC is increasing generally. While the SEC litigation division had eight to ten lawyers some five or six years ago, SEC litigators now number seventeen and have some eighty to ninety cases in some stage of the litigation process (McLucas, quoted in *Securities Regulation and Law Report* 1992).

A. Mandate of Enforcement

Although state securities laws prohibit insider trading, the bulk of insider trading enforcement rests within the jurisdiction of the federal government, specifically the Securities and Exchange Commission and the U.S. attorneys' offices. Most of the nation's stock exchanges and self-regulatory agencies have prohibitions against insider trading and internal mechanisms for controlling abuse, but these are more limited in scope; they focus their attention only on transactions and parties connected to their particular trading forum or organization. Private actions may be undertaken in response to insider trading; for example, individuals harmed by insider trading may privately sue the violator.

The remainder of this essay focuses on the federal government's response to insider trading. The Securities and Exchange Commission has the "power to conduct investigations, discipline persons subject to its jurisdiction, initiate injunctive actions and refer cases to the Justice Department. One extremely important aspect of the Commission's enforcement program is its ability to seek ancillary remedies [e.g., disgorgement of illegal gains] from the federal courts in injunctive actions" (Ruder 1991, p. 610).

B. Detection

The first problem for regulators is detection. As Shapiro (1984) reports, the Securities and Exchange Commission has a wide range of detection mechanisms available to it. Tips, computerized market surveillance, inspections, and investigatory spin-offs are just some of the kinds of nets available to catch those unlawfully trading on insider information. Her study of enforcement from 1937 to 1977 disclosed that informants, market surveillance, and spin-offs yielded the most

SEC enforcement cases. Fifty percent of the insider trading cases were detected through these three methods. Although the period of her study does not correspond to the apparent surge in insider trading enforcement actions by the SEC, little written in the last decade suggests that this is any less true today.

Computerized surveillance systems have been adopted by the Securities and Exchange Commission, the New York Stock Exchange, and the National Association of Securities Dealers. These systems use statistical models to detect unusual patterns of activity that might reflect unlawful trading. Despite these kinds of technological advancements, accidental discovery continues to play an important role in regulation. In testimony before the Committee on Energy and Commerce, then–U.S. Attorney Rudolph Giuliani argued that the success of the case usually depends on getting someone to talk: "Because insider trading is so sophisticated and secretive, technical computer surveillance can only go so far in investigating crimes. In order to develop these cases effectively, information provided by other individuals who have relevant knowledge of the circumstances may prove essential" (U.S. House of Representatives 1988). It is noteworthy that the most celebrated violations discussed in the media of the eighties began with a tip from an anonymous source. The bounty program written into the Insider Trading and Securities Fraud Enforcement Act of 1988 explicitly recognized the importance of informants in insider trading cases. Not many informants have come forward out of the bounty program, however (*Securities Regulation Law Reporter* 1992).

C. Legal Action

The SEC can proceed against suspected violators in a number of ways, from administrative proceedings within the agency to civil and criminal proceedings in the federal courts.

1. *Criminal Prosecution.*   Insider trading can be criminally prosecuted under a number of penal statutes. The Insider Trading and Securities Fraud Enforcement Act of 1988 covers any person who "willfully" violates any provision of the Securities Exchange Act or a rule or regulation thereunder. Many charges of insider trading, particularly those involving misappropriation of information from one's employment, have been brought under mail and wire fraud statutes. Langevoort (1991) argues that the use of these statutes represents federal prosecutors' "familiarity with and confidence in these provisions as effective weapons against white-collar crime" (p. 268). A third stat-

ute, an emerging option for criminal prosecution of insider trading, is the Racketeer Influenced and Corrupt Organizations Act (RICO).

The SEC itself has no criminal enforcement authority but can refer cases to the U.S. attorneys' offices, which handle criminal prosecutions of insider trading cases. As Shapiro (1984, 1985) details, the path to criminal prosecution is complex, with many opportunities for cases to drop out. In Shapiro's (1985) sample of enforcement cases between 1937 and 1977, only 14 percent of the offenses that carried possible criminal penalties were referred to the Justice Department for criminal prosecution. In 1986, of the 298 enforcement actions (injunctions, administrative proceedings, and the like) only eighty-five (29 percent) were referred to the Justice Department for prosecution (Stern and Schilfrin 1987). To understand the "road not taken" (Shapiro 1985), one needs to consider the full range of remedial action that can be taken once an investigation reveals that some legal action is appropriate.

2. *Civil Remedies.*   Under the Securities and Exchange Act, the SEC can seek an injunction against any person or entity who they suspect has engaged or is about to engage in a violation of securities law. Injunctions are forward-looking remedies that do not carry direct penalties. They stipulate that further misconduct in violation of the law can be punishable by criminal contempt, itself a potential disqualification from further activity as a securities professional. Because the imposition of an injunction assumes some greedy disposition manifest in on-going behavior, it is applied to insider trading cases only when the trading is conducted over a long period of time and substantial monies are involved.

Civil injunctive action can require substantial changes in the structure and personnel of an offending organization. For example, in the case against Drexel Burnham Lambert, Inc., the terms of the settlement included, among other things, the transfer of the high-yield and convertible bond operation from California to New York, the appointment of new members to the board of directors who had no previous connection to the company, and SEC review of key personnel appointed by the firm (Securities and Exchange Commission 1989).

To penalize offenders for their misdeeds, the SEC may also seek ancillary remedies, typically disgorgement of profits illegally gained. In 1986, for example, the SEC obtained a $50 million disgorgement of illegal profits from Ivan Boesky. Money that has been disgorged is held in escrow, supervised by a trustee or receiver, for the benefit of those who have been harmed.

3. *Administrative Remedies.* Traditionally, a good portion of insider trading enforcement involves an administrative proceeding. Administrative remedies are available when the target of the SEC's enforcement efforts is a registered securities professional, that is, a person or organization with some kind of on-going relationship with the SEC. Included here are securities firms and their employees, stockbrokers and traders, investment advisors, and professionals (primarily accountants and lawyers) who practice before the commission.

Administrative actions are brought before an administrative judge whose sole function is to hear SEC matters. Although these judges are not subject to administrative control by the SEC, they are part of the SEC budget. The commission *staff* is technically the plaintiff in these hearings; the commission itself sits as a court of review. The rules of evidence follow administrative law guidelines and are far less restrictive than in criminal law proceedings. Often a great deal of evidence is presented. When there has been a finding of a violation, the judge might censure the professional, limit the actions of the respondent, or revoke a license: "A sizeable number of well-known insider trading cases . . . have arisen through administrative proceedings, and with the adoption of section 15 (f) [of the Securities and Exchange Act] requiring effective firm-wide supervisory procedures regarding non-public information for broker-dealer firms . . . the bases for such actions have expanded considerably" (Langevoort 1991, p. 276).

The reach of administrative proceedings has expanded with the passage of the 1990 Securities Enforcement Remedies and Penny Stock Reform Act. Under that act, cease and desist orders can be brought against any executive or employee in a company who "causes" a violation of the securities law either by negligence or by failure to perform an act. The act also gives the SEC power to seek monetary penalties in civil proceedings against violators and, most significant, gives the SEC the power to levy monetary penalties in administrative proceedings. Taken together, the provisions of this act give the SEC considerably more flexibility in enforcement actions. Rather than going to federal court, where the propensity to commit a crime must be established before injunctions and ancillary relief can be imposed, the commission can now handle the case administratively.

4. *Dilemmas of Enforcement.* Regulatory enforcement of the securities industry can be best described as a loosely coupled system of legal actions and remedies that combines aspects of prevention and deterrence. Administrative proceedings have traditionally been for-

ward-looking. They attempt to structure the environment, set standards, divert conflicts and neutralize the source of violations. Criminal proceedings are backward looking in the sense that they focus on the apprehension and sanctioning of violators in order to discourage future violations. Civil proceedings and the monetary penalties they can impose combine elements of both.

Adopting Shapiro's (1985) analysis of enforcement options for securities violations generally, we can speculate that the organizational attributes of insider trading violations will conduce to noncriminal enforcement of insider trading laws. Organizational embeddedness influences the access and type of evidence necessary to take legal action, the resources needed to pursue legal action, and the social control options available to regulators. As the examples cited above indicate, the direct evidence of illegal trades is often embedded in sophisticated inter-organizational networks that lie beyond traditional means of surveillance and information access. Organizations provide many avenues of cover-up; networks can be difficult to connect. In the face of these difficulties, administrative and civil proceedings that are more accommodating to indirect and circumstantial evidence gleaned from organizational records may be preferred over criminal action. (For a discussion of information rules and sanctioning choice, see Mann 1992.) Notwithstanding the difficulties of detection and evidence, the rigorous standards of evidence necessary for criminal prosecution require significant expenditures of regulatory resources that are not available. The entire SEC budget in 1986 was roughly equivalent to the $100 million fine imposed on Ivan Boesky. And, finally, when organizations are the violators, administrative and civil remedies may be preferred because those penalties are more likely to repair the damage without unnecessarily harming third parties, for example, the clients of securities firms who may be affected by criminal action that effectively "bankrupts" a firm.

As in other areas of organizational crime, criminal prosecution, when it does occur, may be explained in terms of regulatory failure, "a response to offenses that are discovered too late to prevent substantial harm" (Shapiro 1985, p. 199). Criminal prosecution is a forum of "last resort" used when other strategies for managing the environment are not deemed effective, that is, when business practices cannot be altered in ways to ensure compliance with regulatory rules. This is not to deny its significance in the regulatory program. Criminal prosecution can become a kind of "ceremonial production" that helps legitimate the commission's regulatory authority and the integrity of the market as a whole. In the area of environmental regulation, for example, Hawkins (1984) suggests that a good deal of what is criminally enforced in environmental regulatory regimes is not pollution "but deliberate or negligent law breaking that symbolically assaults the legitimacy of regulatory authority" (p. 205). The energy expended to prosecute notorious instances of insider trading in the 1980s may be explained in this way. Among their many misdeeds, the investment bankers caught up in the Wall Street scandals threatened the traditional power structures of Wall Street: "The country's corporate elite disliked Drexel for a simple reason: The firm was sticking its nose where it didn't belong. Investment bankers were supposed to give advice, gentlemen to gentlemen, on financing and friendly acquisitions; they were supposed to be charming, well bred, and low handicapped. They weren't supposed to raise money for hostile takeover artists. And they sure as hell weren't supposed to think up hostile takeovers and then go looking for someone to replace current managers" (Stone 1990, p. 35). One might hypothesize, then, that criminal prosecution of insider trading was less enforcement of securities law than prosecution of those who appeared to be shaking up the power on "the Street."

5. *Self Regulation.* The Insider Trading and Securities Fraud Enforcement Act of 1988 requires securities firms to "establish, maintain, and enforce written policies and procedures reasonably designed to prevent the misuse of . . . material, nonpublic information." As noted earlier, in many firms this means the construction of Chinese walls, procedural architecture that separates information collection and analysis from its sale, trade, or both. The failure to erect Chinese walls is unlawful and subject to civil and criminal liability. The National Association of Securities Dealers (NASD) has added its regulatory support to the adoption of Chinese walls. In addition, NASD recommends requiring firms to conduct routine audits of policy compliance and to maintain records substantiating such reviews.

Despite achieving official status in the regulatory programs of the SEC and NASD, there have been no regulations establishing the minimum criteria for Chinese wall construction. Commentators (e.g., Doty and Powers 1988; Poser 1990) have proposed that firms constructing Chinese walls create separate organizational structures for functionally distinct units (whether this means separate subsidiaries or simply separate divisions is not clear; there is near consensus that, at the least, separate books and records should be maintained; physical separation between units is also advised and access to unit files must be restricted). Other standard proposals include separate compensation systems: compensation in one division should not be linked to the results that might be obtained by another division, audit systems for monitoring the telephone calls across Chinese walls, and restrictions on transfers of personnel across the wall.

While Chinese walls may organizationally separate potential conflicts, they certainly are not impregnable and may be breached for entirely proper reasons. As described by Poser (1990), the SEC's insider trading case against First Boston Corporation (in 1986) demonstrates the complexity of the issue. The first hole in the wall was driven when a member of the firm's Corporate Finance Division gave a research analyst information about an impending announcement concerning a corporate client. This violation of the wall was entirely proper, according to Poser (1990, p. 112), because the corporate finance department needed advice from the analyst on the likely impact of the announcement. The trouble came to First Boston when the wall was crossed a second time. This second crossing occurred when the analyst gave confidential information about the announcement to First Boston's equity trader, who used that information to trade for the firm's proprietary account.

Most significant, these forms of intraorganizational self-regulation are limited because they do little to change the motives and enabling structures for insider trading. When information is brokered across markets and professional contexts, intracorporate controls are not likely to be effective. Self-regulatory strategies that are market rather than organizationally based may offer better controls.

VII. Conclusions

Inside information is a valuable commodity in the securities market. To have inside information is to have an insight into future stock performance. Insider trading rules are designed to limit the advantages that insiders naturally have in the market so that outsiders feel free to participate. Nonetheless, a certain amount of insider abuse appears to be a constant feature of the marketplace.

This essay suggests that patterns of abuse mirror the changing markets for financial information. Insider trading behavior is part of a dynamic market environment in which innovative ways of raising capital are required for success and survival. Regulations are continually adapted to insure a level of stability in the face of the constant push for innovation. Together the push to innovate and the requirement for regulation expand the demand for new sources of information. As information needs expand or change so do the avenues for abuse.

Insider trading uncovered in the mid-1980s provides the backdrop for understanding both the changing dimensions of the behavior and the structural and cultural vulnerabilities to new forms of abuse. I have suggested that the organizational forms of insider trading that appeared in the 1980s developed out of a changing securities market. New information technologies brought new product possibilities and added new dimensions to investment decisions. Markets became connected as never before. The outlets for exchanging inside information unlawfully increased as the capacity to move and hide information and money became easier.

Changing demographics in the market also enabled new forms of abuse. The continuing institutionalization of the markets combined with increased regulation to bring new kinds of professionals into the market. Information networks expanded to include these new roles and relationships. As the markets became more institutional and professionalized, they appeared more impersonal, technical, and abstract. Reputation and other forms of personalized social control lost some of their effect in controlling abuse.

Organizational adaptations to the changing informational needs enabled abuse, as investment banks, in particular, developed flexible organizational structures to respond quickly to changing product needs. In these self-designing organizations coordination and control were constant problems not easily solved through hierarchies of rules and procedures. Normative controls where they existed were often extraorganizational.

The changed market environment created new incentives as well as new avenues for abuse. Competitive pressures in the securities markets created demands for new products and services that had to be sold to clients who themselves were beginning to shop around. Information, particularly valuable nonpublic information, became an important commodity used to attract new business. As competition signaled the loss of income streams or position in existing systems of firm stratification, pressures to operate at the margins, that is, to take regulatory risks, increased as well. The fear of falling behind in the fast-paced, roller coaster world of securities trading was apparently a strong motivator for engaging in deviant behavior. Ever-changing interpretations of the substance and scope of securities laws further encouraged actors to take legal risks.

The culture of securities work continued to support the formation of deviant subcultures. Sporting metaphors dominated trading practices. The market and its regulation were seen by participants as contests or challenges. Individuals were rewarded for pitting their wits against the system. Inside information was a valuable piece of equipment in this game.

The pressures to engage in insider trading were not balanced by a strong system of control. Organizational controls are problematic in arenas where conflicts of interest are endemic and where so much activity is directed outside the organization or crosses organizational boundaries. Market controls were limited as well. Despite technological advances in market surveillance and an increase in enforcement actions during the 1980s, the regulation of financial transactions appeared to be losing ground. Trading volume more than tripled and the number of brokers/dealers doubled during the same period. The regulatory apparatus simply did not have the flexibility afforded to traders.

The analysis offered above suggests that we must begin to build dynamic models of organizational crime that recognize organizational capabilities to adapt to regulatory environments and to shape the regulatory apparatus that governs their behavior. The observation that insider traders have moved the locus of their work from trades around mergers and acquisitions to trades elsewhere seems to reflect this. There is an important dynamic to insider trading and organizational crime in general that can be missed by static models of organizational behavior.

REFERENCES

Adler, Patricia, and Peter Adler, eds. 1984. *The Social Dynamics of Financial Markets*. Greenwich, Conn.: JAI Press.

Auerbach, Joseph, and Samuel Hayes III. 1986. *Investment Banking and Diligence—What Price Deregulation?* Cambridge, Mass.: Harvard University Press.

Auletta, Ken. 1986. *Greed and Glory on Wall Street: The Fall of the House of Lehman*. New York: Warner Books.

Beck-Dudley, Caryn L., and Alan A. Stephens. 1989. "The Efficient Market and Insider Trading: Are We Headed in the Right Direction?" *American Business Law Journal* 27:441–65.

Benson, Michael L. 1985. "Denying the Guilty Mind." *Criminology* 23:583–607.

Bianco, Anthony. 1986. "The Power on Wall Street." *Business Week* (July 7), pp. 56–62.

Bloch, Ernest. 1986. *Inside Investment Banking*. Homewood, Ill.: Dow Jones-Irwin.

Burk, James. 1988. *Values in the Marketplace: The American Stock Market under Federal Securities Laws*. New York: de Gruyter.

Carosso, Vincent P. 1970. *Investment Banking in America*. Cambridge, Mass.: Harvard University Press.

Carrington, Tim. 1986. "Arbitragers, Investment Bankers Increasingly Rely on Each Other." *Wall Street Journal* (May 23), p. 8.

Chandler, Alfred. 1962. *Strategy and Structure: Chapters in the History of Industrial Enterprise*. Cambridge, Mass.: MIT Press.

Clinard, Marshall, and Peter C. Yeager. 1980. *Corporate Crime*. New York: Free Press.

Coffee, John, Jr. 1988. "Hush! The Criminal Status of Confidential Information after *McNally* and *Carpenter* and the Enduring Problem of Overcriminalization." *American Criminal Law Review* 26(1):121–54.

Coleman, James W. 1987. "Toward an Integrated Theory of White Collar Crime." *American Journal of Sociology* 93:406–39.

Doty, James R., and David N. Powers. 1988. "Chinese Walls: The Transformation of a Good Business Practice." *American Criminal Law Review* 26: 155–79.

Eccles, Robert G., and Dwight B. Crane. 1987. "Managing through Networks in Investment Banking." *California Management Review* 30(1):176–95.

———. 1988. *Doing Deals*. Cambridge, Mass.: Harvard University Press.

Ferrara, Ralph C., and Robert E. Dozier. 1988. "Prohibiting and Preventing Insider Trading." Study materials prepared for the American Law Institute–American Bar Association course held in Washington, D.C., February 25–26. Philadelphia: American Law Institute–American Bar Association Committee on Continuing Education.

Frantz, Douglas. 1987. *Levine and Co.: Wall Street's Insider Trading Scandal*. New York: Holt.

Gross, Edward. 1980. "Organizational Structure and Organizational Crime." In *White Collar Crime: Theory and Organization*, edited by G. Geis and E. Stotland. Beverly Hills, Calif.: Sage.

Hawkins, Keith. 1984. *Environment and Enforcement: Regulation and the Social Definition of Pollution*. Oxford: Clarendon.

Hawkins, Keith, and John Thomas, eds. 1989. *Making Regulatory Policy*. Pittsburgh: University of Pittsburgh Press.

Hayes, Samuel, III, A. Michael Spence, and David Van Praag Marks. 1983.

Competition in the Investment Banking Industry. Cambridge, Mass.: Harvard University Press.

Herlihy, Edward. 1987. "Chinese Walls and Insider Trading: How Well Does Self-policing Work?" *National Law Journal* (May 18), pp. 39–49.

Hirsch, Paul. 1986. "From Ambushes to Golden Parachutes: Corporate Takeovers as an Instance of Cultural Framing and Institutional Integration." *American Journal of Sociology* 91:800–37.

Jackall, Robert. 1988. *Moral Mazes.* New York: Oxford University Press.

Katz, Jack. 1988. *The Seductions of Crime.* New York: Basic.

Keenan, Michael. 1979. "The Scope of Deregulation in the Securities Industry." In *The Deregulation of the Banking and Securities Industries,* edited by Lawrence G. Goldberg and Lawrence J. White. Lexington, Mass.: Lexington.

Langevoort, Donald C. 1991. *Insider Trading Regulation.* New York: Clark Boardman.

Lawrence, Paul R., and Jay W. Lorsch. 1969. *Developing Organizations: Diagnosis and Action.* Reading, Mass.: Addison-Wesley.

Levine, Dennis B. 1991. *Inside Out: An Insider's Account of Wall Street.* New York: Putnam.

Light, Jay O., and Andre F. Perold. 1987. "The Institutionalization of Wealth: Changing Patterns of Investment Decision Making." In *Wall Street and Regulation,* edited by Samuel L. Hayes III. Boston: Harvard Business School Press.

Lipton, Martin, and Robert B. Mazur. 1975. "The Chinese Wall Solution to the Conflict Problems in Securities Firms." *New York Law Review* 50(3):459–511.

McLucas, William R., Stephen M. DeToe, and Arian Colachis. 1991. "SEC Enforcement: A Look at Current Programs and Some Thoughts about the 1990s." *Business Lawyer* 46(3):797–848.

Mann, Kenneth. 1985. *Defending White Collar Crime: A Portrait of Attorneys at Work.* New Haven, Conn.: Yale University Press.

———. 1992. "Procedural Rules and Information Control: Gaining Leverage over White Collar Crime." In *White Collar Crime Reconsidered,* edited by K. Schlegel and D. Weisburd. Boston: Northeastern University Press.

Manne, Henry. 1966. *Insider Trading and the Stock Market.* New York: Free Press.

Mayer, Martin. 1955. *Wall Street: Men and Money.* New York: Collier.

Mergers and Acquisitions. 1991. "1990 Profile." *Mergers and Acquisitions* (May/June), p. 13.

Metz, Tim. 1987. "Trading Abuses Run Deep on Wall Street." *Wall Street Journal* (February 17), p. 27.

Mizruichi, Mark S., and Michael Schwartz, eds. 1987. *Intercorporate Relations: The Structural Analysis of Business.* New York: Cambridge University Press.

Moran, Michael. 1984. *The Politics of Banking: The Strange Case of Competition and Credit Control.* New York: St. Martin's.

Parsons, David. 1987. "The SEC and Foster Winans: Different Perspectives on Financial Fraud." Paper presented at the annual meeting of the Law and Society Association, Washington, D.C., June.

Pfeffer, Jeffrey, and Gerald R. Salancik. 1978. *The External Control of Organizations: A Resource Dependence Perspective.* New York: Harper & Row.

Poser, Norman S. 1990. "Conflicts of Interest within Securities Firms." *Brooklyn Journal of International Law* 16(1):111–23.

Rose, Arnold. 1966. "A Social Psychological Approach to the Study of the Stock Market." *Kyklos* 19:267–87.

Ruder, David S. 1991. "SEC Enforcement Practice." *Northwestern University Law Review* 85(3):607–12.

Russell, George. 1986. "Manic Market." *Time* (November 10), pp. 64–70.

Schotland, Roy A. 1980. "Introduction." In *Abuse on Wall Street: Conflicts of Interest in the Securities Market—Report to the Twentieth Century Fund Steering Committee on Conflicts of Interest in the Securities Market.* Westport, Conn.: Quorum.

Securities and Exchange Commission. 1989. "Securities and Exchange Commisson v. Drexel Burnham Lambert, Inc., Drexel Burnham Lambert Group In., et al. 88 CIV 6209 (MP) (SDNY 1988)." Securities and Exchange Commission Litigation Release no. 12061, April 13. New York: Securities and Exchange Commission.

———. 1991*a*. "Securities and Exchange Commisson v. Anthony R. Tavani, 91, CIV 3541 (DNE) USDC SDNY." Securities and Exchange Commission Litigation Release no. 12865, May 28. New York: Securities and Exchange Commission.

———. 1991*b*. "Securities and Exchange Commission v. Robert H. Willis, Martin B. Sloate, Howard Kane, and Kenneth Stein, 91 CIV 0322 (WCC) (USDC SDNY)." Securities and Exchange Commission Litigation Release no. 12754, January 14. New York: Securities and Exchange Commission.

Securities Regulation Law Report. 1992. "McLucas Says Remedies Act Could Mean More Good Soldier Cases." *Securities Regulation Law Report* 24(19): 694–701.

Seyhun, H. Nejat. 1992. "The Effectiveness of the Insider-Trading Sanctions." *Journal of Law and Economics* 35:149–82.

Shapiro, Susan P. 1984. *Wayward Capitalists: Targets of the SEC.* New Haven, Conn.: Yale University Press.

———. 1985. "The Road Not Taken: The Elusive Path to Criminal Prosecution for White Collar Offenders." *Law and Society Review* 19:179–218.

———. 1987. "The Social Control of Impersonal Trust." *American Journal of Sociology* 93:623–58.

Sharpe, William F. 1985. *Investments.* Englewood Cliffs, N.J.: Prentice-Hall.

Smith, C. W. 1981. *The Mind of the Market.* Totowa, N.J.: Rowman & Littlefield.

Standard and Poor's Statistical Service. 1990. *Basic Statistics: Banking and Finance.* New York: Standard and Poor's Corporation.

Staw, B. M., and E. Szwajkowski. 1975. "The Scarcity Munificence Component of Organizational Environments and the Commission of Illegal Acts." *Administrative Science Quarterly* 20:345–54.

Stein, Benjamin. 1987. "The Reason Why: What Motivated the Insiders." *Barron's* (February 23), pp. 16, 22.

Stenning, Philip, Clifford Shearing, and Susan Addario. 1986. "Insider Policing: Securing Compliance and Monitoring Trust in a Financial Market." Unpublished paper. Toronto: University of Toronto, Centre of Criminology.

Stern, Richard L., and Matthew Schilfrin. 1987. "Crime Wave." *Forbes* 139(14):67–70.

Stevens, Mark. 1987. *The Insiders: The Truth behind the Scandal Rocking Wall Street*. New York: Putnam.

Stewart, James B. 1992. *Den of Thieves*. New York: Simon & Schuster.

Stewart, James B., and Daniel Hertzberg. 1986. "Fall of Ivan F. Boesky Leads to Broader Probe of Insider Information." *Wall Street Journal* (November 17), p. 1.

———. 1987. "The Wall Street Career of Martin Siegel Was a Dream Gone Wrong." *Wall Street Journal* (February 17), p. 1.

Stone, Dan G. 1990. *April Fools: An Insiders' Account of the Rise and Fall of Drexel Burnham*. New York: Donald Fine Company.

Sykes, Gresham, and David Matza. 1957. "Techniques of Neutralization: A Theory of Delinquency." *American Sociological Review* 22:664–70.

Szockyj, Elizabeth. 1990. "The Inside Story of Insider Trading: The Genesis of a Social Problem." Paper presented at the forty-second annual meeting of the American Society of Criminology, Baltimore, November.

Taub, Stephen. 1989. "The Shootist: Stanley Sporkin Would Shake Up and Shape Up the Markets." *Financial World* 158(9):30–31.

Thompson, James. 1967. *Organizations in Action*. New York: McGraw-Hill.

Tidwell, Gary L., and Abdul Aziz. 1988. "Insider Trading: How Well Do You Understand the Current Status of the Law?" *California Management Review* 30(4):115–23.

Tomasic, Roman, and Brendan Pentony. 1989. "Insider Trading and Business Ethics." *Legal Studies Forum* 8(2):151–69.

U.S. Bureau of the Census. 1988. *Statistical Abstract of the United States, 1988*. Washington, D.C.: U.S. Government Printing Office.

———. 1990. *Statistical Abstract of the United States, 1990*. Washington, D.C.: U.S. Government Printing Office.

U.S. General Accounting Office. 1988. *Securities Regulation: Efforts to Detect, Investigate and Deter Insider Trading*. Washington, D.C.: U.S. General Accounting Office.

U.S. House of Representatives. 1988. *Insider Trading and Securities Fraud Enforcement Act of 1988*. 100th Cong., 2d Sess. Report 100-910. Washington, D.C.: U.S. Government Printing Office.

Vaughan, Diane. 1983. *Controlling Unlawful Organizational Behavior*. Chicago: University of Chicago Press.

———. 1992. "The Micro-Macro Connection." In *White Collar Crime Reconsidered*, edited by Kip Schlegel and David Weisburd. Boston: Northeastern University Press.

Weisburd, David, Stanton Wheeler, Elan Waring, and Nancy Bode. 1991. *Crimes of the Middle Classes: White Collar Offenders in the Federal Courts.* New Haven, Conn.: Yale University Press.

Welles, Chris. 1987. "The Case against Drexel: Will the Government Come Up Short?" *Business Week* (August 10), pp. 56–60.

Winans, R. Foster. 1986. *Trading Secrets: Seduction and Scandal at the Wall Street Journal.* New York: St. Martin's.

Wolfson, Nicholas. 1980. "Investment Banking." In *Abuse on Wall Street: Conflicts of Interest in the Securities Market—Report to the Twentieth Century Fund Steering Committee on Conflicts of Interest in the Securities Market.* Westport, Conn.: Quorum.

Worthy, Ford S. 1987. "The Coming Defaults in Junk Bonds." *Fortune* (March 16), pp. 26–34.

Peter Cleary Yeager

Industrial Water Pollution

ABSTRACT

Twenty years' experience with Environmental Protection Agency efforts
to enforce the 1972 Clean Water Act's controls on water pollution have
demonstrated the scientific, bureaucratic, political, and organizational
complexities of regulating industrial organizations. Industrial
representatives play much more active and influential roles in standard
setting and rule enforcement than do environmental and other public
interest groups. Political ideology and political influence play an
important role in the process. Enforcement efforts have relied more on
consensual and negotiative strategies than on deterrent and civil or
criminal law enforcement strategies. This results from trade-offs between
concerns for economic viability and public benefit, from the ability of
large organizations to deploy human and financial capital, from
insufficient funding of environmental regulatory agencies, and from
scientific uncertainties about appropriate standards and feasible
amelioration methods.

On October 5, 1976, the U.S. government fined the large, multinational Allied Chemical Corporation $13.24 million for criminal discharges of the toxic pesticide Kepone and other chemicals into Virginia's James River.[1] Not only was this single fine greater than the

Peter Cleary Yeager is associate professor of sociology, Boston University. He is
grateful to Kathy Kram (as always), to Jason Kram Yeager (for patience beyond his
years), and Gary Reed (for his spirited assistance); to Albert J. Reiss, Jr., for his keen
analytic and editorial eye; and to Michael Tonry for his encouragement and patience.
He acknowledges the gracious and civic-minded assistance of officials at the U.S. Environmental Protection Agency, the Department of Justice, Congress, and the U.S. General Accounting Office. Naturally, the views and any errors found in this essay are the
author's responsibility alone.

[1] The court later reduced the fine to $5.24 million when Allied Chemical agreed to
donate $8 million to a new, nonprofit corporation that would fund research projects and

total fines and penalties imposed in all other cases initiated by the Environmental Protection Agency (EPA) to that date (through September 1976), but only seven years earlier neither criminal fines nor civil penalties were part of the federal government's general response to the increasingly threatening environmental degradation resulting from water pollution.[2]

Seven years later the EPA's regulatory program was in disarray. Weakened by deep budget cuts and directed by a leadership eager to relieve industry of regulatory costs, the agency's enforcement efforts were in serious decline in all areas of environmental protection. This was a result of the Reagan administration's wide-ranging policy to free private enterprise from public regulation as part of a "supply-side" strategy to stimulate economic growth. But the results proved more dramatic at EPA than in any other regulatory arena. By early 1983 the agency was enmeshed in public scandal amid charges that its rule making and enforcement had become corrupted by a pattern of secret negotiations with industry representatives and improper influence exerted from the upper reaches of the Executive Branch (Yeager 1991, pp. 227–30, 312–20). By April most of the president's appointees to leadership positions in the agency, including top administrator Anne Burford, had resigned under fire as the administration sought to limit the political damage occasioned by the revelations.

If the relatively aggressive prosecution of the Allied Chemical case did not represent the government's typical enforcement vigor in the 1970s (criminal prosecutions were very uncommon, multimillion dollar fines very rare), neither did the administration's efforts to deregulate the economy in the 1980s signal the end of environmental controls. Indeed, by the 1990s another Republican administration was heralding its commitment to stiffened prosecution of environmental crimes, a claim generally supported by developments in law and by Justice Department data on criminal cases (e.g., Moretz 1990; Adler and Lord 1991; Starr 1991; Strock 1991; Thornburgh 1991).

These substantial policy shifts and reversals over the relatively short span of twenty years indicate the volatility in the environmental regula-

---

implement remedial activities to mitigate Kepone damage. This had the effect of reducing the true, after-tax cost of the penalty by about $4 million, since Allied was able to claim the donation as a tax-deductible expense. The company also made a contribution to fund Kepone-related medical research and paid some of the cleanup costs, and in 1977 it faced more than twenty lawsuits for health-related damages, one of them a class action seeking more than $26 billion (Yeager 1991, p. 1).

[2] See, e.g., U.S. Environmental Protection Agency (1977, p. 1).

tion of business as the state—through law—endeavors to balance the tensions between economic growth and environmental protection. The instability and tension also underscore the importance of key processes that commonly attend the legal regulation of corporate behavior. Because regulation constrains profit, such legal controls are beset by a certain moral ambiguity as values underlying concerns for consumer, environmental, and worker protection compete with those of economic growth and well-being. As a result, such regulatory lawmaking often requires careful public deliberation at all of its phases to determine the appropriate balances, certainly in democratic, rule-of-law societies. But such deliberations often prove difficult to provide, especially when complex legal processes combine with a virtual industry monopoly on the necessary technical information to screen out the voices of wider public interests.

To the extent that formally neutral, egalitarian legal procedures advantage some policy influences over others, regulatory processes are central to shaping patterns of compliance and lawbreaking by businesses. In other words, the analysis of regulatory compliance requires a precise understanding of *law* as much as it does an understanding of the compliance orientations of regulated populations.[3] Indeed, it is the thesis of this essay that regulatory law and compliance are so systemically intertwined that neither can be understood without understanding both. This is surely the case with environmental protection law, an area of regulation that—for all its limitations—receives wide and consistent public support, including that of business leaders.[4]

To make this series of arguments, the essay focuses on the federal regulation of industrial water pollution. The case illustrates several processes that commonly attend the legal regulation of business, particularly where complex rule-making procedures aim at controlling the industrial processes of often powerful corporate organizations (Stryker 1991). Here I have in mind the processes of negotiation and discretionary regulation and enforcement that shape both law and patterns of compliance and offending. These processes are contingent on factors

[3] For a more detailed development of this general argument, see Yeager (1993).

[4] Survey data continue to demonstrate wide support for environmental protection. For example, a recent survey of citizens and 500 executives from large companies found that both groups viewed corporate environmental crimes as serious illegalities (Stipp 1992). While a greater percentage (75) of the public sample felt executives should be held personally liable for such offenses, it is noteworthy that 49 percent of the sampled executives agreed with this proposition. In general, these views represent a dramatic cultural shift in post–World War II American life, a shift that both shapes and reflects legal developments during this period.

such as political and economic climates and the relative resources of the parties involved, including government, businesses, and the public. But the effects of such factors tend not to be random. Rather, such legal processes tend to privilege the views and behaviors of more powerful and organized parties in the regulatory effort, in much the same way (and for many of the same reasons) as Galanter (1974) has identified in civil litigation. The result is not merely a gap between the "law-in-the-books" and the "law-in-action," long ago noted by the legal realists, but a systematically distorted gap that skews and limits regulatory outcomes in characteristic patterns.

While representative of regulatory processes, the regulation of industrial water pollution manifests its own special characteristics, differentiating its processes and outcomes to some extent even from those in other areas of environmental law, such as the efforts to control air and solid waste pollution. This is because the terms of environmental statutes covering air, water, and ground pollution structure regulation and enforcement differently, with the consequence that these laws differentially shape the dynamics not only of legal processes but also of compliance (Marcus 1980; Yeager 1991, pp. 191–202). Adequate explanations of the patterns of offending and sanctioning vary accordingly, requiring close specification of underlying legal logics that shape and constrain these patterns. In short, what is common to much complex regulation is the privileging of select voices and general tendencies toward systematically skewed regulatory outcomes; what is often specific to separate regulatory schemes are the numbers and places in the legal process where interested voices may or may not be heard and the consequent extent to which outcomes deviate from law's formal goals and from principles of distributive justice.

Finally, in this essay the focus is on violation of federal water pollution law by *industrial organizations*, rather than by other types of organizations or by individuals. This focus is not meant to suggest that serious water pollution is the business only of private-sector corporations. To the contrary: much of the worst pollution is discharged into waterways by *units of government*, such as municipal waste treatment plants and military installations—the latter being responsible, for example, for much of the contamination due to highly toxic wastes associated with weapons manufacture. Moreover, government's "dirty hands" in this regard arguably complicate its efforts to regulate private sector pollution: the aggressiveness of any such efforts is undercut by the example of the state's inability or unwillingness to control its own discharges, or those of the companies it permits to discharge through municipal waste treatment systems. And, of course, *individuals* occasion much serious pollution, whether through small businesses (and even households) or through mishandling their environmental responsibilities in corporate organizations.

Instead, pragmatic considerations have driven this choice. On the analytic side, it is necessary to choose between public and private pollution sources because the issues underlying the control of each are to some extent unique, for example, involving distinct roles for political forces, fiscal constraints, and the like. And from the standpoint of law, most regulatory efforts are directed at organizational entities rather than at their individual members. In part, this aim reflects the difficulty in isolating mens rea in the face of often complex regulatory violations, and in part (and relatedly) the regulators' recognition that compliance with environmental laws more often entails corporate policies and procedures than individual recalcitrance, especially at lower managerial ranks where most of the hands-on control of pollution exists (Reiss 1985).

Given these various links between legal process and patterns of compliance and lawbreaking, this essay approaches industrial water pollution through an emphasis on law and regulatory procedures. Section I explains the relevant law, the Clean Water Act of 1972, and subsequent amendments passed in 1977 and 1987. Section II illustrates the regulatory dynamic underlying compliance and enforcement and offers the example of toxic water pollution, the control of which was the highest priority in the 1972 Clean Water Act, but which twenty years later remains an incomplete regulatory program some seventeen years behind the original schedule. Section III examines some industrial offense patterns found through research and discusses explanations for them. Section IV reviews federal government enforcement policies and practices, not always one and the same. The discussion focuses on the sociolegal forces that shape and limit environmental law enforcement and on their consequences for both the profile of violators and the reach of public policy. Finally, the last section draws implications for theory, research, and policy from the various findings.

I. A Watershed in Law: The 1972 Clean Water Act and Its Amendments

After two decades of virtually complete futility in the federal government's efforts to stiffen the states' resolve to control industrial water pollution, in 1972 Congress finally claimed the regulatory responsibility with a dramatic new law. The strength of the national environmental movement's political impulse is indicated in the respective votes for it: 74–0 in the Senate and 366–11 in the House. When President Nixon vetoed the bill two weeks later on the argument that its program was too costly to implement, the Senate overrode the veto 52–12, the House, by a vote of 247–23 (Yeager 1991, pp. 164–73).

In form, the new law was technically a series of amendments to the long-frustrated Federal Water Pollution Control Act, first passed in 1948 and amended in 1956, 1961, 1965, 1966, and 1970; it would later be amended twice again, in 1977 and 1987.[5] But the 1972 amendments contained an unprecedented, detailed, and ambitious environmental program aimed at the eventual *elimination* of both industrial and municipal water pollution by 1985.[6] Among numerous provisions in eighty-eight pages of legislation, the law included a radically new system of pollution controls and penalties for infractions, broad public participation in the law's administration, and "whistle-blower" protection for employees reporting violations of the law. In establishing this regulatory system, the law set in motion key interorganizational processes of rule negotiation and discretionary enforcement that continue to shape patterns of compliance and lawbreaking.

The statute's centerpiece was a national permit program mandating technology-based standards of water pollution control for all industrial facilities.[7] The law's logic was to "level the playing field" for polluting plants: all facilities within defined industry categories were minimally to achieve the same levels of pollution reduction. The advantages to some firms of "pollution havens," as had been historically provided by states fearful of industry flight from stiff controls, were thereby eliminated.

[5] For a discussion of the earlier versions of the law and their systematic failures to contain water pollution, see Yeager (1991, chap. 3).

[6] Federal Water Pollution Control Act Amendments of 1972, Pub. L. No. 92-500, Secs. 101–518; 33 U.S.C. 1251–1376. See the statute's "Declaration of Goals and Policy," Pub. L. No. 92-500, Sec. 101(a)(1): "It is the national goal that the discharge of pollutants into the navigable waters be eliminated by 1985." Needless to say, implemented policies have fallen well short of this goal to date.

[7] The 1972 amendments also regulated discharges from municipal sewage treatment plants and provided for billions of dollars in federal subsidies for the construction of new pollution controls in them. In addition to regulating industrial discharges directly into receiving waters, the law also regulated industrial discharges into municipal treatment plants. Given several policy and analytic complications involved in the latter form of regulation, mediated as it is by the behavior of the municipal authorities, such industrial discharges are not considered in detail in this essay.

The law required the EPA to formulate two progressively stringent levels of pollution reduction by writing specific regulations for each industry category. The agency was then to apply these regulations equally to all plants in each category by means of pollution discharge control permits that set out required reductions and timetables.[8] The agency was to accomplish its rule-making and permit tasks so that all industrial plants were to reduce pollution by mid-July 1977 to levels that reflected "the application of the best practicable control technology currently available" (BPT) and by mid-1983 to that greater level indicating the use of "the best available technology economically achievable" (BAT). In practice, these two levels of reduction correspond roughly to the better and best control technologies already demonstrated in the various industry categories at the respective stages of regulation. Periodically thereafter, the agency is required to review the state of control technologies with a view toward promulgating ever-more stringent pollution control rules.

The law was uncompromising with respect to toxic pollution, which now poses the greatest risks to the environment and human health: in its first section, the statute states that "it is the national policy that the discharge of toxic pollutants in toxic amounts *be prohibited.*"[9] Instead of the technology-based (and cost-constrained) standards to be applied to the conventional pollutants (such as suspended solids, pH concentrations, and the biochemical oxygen demand of organic wastes), the 1972 amendments sought to regulate toxic discharges (e.g., heavy metals, organic chemicals) on the more stringent criteria of their broad environmental effects on water and water-based organisms, and up the food chain to human health, making no mention of the limits of control technologies or costs.[10] Within fifteen months of the law's passage the EPA was to publish a list of toxic pollutants (both singly and in their myriad toxic combinations) and to finalize the multitude of discharge regulations controlling them "with an ample margin of safety" to protect the environment. Industrial firms were to be in compliance with

[8] See Federal Water Pollution Control Act Amendments of 1972, Pub. L. No. 92-500, Sec. 301 ("Effluent Limitations"); Sec. 402 ("National Pollutant Discharge Elimination System").

[9] Pub. L. No. 92-500, Sec. 101(a)(3); emphasis added.

[10] The law authorized the EPA to promulgate toxic effluent standards that "shall take into account the toxicity of the pollutant, its persistence, degradability, the usual or potential presence of the affected organisms in any waters, the importance of the affected organisms and the nature and extent of the effect of the toxic pollutant on such organisms" (Sec. 307[a][2]). Unlike the statements for establishing BPT and BAT, no mention at all is made of the costs of controls (Schroeder 1983, pp. 27–28).

the new limits no more than one year after their promulgation or by mid-1975.[11] But because of numerous difficulties—legal and scientific uncertainty, industrial resistance to controls, restrictive agency budgets, and so on (see Yeager 1991, pp. 216–42)—final regulations for toxic water pollution were being put into place only by 1990, presaging further years before completion of government-permitting procedures and companies' eventual compliance or evasion.

The new law also represented a dramatic change from previous enforcement efforts. Whereas prior law had emphasized long conferences to negotiate compromise solutions to specific pollution problems (Yeager 1991, pp. 51–83), the language in the new statute made regulatory enforcement *mandatory* for any and all violations, at least through administrative compliance orders. For willful or negligent infractions, the law mandated criminal enforcement and fines of between $2,500 and $25,000 per day of violation, imprisonment of up to one year, or both; on a second conviction, the maximum penalties rose to $50,000 per day and two years' imprisonment. Alternatively, violators might be assessed up to $10,000 in civil penalties per day of violation.[12]

Finally, the statute also provided for citizens' rights to sue violating companies if the government took no enforcement action and to sue the EPA itself when the agency failed to perform nondiscretionary duties under the law (e.g., promulgation of regulations on a timely basis).[13]

Subsequent amendments to the law made significant changes in the regulatory program, relaxing some pollution controls while stiffening

[11] Pub. L. No. 92-500, Secs. 307(a)(1)–(6).

[12] The 1972 amendments' enforcement provisions are found in Pub. L. No. 92-500, Sec. 309. The issue of mandatory enforcement in this law has an interesting legislative and judicial history (see Yeager 1991, pp. 163, 170, 253–57). While the congressional conference report on the House-Senate negotiations to work out the terms of the final bill indicates that both civil and criminal enforcement were to be discretionary (U.S. Senate, 1973, pp. 314–15), the final version of the amendments simply states that "any person who willfully or negligently violates section 301, 302, 306, 307, or 309 or this Act, or any permit condition or limitation implementing any of such sections in a permit issued under section 402 of this Act by the [EPA] Administrator or by a State, *shall* be punished by a fine of not less than $2,500 nor more than $25,000 per day of violation, or by imprisonment for not more than one year, or by both" (Sec. 309[c][1]; emphasis added). While discretion certainly remained in the determination of willfulness or negligence, the phrasing appears to make criminal charges mandatory on such a finding. As noted below, the courts finally decreed that even administrative enforcement against violations was discretionary with the EPA, despite the Congress's clear directive to the contrary.

[13] Pub. L. No. 92-500, Sec. 505.

penalties for violations. The 1977 amendments permitted the lowering of BAT standards for conventional pollutants to a level of control defined as "the best conventional pollutant control technology" (BCT) and also provided that the control standard for toxic pollutants could be set at "best available technology" levels, as originally provided for the conventional pollutants.[14]

The 1987 amendments strengthened the government's enforcement options, enlarging both criminal and civil penalties and for the first time providing that the EPA could issue its own administrative fines for violations.[15] The Clean Water Act now distinguishes three types of criminal violation. It provides the same minimum and maximum penalties for *negligent* offenses as did the 1972 amendments. For *knowing* violations, however, the specified fines now range between $5,000 and $50,000 per day, with up to three years incarceration, or both, with the maximums set at $100,000 and at six years for second convictions. The maximum penalties for violations involving *knowing endangerment* of persons are now $250,000, fifteen years incarceration, or both, and $1,000,000 for organizational offenders. Second convictions for such offenses double the maximums.

Interestingly, for knowing endangerment cases the 1987 amendments explicitly recognize the role of corporate organization in distributing and screening culpable knowledge. The act now provides that "knowledge possessed by a person other than the defendant but not by the defendant himself may not be attributed to the defendant; except that in proving the defendant's possession of actual knowledge, circumstantial evidence may be used, *including evidence that the defendant took affirmative steps to shield himself from relevant information.*"[16]

In addition, the 1987 amendments added the potentially forceful option of administrative penalties, which can be issued by the EPA without adjudication in the courts (however, such fines may be appealed to the courts). This mechanism had long been proposed by members of the legislature but heretofore denied by Congress, presumably on the grounds that it would allow the agency too much discretion in penalizing violators; before 1987, the EPA was essentially

[14] Pub. L. No. 95-217, Sec. 301(b)(2)(E) (conventional pollutants); Sec. 307(a)(2) (toxic pollutants).

[15] Pub. L. No. 100-4, 33 U.S.C. 1251 et seq. (1988 ed.). Criminal penalties are set out at 33 U.S.C. 1319(c)(1)–(3), civil penalties at 33 U.S.C. 1319(d), and administrative penalties at 33 U.S.C. 1319(g).

[16] 33 U.S.C. 1319(c)(3)(B); emphasis added.

limited to civil and criminal referrals to the Justice Department if it sought monetary penalties and other punishments.[17] In any event, the 1987 change constrains the agency's discretion within relatively tight limits: administrative penalties range from $10,000 per day or per violation up to a maximum total penalty of only $125,000, which in some cases arguably will be less than the corporate savings realized by offending. Finally, the 1987 amendments raised the maximum civil penalties from $10,000 to $25,000 per day for each violation.

In sum, the 1972 amendments to the Clean Water Act gave water pollution enforcement its first real bite. After a period of desultory enforcement in the Reagan administration, Congress upped the ante for environmental crimes of this sort, seeking both to deter offenses and to ensure that environmental crime did not pay, in the literal sense of the term. The latter is a basic matter of fairness: business violators should not gain a financial advantage over companies complying with the law in good faith.

II. The Regulatory Nexus: On Deliberating
the Legal Constraint

Implementation of regulatory law is inevitably uncertain and changing when the statutory guidance threatens long-established patterns and relations and poses technically complex issues at law, in science, for administration, or by any combination of these. The complexity of law assures the vital play of discretionary judgment, while its novelty promises a key role to relations of power in the exercise of that judgment.

The roles of complexity, discretion, and power in regulation are basic to an understanding of legal compliance and violation. This is because the regulatory process that implements statutes typically links legal administration to private interests in ways that define the law's requirements and condition its enforcement. In relation to water pollution, federal environmental regulation officially links the interests of rational legal administration (as seen from the state's vantage point), environmentalists, industry, and other interested parties in defining the extent of law's reach. But this effort at formal legal equality and democratic legitimacy will be undercut to the extent that systemic

[17] As with all other regulatory agencies, the EPA must refer all potential criminal cases to the Justice Department for prosecution. While the agency can bring its own civil cases, as a practical matter it has generally preferred to refer these as well to the Justice Department for processing.

biases pervade regulatory administration and legal outcomes. Given the complexity of the Clean Water Act, its radical redefinition of industrial behavior, and the relative positions of vested interests in the political economy, it is perhaps unsurprising that such biases operate in this regulatory domain.

For the EPA, the scope of its duties under the Clean Water Act was immense by itself, let alone in combination with all of the other environmental laws under the agency's jurisdiction, including the Clean Air Act; the Resource Conservation and Recovery Act; and the Comprehensive Environmental Response, Compensation, and Liability Act ("CERCLA," also known as the "Superfund" law), among many others. These statutes require the agency to write the hundreds of separate regulations that translate broad statutory directives into specific legal requirements, to hear countless administrative appeals, and to provide the bulk of the enforcement of the law against violators—by monitoring thousands of pollution sources for compliance, issuing warnings and orders, and compiling evidence for the filing of any criminal (and most civil) cases with the Department of Justice. Moreover, the EPA does much of this work under the suspicious supervision of industry, environmental groups, Congress, the White House (particularly its Office of Management and Budget), and the federal courts, which hear numerous appeals against agency actions by both environmental and industrial interests.

The Clean Water Act required the agency to make complex and politically sensitive (because of their high costs) determinations of BPT and BAT for all types of industry within a year of its passage and to issue water pollution control discharge permits implementing the regulations to tens of thousands of individual polluting facilities within two years. While Congress had identified twenty-eight basic categories of industry to be so regulated, the EPA eventually identified more than five hundred subcategories for which separate technology-based control regulations had to be formulated (Yeager 1991, p. 179). Given the resource constraints that always limit regulatory agency effectiveness, and that certainly limited the EPA (Clinard and Yeager 1980; Yeager 1991), it is not surprising that the agency quickly fell behind its schedule, particularly with respect to the top priority toxic pollutants.

This regulatory process alone included countless key decision points, from the writing of regulations, through the numerous appellate court challenges to regulations made by both industry and environmental law groups, to the issuance of individual plant permits implementing them, to the hearing of thousands of business appeals of the terms of the permits (Yeager 1991, pp. 190–91, 206). Given the importance to pollution control of these many decisions, and the discretion necessarily involved in them, Congress provided for wide public input in each.

But in the nature of things, the content of the input into regulation has always been slanted toward industry's arguments and toward certain segments of industry, however subtly. Indeed, the legal regulation of business in the United States commonly features imbalances that favor industry, as discovered in a congressional study:[18]

At agency after agency, participation by the regulated industry predominates—often overwhelmingly. Organized public interest representation accounts for a very small percentage of participation before Federal regulatory hearings. In more than half of the formal proceedings, there appears to be no such participation whatsoever, and virtually none at informal agency proceedings. In those proceedings where participation by public groups does take place, typically it is a small fraction of the participation by the regulated industry. One-tenth is not uncommon; sometimes it is even less than that. This pattern prevails in both rulemaking proceedings and adjudicatory proceedings, with an even greater imbalance occurring in adjudications than in rulemaking. [U.S. Senate 1977, 3:vii]

In thus shaping in characteristic ways what the law-in-action will be, such systemic processes necessarily shape the profile of offenders and the nature of sanctions.

A. The Structures of Deliberation

The very *substance* of legislation structures influences on policy-making and the weighing of factors in decision making. In effect, the language of statutory law often differentially distributes access to (and relative advantage in) regulation to the various interests in its outcomes.

---

[18] The congressional study of imbalances in public participation was based on information on rule making and adjudicatory proceedings from eight regulatory agencies variously responsible for both economic and social regulation: Federal Communications Commission, Federal Power Commission, Federal Trade Commission, Interstate Commerce Commission, Civil Aeronautics Board, Food and Drug Administration, Nuclear Regulatory Commission, and the Securities and Exchange Commission. For no apparent reason other than simple sampling and resource constraints, this aspect of the study did not include the EPA. Nonetheless, the report clearly suggests that the findings of imbalances applied to federal regulatory agencies of all sorts.

Moreover, statutes and regulatory standard setting together shape the moral tone of legal deliberations and their consequences for the reach of law.

With the Clean Water Act, the emphasis on *extant technologies* shaped the distribution of access to such key legal determinations as the writing of industry-wide regulations and the inscribing of the specific limitations into individual pollution discharge permits (which draw the lines of compliance and infraction for specific polluting firms). This emphasis tends to favor the perspective of industry over that of competing environmental interests because of the combination of industry's control over vital technical knowledge and the agency's dependence on that knowledge for numerous and complex rulings.[19]

In theory, under the 1972 amendments the EPA could establish "best available technology" on the basis of model plants privately or publicly funded, or on that of the single best plant in an industry. But as a practical matter the agency chose not to develop novel approaches (in part because of budget constraints) and instead focused its regulatory search on existing technologies in industry with a view toward bringing all firms up to the standard of the better (BPT) and best (BAT) of the control techniques already demonstrated in their respective industries. In addition, this focus was complemented by the law's "end-of-line" approach to pollution control: the law and the agency implemented the position that the government would only seek to control pollution outside of the factory, at the point of discharge to the environment. The law would not endeavor to force specific changes in manufacturers' production practices, just as the government would not itself work to develop new, less polluting production methods. In these twin respects, then, the law deferred both to the autonomy of industrial processes and to the salience of management's views on available technologies.

In the second place, the 1972 statute shifted legal liability for infractions away from considerations of harm to the receiving waters or human health. The government then needed only to show violation of the technology-based permit limits to pursue sanctions against offenders. Congress took this "harm-irrelevant" approach in order to avoid the complexities entailed in proving various levels of harm to the eco-

---

[19] Compare Hawkins's (1984; Reiss 1985) account of the regulation of water pollution in Great Britain. There, the controlling statute requires no implementing regulations prior to enforcement, leaving great discretion and (as Hawkins points out) moral judgments to the government's field inspectors.

system and arguably to avoid the natural inequities that follow from the location of specific plants in the same industry: depending on such factors as water flows and levels, other pollution sources on the river, and so on, the same polluting discharges may or may not involve demonstrable harm.

But these reasonable purposes aside, the focus on technologically determined limits and violations produces the unintended consequence that debates over the terms and application of standards tend disproportionately to attract and to favor industrial over environmental concerns. (It also undercut the prosecution of criminal cases, as detailed in a later section.) Couched in the dry terms of the limits of engineering technologies rather than in the environmentally and morally compelling language of the limits of nature, all of the key decisions—from writing standards to the permitting of individual plants to the making of enforcement decisions—present themselves as technical, depoliticized matters that seldom evoke the moral drama of rights discourse that had originally motivated the 1972 law (Yeager 1991).

In addition, this separation of moral considerations from regulatory deliberations has the effect of increasing the weight given to cost considerations at every decision point. In other words, the focus on technical potentials enhances the tendency in utilitarian (or equity) calculations to favor the "hard" estimates of industry costs over the "soft" determinations of public benefits.

As McGarity (1983, p. 208) has observed when comparing technology-based standards with those based on the quality of the receiving media (e.g., air or water): "The regulated firms may feel more comfortable with a process that gives them room to bargain with the agency in low visibility proceedings that depend heavily on industry-supplied information, especially when the agency may be sympathetic to their plight." Because the water law was implemented by often inexperienced discharge permit writers in EPA regional offices and various state agencies (under EPA delegation), who issued tens of thousands of permits against tight deadlines to often complaining businesses, and under a variety of legal frameworks (e.g., to meet deadlines, permits were sometimes issued under preliminary regulations, and even in the absence of regulations), the playing field was all the more likely to be tilted—toward industry's views and toward those firms able to make the more convincing arguments for limited controls.

The evidence on public participation in the regulation of industrial water pollution suggests structured imbalances in input. At the broad levels of law making and appellate court review, environmental interests have enjoyed a rough parity with industry groups in bringing their positions to bear on policymakers' deliberations (Yeager 1991). In the formulation and application of industry-wide standards to dischargers, however, the balance swings toward the regulated. For example, the most successful public-interest environmental law firm, the Natural Resources Defense Council (NRDC), has only infrequently been able to participate in the agency discussions leading to industry discharge standards. By 1977 the NRDC docket listed the council as having fully participated in the formulation of just five of the numerous sets of regulations the EPA had then written. Passion and commitment are not in short supply; resources are. And the narrower the decision matter, the more limited is the voice of environmentalists. An NRDC official noted that his group was rarely able to participate in such matters as EPA's formal adjudicatory hearing procedures, in which individual polluters seek favorable alterations in the terms of their permits (to allow greater discharges or longer compliance timetables) in courtlike proceedings before administrative law judges or other (less formal) permit modification proceedings. These key determinations, which determine the application of law in individual cases, were left largely to the deliberations of agency and industry experts. And even when his organization intervened, as in a case challenging several offshore oil permits, an NRDC official reported that it was often "ill-equipped" from a resource standpoint to engage in such numerous "wars of experts."[20]

In sum, the processes thus far described shape law not only independently but synergistically. The tendency of technology-based standards to evoke equity considerations at all stages underscores the importance of representative public participation in each of them, at the same time as their highly technical nature renders such participation increasingly difficult as laws are transformed into applicable rules and applied to firms. Similarly, the heavy regulatory burden the water amendments placed on the EPA forced it to enlarge on the law's discretionary realms—such as writing permits on the basis of incomplete standards to meet statutory timetables—again increasing the need for wide public participation while, because of the proliferation of decision points, making such participation more difficult to insure and provide.

B. Constraints on Regulation: The Case of Toxics

In the 1972 amendments Congress had taken its most stringent stance on the matter of toxics regulation, going so far as to divorce

[20] Interview with author, 1981.

toxic pollution controls from the cost considerations that were to be made for conventional pollutants and providing for industrial compliance by 1975 with these uncompromising standards.[21] Ironically, however, this topmost priority was relegated to the regulatory "backseat" by the federal government. In the early years federal regulation focused instead on the more tractable problems of the less threatening conventional pollutants. Only by 1990—fifteen years past the original deadline—were final regulations being formulated, thereafter to be implemented in factory discharge permits and enforced.

The consequence was that by the end of the 1980s American industry was still discharging billions of pounds of toxic wastes into the nation's surface waters, among more than twenty-two billion pounds of toxic discharges into the land, air, and water, a level the EPA itself called "startling and unacceptably high."[22] Most important, much of this was being done legally by virtue of long delays in formulating and implementing the relevant discharge standards and by virtue of fundamental change in the stringency of the standards as against the original statement of legislative intent.

Regardless of legality, the environmental effects remain significant. EPA tests in two of its ten regions found, for example, that in about 62 percent of samples taken at 551 industrial sites during the 1975–82 period, "the toxic chemicals in the discharge were sufficient to have a lethal effect on the aquatic environment in the stream" (U.S. General Accounting Office 1983, p. 39). In addition to toxic effects on aquatic life and human health, the agency has estimated that toxic discharges to the nation's surface waters (e.g., rivers, streams, oceans) "cause losses of approximately $800 million per year in recreational fishing, swimming, and boating opportunities" (U.S. General Accounting Office 1991a, p. 8).

The reasons for this shortfall in environmental policy range from the statute's regulatory logic to the more familiar problems of the agency's budgetary constraints and the resistance of often powerful business interests.

[21] For a more detailed discussion of the politics and logics of toxics regulation under the Clean Water Act, see Yeager (1991, pp. 216–42).

[22] Studies released by the federal government in 1989 revealed for the first time the massive amounts of toxics being released into the environment (Yeager 1991, pp. 245–46). The EPA reported in April 1989 that American industry had released or disposed of at least 22.5 billion pounds of hazardous substances in 1987, including 9.7 billion pounds of toxics released into surface waters, 3.2 billion pounds injected into underground wells, 2.7 billion pounds into landfills, and 2.7 billion pounds into the air. See also the articles by Philip Shabecoff (1989a, 1989b).

1. *The Logics of Technology.*   A basic feature of this regulatory enterprise underlies the continuing threat of toxic industrial pollution, including the fact of its commonplace and continuing *legality* even in the
face of stringent legislation that outlaws it in principle and despite
significant environmental damages. This is because, in general, technology-based rules can drive industrial laggards to match the standards
of the pollution control leaders in their respective industries but cannot
force the leaders to create new technologies to improve environmental
protection (McGarity 1983, p. 222).

In theory, such a constraint should have mattered less for the toxics
because by statute they were to have been regulated not on the basis
of industrial technologies but on the less cost-conscious basis of toxic
risks to the environment and human health. However, the uncertainties inherent in the law's mandate for toxics—scientific, administrative,
legal (e.g., judicial review of standards), and ultimately political (stem-
ming from the high costs of controls to business)—drove the EPA
administratively to amend the 1972 law. The administrative amendments were later given the imprimatur of the federal courts, the Congress (in the 1977 amendments to the law), and even the organized
environmental public interest groups (Yeager 1991, pp. 219–22).[23]

The key feature of these changes was to have toxics regulated by
the same technological determinations (BPT, BAT) that were being
made for the conventional pollutants. In some ways, the result is understandable: it allowed the agency to proceed surefootedly on the
basis of real technologies rather than on its suspect abilities to penetrate
the obscure mysteries of nature. However, this approach was certain
to limit the control of toxics, arguably even short of manageable cost
constraints in industry. The ironic consequence is that higher levels of
pollution are joined by higher rates of business compliance with the
law.

This consequence was revealed when, for a number of industrial
categories, the EPA rejected the second-stage "best available technol-

[23] On the federal courts, see *Natural Resources Defense Council v. Train* (D.D.C. 1976;
8 ERC 2120). In this 1976 case, the federal district court for the District of Columbia
approved a consent decree (known as the Flannery Decree after the presiding judge)
establishing the new regulatory framework and timetables for compliance for the control
of toxic water pollution. The court ordered that the regulations be finalized no later
than the end of 1979, with industry to achieve compliance no later than June 30, 1983.
But because of factors such as those described in this essay, many additional extensions
became necessary, and the decree was modified by the court in 1979, 1982, 1983, 1984
(twice), 1985, 1986, and 1987 (Yeager 1991, p. 222). On the Congress, see Pub. L. No.
95-217; see 33 U.S.C. 1251 et seq. (1982 ed.).

ogy" altogether, settling for the less stringent "best practicable technology" for the control of toxics. For example, after initially proposing BAT for the leather tanning industry, in response to industry criticisms the agency issued a final rule in 1982 setting controls at BPT because, it said, *the proposed BAT controls had not yet been demonstrated in the industry and were not economically achievable.* This result follows from a problem in the core logic of the 1972 amendments. The risk in the two-stage sequence of controls—from BPT to BAT shortly thereafter—was that the heavy investment in the first-stage controls might prevent the establishment of more advanced control technologies, either because the first would be incompatible with the second (rendering the latter too costly) or because past the first stage the law's logic would not promote the development of yet more advanced BAT controls in some industries. When this occurred, it strengthened industries' arguments that the latter controls were therefore not economically achievable.[24]

In another example of the limits of this technology-based approach, the EPA in 1982 also revoked its proposed BAT regulations for the petroleum refining industry and instead promulgated final regulations setting the controls on toxics at BPT (Bureau of National Affairs 1983). That powerful industry had successfully resisted the agency's original proposal that would have greatly restricted the flow of wastes by mandating recycling and reuse of waste streams. Unlike typically end-of-pipe and less effective BPT controls, the proposed rule apparently intruded too forcefully on the industry's traditional production practices.

Two final points warrant mention. First, in addition to the implied reduction in environmental protection, this policy shift emphasizing extant controls—made long after the public and impassioned stands for the elimination of toxic pollution—necessarily results in higher compliance rates as many businesses are commonly asked to make relatively few changes to comply with standards. Second, there is no small measure of historic irony in this approach. Just as the very first, turn-of-the-century federal water pollution laws were passed to protect commerce by providing for clear river routes for industrial transporta-

[24] Compare McGarity (1983, p. 205): "The technology-based approach in practice can bias pollution control in favor of capital-intensive 'white elephant' technologies which may be ineffective in the long run" (e.g., Tripp 1977). Interestingly, this problem had been foreseen by some members of the House of Representatives prior to the law's passage, but their arguments for a more effective system of controls went unheeded (Yeager 1991, pp. 158–59).

tion, rather than to meet the public health needs of citizens (Yeager 1991, pp. 225–26), so too did the present-day technological "needs" of industry tend to relegate environmental health criteria to the shadows of public policy.

2. *The Limits of Regulation.*   More mundane and familiar features of government regulation also constrain the effectiveness of toxics controls, again with the simultaneous effect of elevating compliance rates in industry. These include agency resources far short of those needed to implement the law, and the resistance of often powerful corporate polluters.

These are, of course, related phenomena. For example, budget constraints limit the government's monitoring of the environment and the adequacy of its rule making, thereby exacerbating the large scientific uncertainties regarding the impacts of toxic pollutants and increasing the likelihood that industry will challenge pollution controls in administrative or judicial forums.[25] Meanwhile, the same fiscal limitations make the agency reluctant to engage in lengthy legal battles with industry that can greatly frustrate both the appearance and reality of regulatory progress.

The operation of these limiting features in EPA's toxic water pollution program was highlighted in an audit of the program by the U.S. General Accounting Office (1991a) in 1991. In a number of respects the study reproduced findings and consequences that the General Accounting Office (GAO) had pointed to in a previous audit published in 1983.[26] The 1991 GAO study identified problems in the toxics program ranging from insufficient monitoring of water quality, to revised ("updated") permits that make little progress in controlling toxic pollution, to reduced standards that elevate corporate compliance rates.

[25] Some 65,000 chemicals are manufactured in the United States every year, and for many there is simply little knowledge of their toxic effects, either alone or in myriad combinations (Conservation Foundation 1982, pp. 119–22; Schneider 1985, p. 15). In 1977 the EPA estimated that the nation's drinking water contained between 3,000 and 5,000 different chemicals and the waterways some several hundred thousand chemical compounds. The agency also noted that the ability to identify such compounds was far outstripping scientists' abilities to determine their toxic effects (for humans and other organisms) and at what levels of concentration they occur (U.S. House of Representatives 1977, p. 24).

[26] See *Water Pollution: Stronger Efforts Needed by EPA to Control Toxic Water Pollution* (U.S. General Accounting Office 1991a); *Wastewater Dischargers Are Not Complying with EPA Pollution Control Permits* (U.S. General Accounting Office 1983). Also see the GAO reports, *Water Pollution: More EPA Action Needed to Improve the Quality of Heavily Polluted Waters* (U.S. General Accounting Office 1989a), and *Water Pollution: Improved Monitoring and Enforcement Needed for Toxic Pollutants Entering Sewers* (U.S. General Accounting Office 1989b).

In an effort to remedy the lack of progress in toxics regulation, the 1987 amendments—also known as the Water Quality Act of 1987— required the EPA and the states to identify and list surface waters that are either impaired or threatened by toxic and nontoxic pollutants, whether from point or nonpoint discharges (such as runoff from agricultural or mining operations).[27] For these waters and their polluters, the EPA and the states were to develop individual control strategies (ICS) to get them to meet pollution control standards by June 1992.

The difficulties begin with the monitoring of water quality in the nation's rivers, streams, lakes, estuaries, and oceans. By 1991, the GAO found, most states had assessed the quality of less than half of their total surface miles of water. Moreover, because there is no national requirement that the states use specific methods to monitor their water quality, the commonly resource-strained state agencies often use only descriptive information on water quality, such as citizen reports. Less often do they conduct actual tests of water samples, which are more expensive but necessary to identify specific pollutants and their sources.[28] In sum, the requisite first step toward effective toxics regulation—the identification of impaired waters and pollution sources—has been small and tentative, a halting stride toward locating polluters and enforcing toxics standards.

Nonetheless, the inventory still identified some 18,770 waters nationwide that are impaired by toxic or nontoxic pollutants or both. But instead of developing ICSs for all of these segments and their polluters, the EPA's regulations require ICSs for only the 529 segments (2.8 percent)—which include 686 polluting facilities—that are impaired largely because of point source discharges of any of 126 priority toxic pollutants identified by the agency. According to the GAO audit, however, even this limited approach to industrial water pollution falls well short of the law's intended reach. This is because, in many cases, toxics standards are not being firmly applied to industrial polluters. The regulatory shortfall manifests itself in a number of ways and for a number of reasons, from those having to do with corporate power to those having to do with the EPA's regulatory burden.

[27] Pub. L. No. 100-4, Sec. 304(l); 33 U.S.C. 1314(l) (1988 ed.).

[28] Regardless of the methods used, EPA data for the late 1980s show that states have assessed the water quality of 519,413 miles of rivers and streams, only 29 percent of the nation's total, and for 16.3 million lake acres, or 41 percent of total lake acres (U.S. General Accounting Office 1991a, p. 23). And of the assessed rivers and streams, only 40 percent were evaluated using actual water samples; for the other 60 percent, only descriptive data were used.

As an example of the role of corporate power, consider the processes by which many industrial dischargers, initially identified on the required lists of toxic pollution sources in impaired waters, were removed from the lists of violators; overall EPA deleted some 309 facilities from the states' original lists. In one variant, firms pressured state governments to make their water quality standards less stringent so that the companies would not suffer public identification as toxic polluters, or be required to take additional steps to clean up pollutants. For example, in Alabama nine of ten paper mills were deleted from the violators' list after the paper and pulp industries pressured the state to reduce its standard for dioxin pollution (U.S. General Accounting Office 1991a, pp. 18–19). In another variant, some companies escaped the violators' lists by tying their discharges into municipal sewage treatment systems. This had the dual effects of deleting such firms from the toxics dischargers' list because it covered only polluters discharging directly into surface waters, while subjecting the companies to the less rigorous regulation governing the separate municipal waste regulatory program.[29]

Such practices indicate the operation of law in shaping the profiles of both compliance and what might be called "designated noncompliance."

Resource constraints in government combine with industry opposition to stringent controls to shape these profiles in another way. Despite the law's clear instructions, the 1991 GAO audit found that the EPA's national regulations are controlling only a limited number of toxic and other nonconventional pollutants. For example, of the thirty-five sets of toxics regulations for the same number of industrial categories, nineteen had not been revised to reflect advances in treatment technologies in over five years, the time frame for review and revision set forth in the statute; nine of the nineteen sets of regulations date to the 1970s. In addition, for some industries national rules regulating toxics had not even been formulated, while other existing rules failed to regulate at least some types of toxics.

The audit cited limited and declining agency resources as the principal reason for these shortfalls. The decade of the 1980s brought large

---

[29] For example, the GAO cited a 1986 EPA report showing that extant regulations still failed to regulate a number of industries discharging toxics into publicly owned treatment works, as well as a number of "nonpriority" toxic pollutants such as methanol and xylene that are discharged into such works in "significant concentrations" (U.S. General Accounting Office 1991a, p. 28).

budget and personnel cuts to the agency and high turnover among staff responsible for developing national regulations for categories of industry. As the GAO study notes, the result is daunting (1991*a*, p. 28): "Because of limited staff, one person is usually responsible for all aspects of reviewing, revising, or developing a number of guidelines, which can involve numerous facilities, products, and complex production processes."

The 1991 GAO study found that the EPA had been similarly slow to develop and revise separate rules limiting the concentrations of toxic pollutants in waterways. The Clean Water Act required these water quality criteria as further protection for human health and aquatic life; they were to regulate industrial discharges more strictly when the technology-based rules failed to adequately protect these interests.[30] And even where these rules had been established, states have commonly been reluctant to impose them on businesses.[31] The states variously challenge that the criteria are insufficiently supported scientifically—so that adoption of them may lead to increased industry challenges, further straining state governments' spare regulatory resources—and that the discharge permit limits based on the criteria are too stringent.

In addition to the result that compliance rates are "artificially" elevated, the failure of national regulations to address key toxic pollution problems has another ironic consequence: an increase in bureaucratic discretion in the development and application of regulatory standards. In the absence of specific regulations, government officials charged with writing the individual pollution control permits often found themselves relying on their "best professional judgment" to set specific pollution discharge limits for individual factories. Predictably, highly discretionary calls in bureaucracies are commonly made by individuals of variable technical expertise, who are therefore often intimidated by industry's experts. In addition, such regulatory decisions are more likely than carefully promulgated national standards to be challenged by businesses if they find the limits too stringent.[32] The ultimate regu-

[30] The water quality control requirement in the statute is set out at 33 U.S.C. 1313(c)(2)(B) (1988 ed.).

[31] Only twenty-four states were in compliance with the national criteria as of March 1991 (U.S. General Accounting Office 1991*a*, p. 30).

[32] "EPA and state officials told us, however, that some [permit] writers do not have the technical expertise to write effective permits in the absence of national discharge limits. They also believe that some writers may be intimidated by industry representatives and fear possible legal challenges if they include very stringent limits in permits. The officials added that if writers choose to incorporate stringent limits using their

latory result is an uneven playing field for compliance with the Clean Water Act, just the sort of "irrationality" and "randomness" that the law had been designed to overcome.[33]

III. Patterns in Lawbreaking, Structures of Compliance

The preceding sections have sought to establish the key role of law in shaping the rates and distributions of compliance and offenses. This analysis is a corrective to the standard approach in much criminological research, in which the nature of law is taken as given and criminologists are free to investigate violations as "pure" behavioral phenomena unconfounded by the form of law or the processes of its enforcement. While the approach is sensible for some types of questions, and to a point (Yeager 1993), taken without proper caution it can play havoc with researchers' interpretive work and lawgivers' policy work. The case of environmental law is illustrative of the risks of avoiding careful analysis of legal and political processes. As an assistant attorney general for New York State once noted of its environmental laws, "Enforcement [has become] a process of whittling down the obligations of the polluter to the point where he can meet them" (quoted in DiMento 1986, p. 28). If rather overstated as the general case, this sentiment should nonetheless give pause to researchers attracted to the standard approach, at least for many important criminological problems.[34]

The caution duly noted, in this section I turn to the empirical evidence on business violations of environmental law, focusing again on

---

judgment, some industry representatives believe that these limits are inherently less legally defensible and may challenge them in court.

"This assertion was substantiated by some of the officials we visited. For example, Michigan officials told us that at least 24 permittees appealed permits whose toxic discharge limits were largely based upon best professional judgment. Michigan officials said far fewer permits based on the national effluent guidelines have been challenged in their state" (U.S. General Accounting Office 1991a, p. 31).

[33] Another matter further complicates the regulatory playing field according to the 1991 GAO audit (1991a, pp. 32–33). This is the granting to polluting companies of variances and exceptions to the original permit limitations. The audit, citing a 1990 report entitled *National Assessment of State Variance Procedures*, notes that regulatory officials find that the states grant variances and other exceptions on an inconsistent basis, an unsurprising result inasmuch as the EPA has no clear national policy for the granting of legitimate variances. The officials also predicted that when more stringent water quality criteria and industry guidelines are finally implemented, states will increasingly grant variances to polluting companies unable to meet the new limits, again shaping the profiles of compliance and infraction.

[34] Compare, for example, Reichman (1992) on the case of securities regulation: "Regulatory compliance is a fluid process that involves negotiated interpretations of both rules and facts." For a discussion of the more general case in white-collar crime enforcement and defense, see Mann (1985); also McBarnet (1991).

the Clean Water Act. There are surprisingly few empirical studies in this area. Given the importance of this policy area, this dearth is something of a conundrum. Perhaps this neglect is owing to the methodological challenges often encountered in such investigations, or perhaps to a moral ambivalence toward "technical" offenses. Both problems are encountered in the study of environmental regulation, but the methodological difficulties can be overcome by those curious to look past—or at—the moral ambivalence of such violations.

A. Explaining Offenses: The Standard Approach

The effort to analyze regulatory lawbreaking is complicated by a number of methodological challenges. Among these is the standard criminological problem of the limitations of official data on offending. But here the matter goes beyond the problem of the unknown "dark figure of crime" that results from undetected and unreported violations. As just suggested, reliance on the official data of *regulatory* infractions risks the result that analyses will unwittingly incorporate systemic biases that are built into the legal apparatus, shaping distributions of offenses, offenders, and official sanctions.

Another challenge in some regulatory arenas, certainly including environmental law, is the problem of conceptualizing compliance and offenses. In theory there is no problem: either a firm is meeting standards or it is not. But in practice there are complications. Rather than being an either-or matter, compliance may be seen as a *process* in which companies are categorized as making adequate progress toward pollution reduction or as failing to do so. As DiMento (1986, p. 111) has pointed out, there is arguably a completeness dimension to compliance: should good faith efforts at compliance be accorded the same status as compliance now, in fact, or essentially as manifesting the same phenomenon as the willful noncomplier? As a practical matter, the EPA commonly recognizes the distinction by granting deadline extensions to polluters that demonstrate good faith efforts to reach pollution control goals. In this case, technical noncompliance is transformed into technical compliance, at least for the duration of such extensions.

Researchers have handled these and other complications in various ways.[35] But regardless of the methodological approach taken, most investigations of business noncompliance with environmental laws

---

[35] For additional discussion of other methodological issues and the ways in which they may be handled, see Yeager (1991, pp. 296–301).

have found significant rates of offending, both in the 1970s and in the 1980s. While significant, the rates are not always high, and it must be kept in mind that noncompliance constitutes events ranging from the refusal even to apply for discharge permits, and the failure to install pollution abatement equipment on the legally required schedule, to failure to submit accurate self-monitoring reports and periodic discharges over permit limits. Thus, even noncompliers in our typically static data bases may more often be in compliance than out of it with respect to continuous discharge limitations.

Available studies include the federal government's own efforts to estimate noncompliance rates and identify proximate causes of environmental lawbreaking and those of academic social scientists that identify and explain the profiles of offenses using predictive statistical models.

1. *Counts and Measures.*   Over the years studies of business compliance with water pollution laws have found significant noncompliance. For example, U.S. General Accounting Office surveys in 1978 and 1980 found that 55 percent of industrial waste dischargers had committed "serious" offenses against their permit requirements at some time in the previous year (cited in Harrington 1988, p. 31). Similarly, in a random sample survey in the latter 1980s, the GAO found that about 41 percent of industrial dischargers that send their wastes to publicly owned treatment plants had violated one or more of their discharge limits during a twelve-month period (U.S. General Accounting Office 1989b; Adler and Lord 1991, p. 789). Many of these wastes are toxic and cause treatment plants to break down, resulting in the discharge to waterways of untreated toxics and sewage and exposing municipal plant workers to health and safety risks. For example, at the Bergen County Utilities Authority in New Jersey, a worker died from inhaling toxic fumes at the publicly owned treatment plant. The authority's principal engineer reported that a number of industrial users of the plant had consistently violated the cyanide limits; when combined with wastes with low pH concentrations, the result can be deadly gas.[36]

A more sophisticated government study not only highlights the methodological and conceptual issues in research of this sort but also demonstrates something of the role of political considerations and interorganizational disputes within government in estimating offense rates

---

[36] According to the GAO, "One firm, we were informed, discharged wastes with 40, 50, or even 100 ppm [parts per million] of cyanide although the local limit is 0.5 ppm. The combination of high levels of cyanide and low pH can produce hydrogen cyanide, a deadly gas that poses a health threat to workers in the sewer system" (1989b, p. 22).

and presents a view of the *proximate* causes of business's environmental violations (U.S. General Accounting Office 1983).

Seeking to exclude counts of minor, episodic violations (such as single-day violations of a discharge limit), the study focused on "significant noncompliance" by major polluters, generally those facilities discharging large amounts of pollutants, often including toxics.[37] The GAO study defined "significant noncompliance" in terms of industrial facilities that had exceeded one or more of the permitted discharge limits by 50 percent or more for at least four consecutive months.[38] Based on a random sample of 257 major industrial dischargers in six states, the study found that 16 percent of the sample (20 percent of the violators) were in significant violation of their permits (1983, p. 9).[39] Significant noncompliance rates ranged from 9 percent in Texas to 24 percent of sampled firms in New Jersey (1983, p. 45).

It is possible that these rates are substantially underestimated because, like most other government and academic investigations of compliance with the Clean Water Act, the GAO study relied on the law's self-reporting system, in which polluters submit periodic self-monitoring reports of their compliance or noncompliance. Naturally such reports may be inaccurate, whether willfully or not. The law polices the system by making false reporting (or failure to report) a punishable offense and by supplementing it with the prospect of periodic field inspections of polluting facilities to check compliance. But both of these means are also severely constrained in practice, most significantly by limited inspectional and enforcement resources.

Recognizing the problem, the GAO attempted to measure the extent of misreporting, at least in the form of failing to report. It found that 6 percent (16 of 257) of the sampled industrial plants failed to submit one or more of the required discharge monitoring reports (DMRs) to the regulatory authorities. This was a significant decline from the 23

[37] The category of "major" discharger is based on the facility's potential for discharging toxic wastes, the volume and type of wastewater, and whether the receiving water is used for drinking (U.S. General Accounting Office 1983, pp. 2–3). So defined, major dischargers have always been top priority at the EPA in the formulation and enforcement of pollution controls (Yeager 1991).

[38] Pollution control permits commonly set discharge limits for both concentrations and quantities of numerous regulated pollutants. A plant that exceeds any one of these limits—even for but a single day—has technically violated the Clean Water Act, regardless of level of harm to the environment.

[39] The six states are Iowa, Louisiana, Missouri, New Jersey, New York, and Texas. The study also included a random sample of 274 municipal treatment plants (POTWs). In this discussion I focus only on the findings pertaining to the industrial dischargers.

percent (38 of 165) found in its 1978 study of industrial water dischargers. But the GAO also found relatively high rates of incomplete
DMR reporting in 1983, ranging from 26 percent of the sampled facilities in Louisiana to 52 percent in Iowa (U.S. General Accounting
Office 1983, pp. 6–17). In these cases, companies fail to report on one
or more of the pollutants they are discharging to receiving waters,
rendering compliance counts suspect. The study also found that missing or incomplete DMRs were not always handled consistently by
either the EPA or state authorities enforcing the law under EPA delegation. For example, EPA's Region 6 (headquartered in Dallas) was
not reviewing for completeness those DMRs submitted by minor dischargers, while "Iowa procedures state that no specific effort is required to review DMRs for completeness because of the time that
would be required for manual review" (1983, p. 17).[40]

Inspections, too, provide at best only an irregular check on and
stimulus to self-reporting accuracy. The EPA's official policy calls for
at least annual inspections of all major dischargers, but resource constraints undercut this aim. In particular, resource-intensive sampling
inspections, which would provide independent checks of discharge violations but which take about thirty days each to complete (Magat and
Viscusi 1990, p. 338), tended to be infrequently conducted, generally
aimed at plants against which regulators are planning or considering
an enforcement action. Between 1979 and 1981, such inspections of
nonmunicipal dischargers declined by 48 percent; only 7 percent of
major dischargers in New Jersey were visited for effluent sampling
inspections in 1982 (U.S. General Accounting Office 1983, pp. 20–21;
Yeager 1991, pp. 270–71).

It is noteworthy that infrequent inspections may not only promote
faulty self-reporting but may also undercut compliance with pollution
controls. In their study of compliance in the pulp and paper industry
in the mid-1980s (but with respect to conventional pollutants only),
Magat and Viscusi (1990) proposed that inspections be considered as
enforcement tools and in multivariate statistical analyses found that

[40] Another difficulty in the accuracy of the DMRs is the reliability of the assessments
made by the independent laboratories to which major industrial and municipal dischargers send samples for analysis (the results of which are reported in the DMRs). The
EPA quality assurance tests in the early 1980s found that laboratory analyses for 58
percent of the industrial dischargers sampled nationwide, and 68 percent of the municipal
dischargers, "did not show acceptable results for one or more pollutants analyzed" (U.S.
General Accounting Office 1983, pp. 17–18).

field inspections tended to produce higher subsequent compliance rates among the inspected plants.[41] They also found that inspections tended to increase the completeness of reporting in the subsequent DMR reports and that, unlike the earlier findings, the sample firms averaged about one inspection per year. Clearly, regular inspections carry the message that regulators are watching, with the implication that continued noncompliance will be sanctioned. But the results must be interpreted cautiously, given the restriction to a single industry (and a sample of seventy-seven facilities), conventional pollution, and a specific time frame. While regulatory policy may focus its resources on particular problem areas at particular moments, such resources are always tightly constrained. And in any event, the extent to which more complete DMR reporting correlates with accurate reporting remains unclear.

Despite its relatively conservative focus on "significant noncompliance," and the likelihood that the measure is underestimated, the GAO study encountered what might be called the "regulatory politics of noncompliance" when the EPA objected that the reported rates seriously *overestimated* noncompliance (U.S. General Accounting Office 1983, pp. 9–12). The EPA argued that by its own measure significant industrial noncompliance for the sample declined from 14 percent to 10 percent between March 1981 to March 1982. Although the EPA had itself characterized the GAO's measure as "conservative" two years earlier when it had been applied to municipal waste dischargers, by 1982 the agency was applying a much more conservative measure (1983, pp. 9–10).[42] Given the timing of this change in the EPA's policy, during a period in which the Reagan administration was endeavoring to show that environmental regulation could be relaxed without substantial costs to the environment, the compliance debate illustrates one

---

[41] "The role of EPA inspections is to raise the expected cost of noncompliance" (Magat and Viscusi 1990, p. 347).

[42] The EPA had decided informally to define significant noncompliance in terms of exceeding a monthly average permit limit by more than 40 percent for conventional pollutants and 20 percent for toxic ones during any two months of a six-month period. But it applied the definition only to factories with final permit limits, rather than also to those with interim limits in their permits; about 25 percent of the sampled plants were operating under interim limits, which are given to facilities that are upgrading to meet more stringent final limits. In addition, in calculating its noncompliance rate the EPA considered out of compliance only those factories that were so in the final month of any quarter; this omits those that were significantly out of compliance during the first two months of a quarter but that achieved compliance during the last month. Given the unevenness, even sporadic nature of much industrial compliance with permit limits, these latter two decision rules appear restrictive.

type of interorganizational dispute in government that may distort official counts of lawbreaking.

Finally, the 1983 GAO report offered an assessment of the proximate causes of industrial noncompliance with the Clean Water Act (U.S. General Accounting Office 1983, pp. 13–14). Among the listed factors were deficiencies in the maintenance and operation of treatment facilities (e.g., limited staffing and inadequate training of pollution control equipment operators), equipment deficiencies, and poorly designed plants.[43] The report also noted another cause of noncompliance: underfunded and lax enforcement efforts that permit industrial lawbreaking to continue in plants over long periods of time. But in addition to problems of noncompliance, the GAO noted that *compliance* could also bring environmentally lethal results, as earlier discussed: because of expired discharge permits that have not been updated with stricter limits, the EPA found that many companies were discharging chemicals that are toxic to aquatic environments (1983, p. 39).[44]

2. *Predicting Offenses: Finance and Organization.* There have been few studies of environmental law compliance rates or counts and even fewer that try to explain such findings on the basis of predictive models of offending. These few investigations have generally examined the possible relations between business financial success (or failure) and corporate and industry structural characteristics and the degree of environmental lawbreaking. In general, these studies have found few significant correlates of such offending in the data and face significant methodological challenges.

In their effort to "update" Sutherland's (1949) pioneering research on white-collar crime, Marshall Clinard and his colleagues examined whether financial and structural variables could predict the levels of

---

[43] Compare Magat and Viscusi (1990, p. 352, n. 27) arguing that inspections enhance compliance "through immediate attention to better plant operation and maintenance, rather than longer-term capital investments"; and Yeager (1991, p. 211) quoting an internal EPA memorandum in 1977 noting that "there is a greater economic incentive to avoid [the expensive] O&M [operation and maintenance] costs than to avoid the capital costs of installing control equipment," and that "the difficulty and cost of enforcing adequate O&M is greater than the surveillance and enforcement necessary to get greater control equipment installed."

[44] "Tests conducted by EPA personnel in two of its regions showed that frequently toxics can have lethal effects on aquatic life. Results of samples taken at 551 industrial sites during the period 1975–82 showed that in about 62 percent of the cases the toxic chemicals in the discharge were sufficient to have a lethal effect on the aquatic environment in the stream. We were told by the chief, Ecological Support Branch, Environmental Support Division, EPA Region 4, that in almost all cases the 551 sites had first-round permits and that second-round permits—if properly developed—would bring the toxic chemicals under control" (U.S. General Accounting Office 1983, p. 39).

environmental offenses and their distributions among firms (Clinard et al. 1979; see also Clinard and Yeager 1980). The effort was part of a larger study of identified violations of numerous federal laws by Fortune 500 industrial corporations during 1975 and 1976.[45] In this research, the category of environmental violations included both air and water pollution cases, and the analyses did not distinguish these two types. Moreover, the study was beset by a number of significant methodological limitations that produced an underestimate of offending rates and imprecision in the statistical tests, about which more is said below.

The study found that 27 percent of the 477 large industrial firms had been charged with environmental violations during the two-year period and that the violating companies averaged almost four such offenses during the period (Clinard et al. 1979, pp. 92–93). In addition, the research found that the chemical, oil, and auto industries had disproportionate shares of the offenses and that the larger of these large firms had more environmental violations than the smaller (Clinard et al. 1979, pp. 283, 285).

To examine possible predictors of corporate environmental lawbreaking, multivariate statistical analyses were conducted using several measures of firms' and their industries' financial health and several indicators of companies' and industries' organizational structures.[46] These latter indicators included, for example, measures of firm size and growth (both measured in terms of a company's assets), diversification in companies' lines of business, the relative dominance of firms in their markets, relative labor intensiveness (vs. capital intensiveness), proportion of sales in foreign markets, and concentration ratios for the industries. These measures were used in statistical equations relating them to firms' records of total environmental offenses.

The principal findings can be simply summarized (see Clinard et al. 1979, chap. 8: app. J, tables 22–24). There was some evidence that poorer financial health led to greater involvement in environmental violations, particularly among companies operating in industries with

[45] The Fortune 500 are the 500 largest industrial corporations in the United States, as identified in the annual listings of *Fortune* magazine (based on annual sales figures). The Clinard et al. (1979) sample comprised only 477 companies, as twenty-three were eliminated from the study on a number of methodological grounds.

[46] The research examined three types of measures of financial health: *profitability*, capital turnover or *efficiency*, and *liquidity* (a measure of working capital relative to a firm's total assets). These were examined in terms of both levels and five-year trends and at both the firm and industry levels of analysis. For more detailed discussion of these and the other predictor variables, see Clinard et al. (1979, pp. 155–62).

capital liquidity and turnover problems. But in some of the analyses there was a very slight tendency for firms in industries experiencing increasing profitability also to violate these laws more often, leaving open the question of the ways in which financial performance might complexly help to determine the likelihoods of environmental offending.

Regarding structural characteristics, firms in more capital-intensive industries were more likely to break environmental laws, while companies with greater assets abroad (as measured indirectly by proportion of foreign sales) committed fewer such infractions. While the dynamic linking capital intensiveness to these violations also remains obscure (although one may conjecture such possibilities as a greater tendency to understaff and undertrain employees, leading to the O&M problems discussed above), the latter relationship may be due to the dedication of regulatory (and labor) savings abroad to compliance with U.S. law in home operations or simply to the fact that overseas operations are not subject to U.S. environmental regulations (so that less of a multinational corporation's total manufacturing output risks falling into violation). Finally, although larger firms tended to have greater absolute numbers of identified offenses, they had no more *per-unit size* of the company (calculated in terms of violations per $100 million in annual sales) than did the smaller of these corporations, suggesting that the greater offending levels are principally a result of greater output at risk of being found in violation (e.g., having more factories under regulation).

But these findings are attended by a number of qualifications. First, even together—let alone separately—these numerous measures explained little of the total variation in offense levels among firms, leaving unexplained 91 percent of the variation (Clinard et al. 1979, pp. 176–77). In separate research (see fuller discussion below), I similarly found that measures of profitability and relative dominance of firms in their markets did not contribute to the explanation of patterns in business violations of the Clean Water Act (Yeager 1981, p. 273). Second, and relatedly, the lack of predictive power in such research may be at least partially due to problems in the level of measurement used. Because of data limitations, the measures of financial health and structure are typically limited to the firm and industry levels of analysis. But many of the decisions (and pressures) relevant to compliance with regulatory laws, certainly including the commonly expensive environmental regulations, are made (and experienced) at lower levels of organization in large, complex firms, such as at the divisional, factory, or other subunit levels, which are often considered by corporate headquarters to "be on their own bottoms" financially.[47]

Finally, incomplete information in the violations data limited the study. The researchers were unable to make distinctions between minor and substantial environmental offenses, and the study significantly undercounted industrial water pollution offenses because it was largely limited to the incomplete data reported in the government's published annual enforcement reports.

B. Explaining Offenses: The Role of Law

It is altogether possible that the predictive models estimated to date fail to perform persuasively because the level of measurement is insufficiently sensitive to the organizational dynamics in business that underlie compliance behaviors. But it is also the case that such models are simply misspecified, because they neglect the basic role of legal process in shaping the profiles of lawbreaking and sanctioning. This role was the object of research I later conducted using Clean Water Act violations and sanctioning data from the EPA's Region 2, headquartered in New York City and responsible for implementing federal pollution control laws in New Jersey, New York, Puerto Rico, and the Virgin Islands (Yeager 1987; 1991, chap. 7).

The data analyzed for the study tracked the EPA's enforcement of the Clean Water Act against industrial polluters in New Jersey from 1973 through early 1978, a period of relatively active enforcement as the agency's program came to maturity. The sample comprised 321 industrial facilities, 117 (36 percent) of which were classified as major dischargers, while the remaining 204 were classified as minor.[48]

[47] At times the federal government is sufficiently persuaded of this fact to base regulatory decisions on it. For example, in promulgating final discharge regulations in 1987 for the "organic chemicals and plastics and synthetic fibers" industry, the EPA set reduced controls for small plants to spare them unduly harsh economic consequences. In doing so, the agency did not distinguish between small plants independently operated and those owned by large corporations. The EPA based this decision on industry comments that small plants owned by larger firms are run as independent profit centers, and on its analytic findings that small plants tend to experience similar levels of regulatory impacts regardless of ownership, and "despite the fact that in our closure analysis the weighted average cost of capital assigned to plants owned by medium and large sized firms was from one to two percentage points lower than the weighted average cost of capital assigned to small single plant firms." See *Organic Chemicals and Plastics and Synthetic Fibers Category Effluent Limitations Guidelines, Pretreatment Standards, and New Source Performance Standards*, 52 Fed. Reg. 42522 (November 5, 1987), at 42551-2.

[48] The analysis was limited to manufacturing plants discharging wastes directly into the state's waterways. For further discussion of the parameters of the sample, see Yeager (1987; 1991, p. 269, n. 26).

1. *The Offense Record.*   Given the dramatic shift in environmental policy represented by the 1972 water law, it is not surprising that 70 percent of the sample had committed nonminor violations of the act by 1978.[49] Moreover, while almost a third of the plants had no nonminor infractions of any type, many of these were facilities only recently permitted (just prior to 1978) or for which no significant new construction was required to meet effluent limits.

Violation rates varied substantially by type of infraction. While half the sample had committed nonminor pollution discharge violations, and 47 percent had violated the self-monitoring, self-reporting requirements at least once, only 14 percent had violated their compliance schedules for installing new pollution control systems. Among facilities found to have violated the water law extensively, such variation continued to exist: 14.5 percent of the sample had five or more nonminor effluent violations, while only .6 percent had as many compliance schedule infractions, and 1.2 percent had five or more reporting offenses.

The high degree of compliance with the construction schedules suggests that the EPA was successful in targeting this facet of the regulatory scheme for attention. The agency consistently emphasized the importance of maintaining compliance in this key aspect of the law, without which pollution control is indefinitely delayed, and typically took its stiffest enforcement stance against such violations. But additional violations of construction schedules were often prevented not by regulatory vigor but by legal forbearance: companies often sought and obtained extensions of schedules when they fell behind the original ones.

Effluent discharge violations, in contrast, were much more common because such offenses can occur on a spot basis (due to such factors as operator error or carelessness or equipment malfunction) and because the EPA's enforcement policies did not aggressively discourage such offenses in the 1970s, a pattern that arguably continues today. Typically, these violations were treated either with no enforcement action at all or with warning letters. Not uncommonly, a company could receive a number of such responses to these offenses, especially if they did not constitute evidence of systematic noncompliance ("bad faith"), without incurring more stringent enforcement responses such as formal administrative orders or referrals to the Justice Department for civil or criminal prosecution.

---

[49] Nonminor violations include all infractions except effluent discharge violations that were designated as minor in the region's data.

2. *Structural Bias.* What animated this research, however, is the question of whether (and how) discretionary decision making in regulatory law becomes systematically distorted, biased in favor of some interests over others because of structured imbalances in power and input. The findings suggest that larger, more powerful companies have both direct and indirect advantages at law over their smaller brethren, advantages that accrue through the routine operations of ostensibly neutral legal procedures.

By hypothesis, the *direct advantages* have to do with what might be called the "regulatory economies of scale" by which larger companies can more easily manage expensive regulatory costs (to the extent that they have larger facilities that spread such costs over larger volumes of production), and therefore generate higher rates of compliance, and with the reluctance (or inability) of regulators aggressively to sanction more powerful adversaries on violation.[50] The *indirect advantages* involve larger companies' greater access (due to their greater resources and expertise) to technical agency procedures by which firms can gain exceptions to the regulatory requirements initially imposed on them, thereby bringing the law more into line with their intent or capacity to comply.[51] These firms should then demonstrate higher rates of compliance.

The results can be briefly summarized as follows. For both types of offenses, it was found that larger firms were more likely to participate in the agency's adjudicatory hearing procedure, a judicial-like process in which technical arguments may be mounted (and countered by the government) as to why compliance with the current regulations is not feasible. When successful, these appeals produced advantages in the experience of violations and sanctions (Yeager 1987; 1991, pp. 288–92, 301–2). For the important compliance schedule requirements, the use

---

[50] As noted earlier, that they have larger facilities that spread costs over production may not always be the case at the plant level. But in general the conventional brief for corporate growth and conglomeration includes an argument that these lead to efficiencies that serve shareholders' interests.

[51] The financial and technical abilities of any given firm to comply with governmental regulation are often quite difficult to disentangle from its philosophical willingness to comply. Thus questions of the perceived appropriateness of state intervention into the economy may be interwoven with arguments concerning the very feasibility of compliance with regulation. Because of private industry's "knowledge advantage" in financial and technical matters often considered proprietary, it is possible to shroud ideological opposition to the fact of regulation itself with arguments couched in the language of feasibility. Since in any case both the fact and *degree* of regulatory intervention are determined by political processes involving matters of power and legitimacy, this private-sector advantage may work against socially efficient and just regulation.

of the hearings was associated with lower violation rates, in some cases because compliance schedules were modified to fit companies' intentions or abilities to comply better, in others because the original schedules were legally stayed during the (often long) periods of appeal as the government anticipated new compromise schedules.

There was also a small direct effect of corporate size on compliance schedule offenses:[52] larger firms were slightly less likely than smaller ones to fall behind the often expensive construction requirements, as suggested by the "regulatory economies of scale" argument. The finding remains only suggestive at present because it is a small effect. But that it appears despite the imprecise level of measurement—size/strength is measured at the level of parent companies, while the legal and compliance measures are made at the facility level—suggests that the role of corporate size and resources may be especially key when regulatory requirements cause significant capital expenditures, as in this case. However, corporate size produces no direct advantage in the sanctioning of firms: regardless of size, firms were very likely to be formally sanctioned by the EPA for violations of original or modified compliance schedules, as the agency considered these to be top priority for (relatively) stringent enforcement once the timetables were in place. Without compliance with the schedules, no substantial pollution control could go forward. As noted in the next section, too, the government reserved the more serious sanctions for such violations.

For pollution discharge violations, the findings were different, and in telling ways. Again, larger firms were more likely to benefit from use of the agency's adjudicatory hearing process, but in this case it acted to insulate companies from sanctions because the agency deferred sanctioning of violations while the permit conditions were under appeal; here, the agency's records continued to consider discharge violations as offenses, but ones not to be acted on. And note that this could be a considerable advantage for companies for two reasons: because of long backlogs in the hearing process many of the appeals lasted two and three years or longer, and because, ultimately, access to the procedure typically leads to altered permit conditions more in line with companies' abilities or intentions to comply.

For pollution discharge violations, however, there were no substantial *direct* advantages accruing to corporate strength: larger companies were not less likely either to violate discharge limits or to receive fewer

---

[52] Controlling for the effect of the hearings process on violations.

sanctions (controlling for violation rates and use of the hearings process) than were smaller firms. That larger companies do not appear to violate the limits less frequently suggests that the incidence of these infractions may be determined less by a company's ability to afford regulatory compliance than by its commitment to the adequate operation and maintenance of pollution abatement technology once in place. If there has been a generalized reluctance on the part of industry to make full compliance with the environmental laws of the 1970s a priority (Yeager 1986), then the distribution of violations reflecting daily operations may be relatively random across firms. This finding also fits the above-mentioned suggestion that firms were more likely to make a show of compliance with the highly visible (and EPA-prioritized) construction of new pollution controls and less likely to worry about the harder-to-police operation and maintenance requirements. Enforcement policies also supported this outcome: unlike compliance schedule violations, pollution discharge offenses were much more likely to be met with agency decisions to take no enforcement action at all, and, when taken, enforcement was largely in the form of warning letters, in some cases several successive letters before stiffer sanctions were likely.

But if larger firms were no more or less likely to be sanctioned than smaller companies for discharge violations, the evidence does suggest that the *types* of sanction may vary by size of company. In particular, the data suggest that smaller violators are more likely to receive stiffer sanctions, including formal administrative orders and civil and criminal referrals.

IV. Enforcement: The Structures and Processes of Policy Enforcement is the capstone of the regulatory process, the set of policies intended to insure law's effectiveness among the amoral calculators and the misguided, as well as to insure fairness in the legal system. Environmental law enforcement has always had among its goals the deterrence of violations (and, therefore, environmental harm) and the achievement of justice, in the forms of both retribution for wrongs and the leveling of the playing field: all violators should be similarly treated at law so that none benefits from noncompliance relative to complying competitors.

But as against the clean theory of enforcement policy, the practices always vary, most commonly for systemic reasons and in systematic ways. One of the dimensions over which enforcement practice varies is time. Some of the variation is based in statutory change (e.g., Adler and Lord 1991; Yeager 1991), as the legislature expands (more rarely, contracts) the executive's enforcement tools and responsibilities. But importantly, it is also rooted in philosophical differences, as when environmental enforcement was virtually vacated during the first term of the Reagan administration (Yeager 1991, chaps. 7 and 8). In what follows, however, I do not focus on the direct role that ideological differences may play. Instead, I concentrate the discussion on more systemic factors shaping enforcement in our political economy and legal organization, factors that appear relatively invariant with respect to the views of administrations in power.

A. Policies and Penalties

As a matter of statutory language and the legislative history, the Clean Water Act makes formal sanctions mandatory on a finding of any violation of the law; at a minimum, administrative orders to comply were to be issued to violators, with more consequential civil and criminal penalties to be sought in the case of more serious offenses, including those involving repeated violations and substantial harm. But very early on in its regulatory history, the EPA determined that formal enforcement would be discretionary, a position later affirmed by the courts.[53] The real range of enforcement responses ran from no action at all through criminal referrals to the U.S. Justice Department. The general approach of the agency has been to use the "jawboning" sanctions of warnings and administrative orders to negotiate and pressure compliance. By policy, civil and criminal penalties have generally been reserved for serious violations within the control of business management. For example, the EPA has considered criminal cases to be appropriate only in situations of willful, reckless, or negligent misconduct and especially when continued noncompliance suggests bad faith on the part of the violator (Yeager 1991, pp. 254–55).

Behind the implied rationale linking sanctioning severity to violation seriousness, however, lies a consistent tension between many enforcers' instinct that negotiation with polluters is the surest way to compliance, as well as a fear of contesting powerful corporate adversaries in court with limited enforcement budgets, and the need to achieve the law's goals of justice, fairness, and integrity or legitimacy.

Civil cases seeking monetary penalties and criminal cases seeking fines, incarceration, or both remain rather infrequent relative to viola-

---

[53] *Sierra Club v. Train*, 557 F.2d 485 (5th Cir. 1977). See also n. 12 above.

tion levels, but recent evidence suggests some increases by the end of the 1980s. For example, my research on EPA's enforcement practices in New Jersey found that civil and criminal cases were quite rare in the latter years of 1970s: they constituted only .6 percent of the agency's responses to violations (Yeager 1991, p. 279). A decade later, however, both the EPA and the Justice Department were more aggressively enforcing environmental laws with criminal sanctions (Adler and Lord 1991). Arguably, this reflects not only the continuing high rates of noncompliance but also ongoing public pressure for greater enforcement, which only accelerated in the wake of the Reagan administration's failure to enforce the environmental laws in the earlier part of the 1980s.

For example, Adler and Lord (1991, pp. 792–97, 843–45, 860–61) report government data showing that between 1985 and 1989 the average number of criminal investigations being carried out by the EPA (for all types of environmental offenses combined) increased from sixty to sixty-five annually to eighty-five to ninety. Similarly, the agency significantly increased the percentage of these cases actually referred to the Justice Department for criminal prosecution during this period, from 43 percent in 1985 to 65 percent by 1989. For its part, the Justice Department increased its prosecutions of referred cases from about ten to fifteen per year to twenty-five to forty per year; the percentage of EPA referrals prosecuted by the Justice Department increased from forty-six in 1983 and fifty-two in 1984 to sixty-six in 1988 and sixty-two in 1989. The department's budget for enforcing the law against environmental crimes increased from $257,000 in 1983 to $3 million in 1989, a tenfold increase (Thornburgh 1991, p. 779).

The penalties on conviction have also increased, for both corporations and individuals. (And note that corporate officers are typically prosecuted when companies are charged with criminal offenses: in 1983 officers were charged in 81 percent of the cases brought against their companies; in 1988 the number was 73 percent. (See Adler and Lord 1991, p. 845.) Under the Clean Water Act, for example, average *corporate* fines *per count* of violation have increased threefold, from $10,750 in 1983–84 to $34,375 in 1989; typically a count represents a single day of violation. Similarly, average fines per count for *individuals* increased from $1,586 in 1983–84 to $4,880 in 1988, while those serving jail or prison terms increased from 0 percent to about 25 percent.

The Clean Water Act penalties remain, however, well below statutory maximums, and their deterrent effects remain to be assessed. The average individual fines in 1988 were only one-fifth of the maximum available, and average sentences served (per count) are measured in days rather than months; for example, the average during 1985–87 was a single day served per count (Adler and Lord 1991, p. 860). For corporations, even in 1989 more than three-fifths of the cases involved fines less than the lowest maximum fine established in the 1987 amendments, $25,000 for negligent violations (for knowing violations, the maximum fine is $50,000; for knowing endangerment, $250,000).

B. Constraints on Enforcement

Adler and Lord (1991) argue that these latter findings indicate that the law has not produced the desired deterrence effects, and will not, especially given that high rates of noncompliance continue and that relatively few corporate violators are criminally sanctioned at all; moreover, they suggested that the improved results for the end of the 1980s represented a new plateau beyond which law enforcement was not likely to go without further budgetary and statutory enhancements. When the likelihood of such sanctions is small, deterrence logic calls for high penalties in the few cases that are brought. Additional evidence that deterrence policy may not be sufficiently operating comes from the civil side. A 1991 GAO study found that enforcement officials do not regularly collect civil penalties that equal the economic benefits firms experience through noncompliance with pollution control laws, despite the EPA's formal policy since 1984 that they do so (U.S. General Accounting Office 1991b). The GAO found this to be true of several major EPA enforcement programs including those under the Clean Water Act.[54] Such limitations on enforcement suggest the operation of systemic limits that constrain it.

[54] The GAO cited its own earlier study of enforcement against the illegal discharge of toxics into sewers (U.S. General Accounting Office 1989b), in which it found that, while 60 percent of municipal treatment plant authorities issued notices of violation to industrial offenders, only about 5 percent used administrative penalties or civil fines; even fewer sought criminal penalties. The GAO concluded that this weak enforcement was commonly premised on the authorities' view that it is politically difficult to impose sanctions on industrial facilities that employ local people and pay taxes; the study also noted that weak enforcement was a plausible cause of high industrial violation rates. The 1991 study of the civil penalty experience (U.S. General Accounting Office 1991b, p. 22) also cites a 1990 report by the EPA's inspector general, who found that "the [four audited] EPA regions and the [11] delegated states [to which EPA had delegated enforcement authority] had not assessed penalties in accordance with EPA's civil penalty policy and had not adequately documented penalty adjustments. In forty-six of the sixty-nine civil cases reviewed, the penalty assessments did not recover the economic benefit of noncompliance."

1. *Systemic Bias.* Although never subjected to adequate empirical examination, the belief of many close observers has long been that serious enforcement efforts, especially criminal cases, are rarely directed at large corporations deserving of them and instead are focused on smaller firms less likely to put up formidable resistance. Indeed, in 1978 a seasoned EPA attorney in the Office of Water Enforcement said, "We're afraid to go after [the big corporations]. We prefer to go after the little guys."[55]

Adler and Lord (1991, p. 796) cite some circumstantial evidence in support of this claim. They note, for example, that of the companies prosecuted under the nation's federal environmental laws since 1984, only 6 percent were among the nation's 500 largest corporations in 1989 and that less than 2 percent of the 500 largest industrial corporations have ever been prosecuted for environmental offenses despite their dominant collective share of industrial production.

My own research on the EPA's enforcement of the Clean Water Act found better, not to say definitive, evidence of such bias. For example, the statistical results showed that the EPA was somewhat less likely to issue formal administrative orders—at the time the dominant "in-house" sanction available to it—to larger companies than to smaller ones, controlling for the level of violations and other relevant factors (Yeager 1991, p. 289). In addition, the overall patterning of sanctions found in the study also suggests that systematic biases may operate, in particular, to favor the largest firms. Table 1 shows the distribution of sanctions, from the agency's decision to take no action to referrals to the Justice Department for civil or criminal cases, for New Jersey firms with annual sales of $10 million or less ("small firms"), and for those with annual sales in excess of $1 billion ("large firms"). Results are shown for total violations and for the most common violation types (Yeager 1991, pp. 281–83).

Although the numbers are small (and relevant controls are not included), the results are nonetheless rather consistent. Except for reporting violations, smaller companies are less likely to experience agency forbearance for violations ("no action") and more likely to receive the serious sanctions, including administrative orders and civil and criminal referrals.[56] It is particularly striking that the large firms were never sanctioned with criminal and civil sanctions over the sev-

[55] Conversation with author, EPA headquarters, Washington, D.C., spring, 1978.

[56] Because of their very small number, it was not possible statistically to model the criminal and civil referrals in multivariate models with the relevant controls.

TABLE 1

Sanctioning Responses by Firm Size in New Jersey

	Small Firms ($N = 125$)		Large Firms ($N = 93$)	
	Percent	No. of Cases	Percent	No. of Cases
Total violations:				
No action	27.8	84	56.2	169
Warning letter	53.6	162	25.6	77
Administrative order	4.3	13	1.7	5
Civil/criminal referral	1.3	4	0	
Compliance schedule violations:				
No action	9.8	4	11.1	2
Warning letter	65.9	27	83.3	15
Administrative order	12.2	5	0	
Civil/criminal referral	2.4	1	0	
Nonminor effluent violations:				
No action	51.1	67	67.6	155
Warning letter	19.8	26	11.4	26
Administrative order	3.1	4	1.8	4
Civil/criminal referral	1.5	2	0	
Reporting violations:				
No action	10.2	13	21.2	11
Warning letter	85.8	109	67.3	35
Administrative order	1.6	2	1.9	1
Civil/criminal referral	0		0	

SOURCE.—Yeager (1991), p. 281.

NOTE.—Percent refers to percentages of violations receiving the indicated sanction. N = number of plants owned by large or small firms.

eral-year period studied, despite many having long records of continued noncompliance. Finally, not shown in the table are the results for the few cases in which companies failed to file for discharge permits under the Clean Water Act, offenses generally considered very serious by the agency. Of the three such offenses committed by small firms, two received administrative orders while the other was referred to the Justice Department for prosecution. Of the two such offenses committed by large corporations, one received no action and the other a warning letter.[57]

[57] It should be noted that the intermediate-size companies in the study, those with annual sales ranging from $10 million to just under $1 billion, do not always fall midway between the two groups considered in the table in terms of sanctioning experience (see Yeager 1981, p. 242). For example, some of the firms in intermediate groupings were

An adequate test of the enforcement bias argument remains to be completed for civil and criminal penalties, one that has sufficient cases to test the argument with adequate controls. But the overall picture is strongly suggestive of such bias. Furthermore, research in related areas suggests the operation of systemic processes that can contribute to such results in environmental regulation.

In their study of the use of enforcement discretion by field inspectors from the U.S. Office of Surface Mining Reclamation and Enforcement, Lynxwiler and his colleagues, Shover and his colleagues (Shover, Clelland, and Lynxwiler 1986), found that larger mining companies, because of their greater resources and technical expertise, were able to negotiate more successfully the characterization of environmental offenses with government inspectors. The inspectors generally viewed the larger firms as more cooperative with regulatory expectations (due in part to their ability to negotiate at the highest technical levels with government experts) and (not so paradoxically) more likely than smaller firms to challenge stringent enforcement through legal appeals. One important result was that smaller companies tended to be assessed higher fines than larger corporate violators because inspectors tended to *interpret* the violations of the former as more serious offenses, quite apart from more objective measures of the harm occasioned by them.

Similar conclusions have been reached by Keith Hawkins (1983, 1984) in his intensive investigation of field inspectors attempting to enforce water pollution regulations in Britain. His analysis indicates that compliance negotiations in the field usually go forward as scientific and technical discussions (rather than as moral affairs) between regulators and the regulated and tend to exclude the concerns and viewpoints of environmental interests. Relatedly, he notes the field agents' perception that enforcement must be patient and "reasonable" lest it produce uncooperative attitudes toward compliance on the part of the regulated businesses.

Most relevant here is that Hawkins finds this process to be skewed in favor of larger, more powerful companies, which are more likely to

---

more likely than the small companies to receive administrative orders for infractions, and one group—the $500 million–$1 billion category—received slightly fewer (26.6 percent) no-action decisions than did the smallest companies. Nonetheless, the sanctioning differences remain impressive at the margins. In particular, the smallest businesses were more likely than any other grouping to receive the harshest sanctions: civil and criminal referrals. At the other end of the scale, the group of the largest companies were, in terms of total sanctions, the least likely of all to receive civil or criminal referrals, orders, and warnings and most likely to receive no-action decisions.

have the relevant technical expertise at hand, and which enforcement agents are therefore more likely to see as socially responsible and as generally more cooperative regarding the agency's aims. Among other results, their pollution episodes are more likely to be viewed as accidents than as evidence of recalcitrance.

In sum, the resource advantages of large companies may insulate them from stringent enforcement of environmental laws in several ways: by enabling compliance with expensive regulations in the first place, by enabling legal exceptions from stringent regulations, by permitting a better show of good faith efforts at compliance through technical and scientific argumentation, and by dissuading resource-starved enforcement offices from taking the risk of prosecuting them in long legal battles and persuading them instead to negotiate compliance.

2. *Organizational Constraints.* Additional constraints on enforcement are commonly rooted in the organization of the function. Here I briefly consider aspects connected to the relations between the EPA and the Justice Department, which share civil and criminal jurisdiction, and to the diffusion of enforcement over federal offices and numerous state agencies.

In the case of shared jurisdiction, problems of both bureaucratic competition and differing enforcement logics may arise, as they have at various times in the enforcement of the Clean Water Act. Regarding the first problem, at least from the standpoint of some Justice Department prosecutors, the agency refrains from referring some prosecutable cases because the EPA does not wish to share credit for the case with the department; instead, it uses its informal and administrative sanctions to negotiate compliance so that the agency will get sole enforcement credit and subsequently have a stronger regulatory record to show its superiors and congressional oversight committees when annual budgets are requested. According to the chief assistant U.S. attorney for Los Angeles, for example,

In fact, many cases by the non-criminal investigative agencies—by that I mean the regulatory agencies—never get presented to the U.S. Attorney's Office. A very significant reason why they don't . . . is because the agency gets no credit for a criminal prosecution. The agency gets credit for civil action [or other compliance-generating actions] that it can file and that its lawyers can handle, but the agency gets no statistical credit at budget time for a criminal case that has been prosecuted.

The best example is that for the last three years the United
States Attorney in Los Angeles . . . has been trying to get the
United States government more actively involved in environmental
prosecutions. . . . But when the EPA takes a look at a case, very
often we never even hear about it. They will handle it either
administratively or civilly and they will not bring the U.S.
Attorney's Office into it for criminal prosecution.[58]

The addition of administrative fines to the EPA's arsenal in the 1987
amendments to the Clean Water Act in theory should improve this
situation because the agency can now collect penalties from violators
without referring cases to the Justice Department. But if the agency
fails consistently to collect fines at least equal to the monetary benefits
of noncompliance, as suggested by the recent GAO study noted above
(U.S. General Accounting Office 1991b), and given the limit on maximum penalties in the statute ($125,000), the improvement will be
slight. And should the availability of monetary penalties result in even
fewer prosecutable cases being referred to the Justice Department,
environmental enforcement will to that extent further lose the horta-
tory support of the criminal sanction and whatever deterrent value it
brings.

In addition to the reason of bureaucratic "turf" protection, another
factor may inhibit the government's use of the criminal sanction, this
one having to do with the varying logics of prosecutions. A principal
advantage of the 1972 amendments over previous water pollution control legislation was that they explicitly eliminated the often difficult
burden of proof of showing harm to the environment (or human
health). Under the current law, criminal violations can be shown by a
simple demonstration of a knowing or negligent violation of a plant's
discharge permit, regardless of the level of damage. This was to permit
and encourage the more vigorous enforcement of environmental standards, and it also has the virtue of evening the playing field for dischargers on bodies of water differentially able safely to absorb pollutants.

However, by 1976—as systematic enforcement of permits was being
established—the EPA discovered that U.S. attorneys were often declining to file its enforcement cases unless there was evidence of actual
environmental damage. Dismayed at this executive "amendment" of

[58] Statement of Richard E. Drooyan, chief assistant U.S. attorney, Los Angeles (California Department of Justice 1988, p. 69).

the statute, the agency asked the Justice Department to inform all U.S. attorneys "of the correct interpretation of our statutes and the importance of prosecuting our enforcement cases without requiring proof of harm" (U.S. Environmental Protection Agency 1976).

The department responded that its official policy recognized that proof of environmental harm was not an essential element in water act prosecutions and that it did not support U.S. attorneys automatically rejecting referrals from the EPA for lack of such proof. However, the department wrote the EPA that in its experience "the only assured way of receiving meaningful relief is a showing by the Government of some adverse effect of the defendant's pollutants, and some courts require it. This is a fact which cannot be ignored" (U.S. Environmental Protection Agency 1976). The department therefore told the EPA that it declined to issue a " 'hard and fast' directive of any sort" (U.S. Environmental Protection Agency 1976) to its prosecutors around the country, leaving the "degree of harm" issue a relevant factor in the discretionary decision to prosecute cases. Again, to the extent that such considerations operate, they will tend to mute the reach and potential impacts of criminal sanctions.

The *organization* of the enforcement function also affects its sufficiency. In an extreme example, in the early years of the deregulation-minded Reagan administration enforcement was virtually eliminated as the EPA subjected the function to a series of confusing and distracting reorganizations (Yeager 1991, pp. 318–19). More generally, the locus and structure of enforcement influences its efficiency, consistency, and accountability. Despite the original logic of centralizing authority for environmental protection in the EPA, and thereby overcoming the patchwork of state and local laws and variable wills to enforce them, enforcement under the federal environmental laws remains largely de-centralized—to the level of both states and localities (as in municipal treatment works enforcement against industrial dischargers to sewers)—and often beset by geographic inequities of the sort that had prompted legal reform twenty years ago.

Precisely this result was found, for example, in the GAO study showing that environmental enforcement often failed to implement the EPA's formal civil penalty policy, established in 1984 to insure that civil penalties at a minimum amounted to the economic benefits from noncompliance enjoyed by business offenders (U.S. General Accounting Office 1991*b*). At the EPA, responsibility for setting and carrying out enforcement policies is spread over fifteen offices, with the result that "no one office is clearly accountable for penalty practices" (1991b, p. 11). The GAO found that EPA headquarters was inadequately overseeing the penalty policies even of its own regional enforcement offices, whose *enacted* policies range from strong endorsement of the headquarters approach to deemphasis of penalties in favor of negotiated compliance strategies (1991b, p. 8). Even more dramatic were the findings for the states, to which the EPA has delegated most of the enforcement responsibilities under federal environmental statutes. The agency has not even required the states to implement an economic benefit penalty policy; it has only recommended they do so. In the two EPA regions studied by the GAO, fewer than half the states have adopted such a policy, and it is common for states not to collect penalties at all for significant violations (1991b, pp. 6–8). This is important because 70 percent of environmental enforcement cases are carried by state authorities.

Rather than suggesting yet another reorganization of the enforcement function, the GAO recommended that the agency establish internal information and control systems to communicate, review, and enforce uniformity in the penalty policies with respect to all enforcement jurisdictions (1991b, p. 16).

3. *Resource Constraints.* One of the limits to adopting effective centralized oversight of enforcement policies is constrained agency budgets, always a factor that hampers regulation. In the case of the civil penalty policy, for example, it is likely that the EPA will find it quite expensive to implement the internal controls over state and regional enforcement recommended by the GAO. And one risk in doing so might lie in finding that states commonly fail to implement recovery of the economic benefits of noncompliance, indicating that the agency should exercise its responsibilities by reclaiming expensive enforcement responsibilities from such states. As the GAO has noted, "While EPA would like to see states adopt an economic benefit policy and have argued strongly in favor of such a move, officials in the Office of Enforcement and in the water and hazardous waste programs are concerned about actually compelling states to do so. Their principal concern is that states will relinquish authority for their programs to EPA, a burden that these officials believe would be too difficult to assume" (U.S. General Accounting Office 1991b, p. 14).

Resource limitations also can constrain effective enforcement more directly. For example, the GAO found that limited enforcement budgets, combined with the pressure to meet targeted enforcement levels, often pressure regional officials to settle cases quickly rather than push for appropriate monetary penalties. But these pressures can contradict the essential aims of enforcement: EPA headquarters officials agreed that, "once violators recognize that EPA is unlikely to take them to court, they are less likely to settle on terms favorable to the government. And, in the long run, this can undermine the goal of having penalties serve as a deterrent to violations" (1991b, p. 8).

Finally, the problem of resource limitations helps explain why EPA's regulatory effort has been consistently hampered by a lack of adequate information. For example, the lack of modern, comprehensive computerized data bases, found in my research (Yeager 1987, 1991) as well as in more recent investigations (Brown 1984, p. 18; U.S. General Accounting Office 1991b, pp. 9–10, 30), is by itself a substantial impediment to effective and rational enforcement of the law. Not only does it hinder the development of consistent, deterrence-maximizing enforcement, but it also prevents the agency from sending to the regulated, regulators, and the courts clear signals regarding the fairness, firmness, and rationality of its enforcement policies.

V. Conclusions: The Limits of Law

Research on the environmental regulation of business suggests a number of conclusions regarding criminological work and public policy. Among other things, it suggests that social regulation both reflects and reproduces inequalities in the political economy, certainly within the social structure of business organization. Arguably, too, it suggests that business defendants generally experience advantages at law not available to conventional criminal defendants. These advantages have to do with the structures and complexities of much regulation, which have the effect of shielding many (especially) corporate offenders from the full weight or moral force of law. At the level of policy, the consequence is often a public benefit that falls short of legislative intentions and even of the limits of economic feasibility.

In terms of criminological theory and research, this work and other research on white-collar crime more generally (e.g., Mann 1985; McBarnet 1991) clearly indicate the problem of "counting what we cannot see." To the extent that our empirical work relies on officially generated counts of offenses, typically indicated only by official enforcement responses, it will unwittingly incorporate any biases that are built into legal processes and that structure both the likelihood of offenses among types of regulated parties and the sanctions aimed (or not) at them. Compared to this vital empirical and theoretical challenge, the old but still current debate about just what constitutes white-collar *crime* is the much simpler problem to solve (Yeager 1986).

The accumulating work on the social regulation of business also clearly indicates the importance of historically informed studies of specific regulatory programs. In the first place, depending on the precise nature of the legal requirements—for example, whether the associated costs and benefits are distributed to diffuse or specific constituencies, and the relative political power of each (see, e.g., Wilson 1980; Stryker 1991)—government regulation will be more or less effective in reaching stated public purposes; conversely, it will be more or less vulnerable to compromise by regulated interests. And these variations will be further shaped by changes in the broader society, such as economic and political trends that generate greater or lesser degrees of class organization around important questions of public policy.

In the second place, regulatory regimes vary considerably in terms of the legal processes used to implement them. These processes are ordained both formally (e.g., by statute) and informally (e.g., by administrative "amendment") and are key in generating the profiles of offenders that are available to public view.

This argument has important implications for the prospects for a *general theory* of crime such as that recently proposed by Gottfredson and Hirschi (1990). In general, to the extent that inequalities are variably "structured into" legal processes, and thereby produce different patterns of offenses and sanctions, criminological theorizing is likely to be confined to typological explanations for various subtypes of crime. And notice that this point applies as well to types of conventional offending as to more complex regulatory matters.

Research on regulatory law also has implications for Gottfredson and Hirschi's specific neoclassical view, which they have applied to white-collar crime to exemplify its generality (Hirschi and Gottfredson 1987). In this argument, these authors tend to marginalize the role of opportunity: "Since crimes involve goods, services, or victims, they have other constituent properties as well: they all require opportunity, and are thought to result in punishment of the offender if he or she is detected. Such properties cannot account for the general tendency of particular individuals to engage in crime, and they are therefore not central to a theory of criminality" (1987, p. 959). The argument instead emphasizes a central role for motivation in the explanation of crime, in particular, the classical view of motivation as involving the self-interested pursuit of pleasure and avoidance of pain. But this argument ignores the ways in which motivation and opportunity may be entailed in each other, perhaps especially as wealthy, organized interests endeavor to shape law itself (Coleman 1987).

This would seem to be especially the case for the legal regulation of business behavior. Here, the relation between law and the regulated is highly dynamic. In particular, not only may *perceptions of law* increase (conversely, decrease) the psychological availability of illegal acts, but the relevant (regulated) parties may be actively involved in shaping both law and the regard with which it is viewed. In addition to increasing psychological availability, this action may also reduce the deterrent effects of law, whether considered in terms of the conventional logic of the calculus of pain and gain or in more expressive moral terms. To the extent that such processes occur, both motivation and opportunity will be dynamically produced and reproduced.

In the case of environmental law, for example, core features in the regulatory process reduce the moral salience of offending, as discussed in this essay, and to that extent expand the "moral opportunities" for lawbreaking. Importantly, the regulated parties commonly participate in actively shaping the moral dialogue that produces such expanded opportunities. It is in this sense that opportunities are socially constructed rather than "naturally" given in the environment, as in the simple availability of goods to steal or gullible citizens to fleece.

REFERENCES

Adler, Robert W., and Charles Lord. 1991. "Environmental Crimes: Raising the Stakes." *George Washington Law Review* 59:781–861.
Brown, Michael A. 1984. "EPA Enforcement—Past, Present and Future." *Environmental Forum* 3(1):12–22.
Bureau of National Affairs. 1983. "Special Report: Effluent Guidelines Rulemaking Nears End; Litigation, Compliance Extensions Expected." *BNA Environment Reporter—Current Developments* 13:1629–31.
California Department of Justice. 1988. *Proceedings of Symposium 87: White Collar/Institutional Crime—Its Measurement and Analysis.* Sacramento: California Department of Justice, Bureau of Criminal Statistics and Special Services.
Clinard, Marshall B., and Peter C. Yeager. 1980. *Corporate Crime.* New York: Free Press.

Clinard, Marshall B., Peter C. Yeager, Jeanne M. Brissette, David Petrashek, and Elizabeth Harries. 1979. *Illegal Corporate Behavior*. Washington, D.C.: U.S. Government Printing Office.

Coleman, James W. 1987. "Toward an Integrated Theory of White-Collar Crime." *American Journal of Sociology* 93:406–39.

Conservation Foundation. 1982. "Water Resources." In *State of the Environment 1982*. Washington, D.C.: Conservation Foundation.

DiMento, Joseph F. 1986. *Environmental Law and American Business: Dilemmas of Compliance*. New York: Plenum.

Galanter, Marc. 1974. "Why the 'Haves' Come out Ahead: Speculations on the Limits of Legal Change." *Law and Society Review* 9(3):95–160.

Gottfredson, Michael R., and Travis Hirschi. 1990. *A General Theory of Crime*. Stanford, Calif.: Stanford University Press.

Harrington, Winston. 1988. "Enforcement Leverage When Penalties Are Restricted." *Journal of Public Economics* 37:29–53.

Hawkins, Keith. 1983. "Bargain and Bluff: Compliance Strategy and Deterrence in the Enforcement of Regulation." *Law and Policy Quarterly* 5:35–73.

———. 1984. *Environment and Enforcement: Regulation and the Social Definition of Pollution*. New York: Oxford University Press.

Hirschi, Travis, and Michael R. Gottfredson. 1987. "Causes of White-Collar Crime." *Criminology* 25:949–74.

Lynxwiler, John, Neal Shover, and Donald A. Clelland. 1983. "The Organization and Impact of Inspector Discretion in a Regulatory Bureaucracy." *Social Problems* 30:425–36.

McBarnet, Doreen. 1991. "Whiter than White Collar Crime. Tax, Fraud Insurance and the Management of Stigma." *British Journal of Sociology* 42:323–44.

McGarity, Thomas O. 1983. "Media-Quality, Technology, and Cost-Benefit Balancing Strategies for Health and Environmental Regulation." *Law and Contemporary Problems* 46(2):159–233.

Magat, Wesley A., and W. Kip Viscusi. 1990. "Effectiveness of the EPA's Regulatory Enforcement: The Case of Industrial Effluent Standards." *Journal of Law and Economics* 33:331–60.

Mann, Kenneth. 1985. *Defending White-Collar Crime: A Portrait of Attorneys at Work*. New Haven, Conn.: Yale University Press.

Marcus, Alfred. 1980. "Environmental Protection Agency." In *The Politics of Regulation*, edited by James Q. Wilson. New York: Basic.

Moretz, Sandy. 1990. "The Rising Cost of Environmental Crime." *Occupational Hazards* (March), pp. 38–41.

Reichman, Nancy. 1992. "Moving Backstage: Uncovering the Role of Compliance Practices in Shaping Regulatory Policy." In *White Collar Crime Reconsidered*, edited by Kip Schlegel and David Weisburd. Boston: Northeastern University Press.

Reiss, Albert J., Jr. 1985. "Compliance without Coercion." *Michigan Law Review* 83(February):813–19.

Schneider, Keith. 1985. "The Data Gap: What We Don't Know about Chemicals." *Amicus Journal* 6(4):15–24.

Schroeder, Christopher. 1983. "Introduction: Federal Regulation of the Chemical Industry." *Law and Contemporary Problems* 46(2):1–40.

Shabecoff, Philip. 1989a. "Industrial Pollution Called Startling." *New York Times* (April 13), national edition, p. D21.

———.1989b. "U.S. Pinpoints Waterways Polluted by Toxic Chemicals." *New York Times* (June 14), national edition, p. A24.

Shover, Neal, Donald A. Clelland, and John Lynxwiler. 1986. *Enforcement or Negotiation: Constructing a Regulatory Bureaucracy*. Albany: State University of New York Press.

Starr, Judson W. 1991. "Turbulent Times at Justice and EPA: The Origins of Environmental Criminal Prosecutions and the Work That Remains." *George Washington Law Review* 59:900–915.

Stipp, David. 1992. "Environment: Execs Get Little Sympathy for Crimes against Nature." *Wall Street Journal* (March 11), national edition, p. B1.

Strock, James M. 1991. "Environmental Criminal Enforcement Priorities for the 1990s." *George Washington Law Review* 59:916–37.

Stryker, R. 1991. "Government Regulation." In *Encyclopedia of Sociology*, edited by E. F. Borgatta and M. L. Borgatta. New York: Macmillan.

Sutherland, Edwin H. 1949. *White Collar Crime*. New York: Henry Holt & Co.

Thornburgh, Dick. 1991. "Criminal Enforcement of Environmental Laws—a National Priority." *George Washington Law Review* 59:775–79.

Tripp, James T. B. 1977. "Tensions and Conflicts in Federal Pollution Control and Water Resource Policy." *Harvard Journal on Legislation* 14:225–80.

U.S. Environmental Protection Agency. 1976. "EPA Headquarters Enforcement Memorandum." Unpublished document regarding correspondence between the EPA and the U.S. Department of Justice on problems in enforcement, December 3. Washington, D.C.: U.S. Environmental Protection Agency.

———. 1977. *EPA Enforcement: A Progress Report—1976*. Washington, D.C.: U.S. Environmental Protection Agency.

U.S. General Accounting Office. 1983. *Wastewater Dischargers Are Not Complying with EPA Pollution Control Permits*. GAO/RCED-84-53. Washington, D.C.: U.S. General Accounting Office.

———. 1989a. *Water Pollution: More EPA Action Needed to Improve the Quality of Heavily Polluted Waters*. GAO/RCED-89-38. Washington, D.C.: U.S. General Accounting Office.

———. 1989b. *Water Pollution: Improved Monitoring and Enforcement Needed for Toxic Pollutants Entering Sewers*. GAO/RCED-89-101. Washington, D.C.: U.S. General Accounting Office.

———. 1991a. *Water Pollution: Stronger Efforts Needed by EPA to Control Toxic Water Pollution*. GAO/RCED-91-154. Washington, D.C.: U.S. General Accounting Office.

———. 1991b. *Environmental Enforcement: Penalties May Not Recover Economic Benefits Gained by Violators*. GAO/RCED-91-166. Washington, D.C.: U.S. General Accounting Office.

U.S. House of Representatives. 1977. *Implementation of the Federal Water Pollution Control Act: Summary of Hearings on the Regulation and Monitoring of Toxic and Hazardous Chemicals under the Federal Water Pollution Control Act (P.L. 92-500)*. July 19, 20, 21, 28, 29; serial no. 95-25. Washington, D.C.: U.S. Government Printing Office.

U.S. Senate. 1973. *A Legislative History of the Water Pollution Control Act Amendments of 1972*. Vol. 1, serial no. 93-1. Washington, D.C.: U.S. Government Printing Office.

―――. 1977. *Study on Federal Regulation*, Vols. 1–6. Committee on Governmental Affairs. Washington, D.C.: U.S. Government Printing Office.

Wilson, James Q. 1980. "The Politics of Regulation." In *The Politics of Regulation*, edited by James Q. Wilson. New York: Basic.

Yeager, Peter C. 1981. "The Politics of Corporate Social Control: The Federal Response to Industrial Water Pollution." Ph.D. dissertation, University of Wisconsin—Madison, Department of Sociology.

―――. 1986. "Analyzing Illegal Corporate Behavior: Progress and Prospects." In *Research in Corporate Social Performance and Policy*, vol. 8, edited by James E. Post. Greenwich, Conn.: JAI Press.

―――. 1987. "Structural Bias in Regulatory Law Enforcement: The Case of the U.S. Environmental Protection Agency." *Social Problems* 34:330–44.

―――. 1991. *The Limits of Law: The Public Regulation of Private Pollution*. Cambridge: Cambridge University Press.

―――. 1993. "Law, Crime and Inequality: The Regulatory State." In *Crime and Inequality*, edited by John Hagan and Ruth Peterson. Palo Alto, Calif.: Stanford University Press (forthcoming).

Peter Reuter

The Cartage Industry in New York

ABSTRACT

The private garbage collection industry, dominated until recently by
numerous very small firms in essentially local markets, has a long history
of customer allocation conspiracies in restraint of trade. In New York
metropolitan areas, these agreements have involved members of the Mafia.
The reputation for racketeering involvement in the New York region has
restricted entry, particularly by the few large national firms; maintained
discipline among the conspirators; and inhibited customers from
complaint. The carters have treated customers as assets to be bought and
sold. Prices for collection of waste from commercial customers have been
raised by as much as 50 percent in these markets. Both law enforcement
and regulation have failed to eliminate customer allocation agreements.

The collection of garbage has been an ill-reputed, though necessary,
activity since the development of a concern with urban public health
in the nineteenth century.[1] There may be a sense that society regards
those whose business centers around the garbage generated by society
as polluted by that contact. Garbage collectors are objects of ridicule
in literature and popular culture—for example, Mr. Doolittle in *Pyg-
malion* or Ed Norton in "The Honeymooners" (though both surprisingly redeem themselves with individualized wit). Garbage collection
often takes place early in the morning (to reduce traffic congestion in
urban areas), is intrinsically messy, employs relatively simple technol-

Peter Reuter is codirector of the Drug Policy Research Center at the RAND Corporation, Washington, D.C. Ronald Goldstock made valuable contributions, as well as providing access to important data.
[1] Defined as solid waste, not classified as hazardous, produced by any residential,
commercial, or industrial activity. It includes both organic and inorganic waste.

ogy, and requires little skill and substantial brawn, all adding to its low social standing.

The reputation has sometimes taken on a more sinister cast. In certain cities, it is widely believed that the industry is run by organized crime, usually (and correctly) meaning the Mafia. This belief is particularly firmly held in the greater New York metropolitan area and a good deal of evidence supports the notion that the industry there has indeed had extensive dealings with organized crime.

The thesis of this essay is that the reputation for racketeer involvement has had highly significant consequences for the performance of the industry in New York and its environs. It helps determine who participates in the industry, how customers and suppliers interact, and the nature of regulation of the industry. Prices have been sharply raised in those sectors of the industry most prone to the conspiracy and increased somewhat in all sectors. The industry has exhibited an extraordinarily long-lived and repetitive pattern of violation of law, which has attracted frequent investigations and prosecutions, as well as extensive economic regulation. Racketeer involvement has allowed an unusual phenomenon, namely, operation of successful conspiracies involving large numbers of participants. But it also turns out that reputation for racketeer involvement presents an unusually difficult problem for those who would reform the industry; indeed, it is likely that most reform efforts have been counterproductive.

The essay relies heavily on data collected between 1978 and 1985 in New Jersey, New York City, and Long Island. Three separate activities were involved. In 1978 the National Institute of Justice (NIJ) funded a study of racketeering in legitimate industries; the garbage collection industry in New Jersey and New York City served as one of the case studies (Reuter, Rubinstein, and Wynn 1982). In 1983 NIJ provided a further grant for extending the work to Long Island (Reuter 1987). Finally, in 1985 and 1986 I worked for the New Jersey Board of Public Utilities (BPU) as an expert witness in lengthy civil proceedings related to the conviction of a carter on antitrust charges; that permitted the continued collection of data on the industry. In the first of these studies I interviewed numerous officials in the relevant regulatory agencies, as well as a small number of persons involved in the carting firms themselves. I also had access to certain investigative reports of New Jersey and New York State investigative agencies.[2] When work-

---

[2] Certain records, notably grand jury materials, were not made available for the research.

ing as an expert witness for the BPU, I was able to initiate file searches and other investigative activities by BPU staff. Newspapers provided a great deal of useful information as well.

Some additional evidence is presented to suggest that little has changed since the original data were collected; a customer allocation agreement still operates in all three areas and the reputation for racketeer involvement also remains. The generality of the phenomenon across locations is unclear, but some evidence is offered to suggest that the garbage collection industry shows a tendency to (probably less effective) conspiracy in other cities, even without the involvement of racketeers.

The essay begins with a brief description of the garbage collection industry and its evolution, giving particular attention to the family orientation of the businesses, which is critical to an understanding of the tendency to conspiracy. The descriptive core of the essay is contained in Section II, which outlines the nature of the violations found in the industry. That description points to the complex role of organized crime; an understanding of that role is attempted through an analysis of the problem of designing effective arrangements for cartels with numerous participants and of the assets and strategies available to organized crime (Sec. III). The next two sections examine efforts to eliminate the racketeers and bring about competitive performance first through prosecution and then through regulation. Section VI examines the consequences of the agreements, while the final section deals with the generality of the findings, over time, spaces, and industries.

I. Industry Structure and Development

Waste *collection* (taking garbage from the generator to some other location where it may be recycled, compacted, or disposed of) is not waste *disposal* (providing a final destination for the waste, typically a landfill before 1980, now increasingly incineration or other more technologically complex transformation). Though some firms may provide both services, the vast majority do not. As environmental concerns have become increasingly important, disposal is now usually either directly provided by local government or operated under contract to such a government, reflecting the government's interest in having control of the waste stream.

The opportunities for illegal activity in the two sectors are very different. Local disposal markets are often monopolies, either natural (a uniquely advantaged site in a congested area) or regulatory (only one license granted for environmental reasons). Control of a disposal facility by a group of "carters" (the term used here for the firms that collect solid waste) was one means for limiting entry and competition in earlier eras; only carters who were in compliance with a cartel agreement were allowed to bring their waste to a given facility. Collection generates cartels rather than monopolies.

The garbage collection industry has at least four component sectors, defined by type of customer and nature of waste; these affect the equipment needed for collection. The distinctions are important because these differences affect the opportunity structure for certain law violations. The four sectors are individual residences, institutions and large apartment buildings, commercial and industrial establishments, and construction sites. Different kinds of equipment are used for collection in the various market segments.[3] Most firms operate in only one or two of these segments.[4] Service to individual residents is usually provided by a truck with a mechanized bucket at its rear (a "rear-end loader") into which the individual garbage can's contents are placed. The service can be provided by local government, by a private carter working for that government ("municipal contract"), or by a private carter directly contracting with the householder ("scavenger"). On Long Island in 1984 municipal contracts applied to about one-third of households. Typically the contract ran for one to three years and applied to 2,000–3,000 households, with annual revenues of about $250,000. One-quarter of Long Island households bought services from scavengers. The rest were serviced directly by local government; towns occasionally move among these different modes of service provision. In this essay, I discuss the individual-reference sector only briefly because, for reasons discussed in Section VI, customer allocation agreements do not generally apply to it.

Service to institutions or large apartment buildings, depending on the size of the establishment, can be provided by rear-end loader or by more specialized equipment, with the carter providing a large container that can be hooked directly into the truck. Most municipal contracts covered large apartment buildings but not other institutions.

[3] The separation is not complete, however; for example, a rear-end loader might be used for individual residences and smaller commercial establishments. But larger commercial customers are usually serviced by specialized equipment.

[4] The definition of product markets in the carting industry has been the subject of litigation in recent years. In a 1984 merger case, the Second Circuit Court of Appeals ruled that the residential and business/industrial customers constituted distinct markets; it did not accept finer distinctions offered by the government (U.S. vs. Waste Management, Inc., 743 F.2d 976 [2d Cir. 1984]).

Commercial and industrial establishments, if large enough, receive "roll-off" service. A large container is picked up at the site, and an empty one is left in its place. Very few municipal contracts provide for service to these establishments.[5] This is the market segment with which this essay is most concerned. It involves establishments such as restaurants, stores, and light industry. These establishments contract directly with the carter. Contracts are generally not written; the arrangement provides for service as required, although, apart from seasonal fluctuations, this is likely to be fairly routinized on a weekly basis.

Roll-off service is usually provided to construction sites, always under direct contract. Construction activities and heavy industry generate distinctive, mostly inorganic, wastes. Construction sites usually require collection service for a relatively short time. However, over time a construction firm will typically have many sites, so that there may be a certain contractual stability; one carter may effectively have a contract to provide pickup at all the sites of a particular construction company within his service territory. The failure of customer allocation agreements to include this segment is also analyzed in Section VI.

Despite the growth of a small number of highly profitable multinational corporations handling solid and toxic waste, the garbage collection industry remains dominated by numerous, small, family-owned businesses, frequently passed on from father to son over three generations. If the Jeffersonian ideal had been extended to cover urban industry, these firms might have been held up as the counterpart to the small yeoman farmer. Often the whole family is involved in the operation of the firm, with the wife handling a variety of office chores and sons working on the trucks.

Entry into the collection industry requires little capital. Though new trucks may cost upward of $100,000, there is an active second-hand market, as well as many leasing firms that facilitate much lower-priced entry. Typically the small firm equipment is garaged either at the owner's home or in a general purpose garage.

These small firms operate in only one metropolitan area; indeed, in large metropolitan areas they may operate in only one region. For example, Long Island, a two-county area (Nassau and Suffolk counties) with a population of about 2.5 million in 1985, had at least 200 garbage

[5] Stevens (1991) reports on a survey of New York State, which found that commercial establishments received garbage collection under municipal contract only in areas with 4 percent of the population. Also see Stevens (1978).

collection firms. New York City in 1979 had about 300 firms; the largest had less than 5 percent of the market. None offered service in every part of the city or Long Island. Many had only one truck, though these accounted for a relatively small share of total capacity—approximately 5 percent on Long Island, 20 percent in New York City. In New Jersey, 755 out of 891 licensees (85 percent) in 1980 had fewer than six employees; most of these were one- or two-truck firms.

In all three areas the business is dominated by males of Italian origin. In looking through files on transactions involving New York carting firms in the late 1970s I came across only two firms whose owners' names were not clearly Italian. In New Jersey a substantial number of the firms were started by Italians living in the Plainfield area; most were descendants of immigrants from a single town in southern Italy who founded these firms in the early part of this century.

There are numerous family connections between firms. A younger son splits off and starts his own firm; in the next generation competition is between cousins, a process still further complicated by intermarriage. Consider New York Carting, one of the firms I examine below. It was founded by Joseph Macaluso in the early 1950s. His two sons, Robert and Charles, joined him. In the late 1960s he retired from active management of the firm, which passed to the two sons and a son-in-law. Charles, the elder son, then began a firm in New Jersey, and the younger son took over. The son-in-law then moved to run another carting firm in Queens.

Ethnic homogeneity is apparently characteristic of the carting market in many cities according to experts in the industry. In Chicago most firms were set up by men of Dutch origin. The Los Angeles industry has long been dominated by two ethnic groups, Armenians and Jews; in San Francisco, Italians dominate.

The ethnic homogeneity is not accidental and has important consequences. A carter cannot afford to allow equipment failure or employee problems to interrupt service for even as long as a day. Yet in their early days most firms could not provide for reserve equipment since the entrepreneur had modest capital and very limited access to external finance. Moreover, mechanical equipment, particularly the trucks, was vulnerable to frequent breakdowns in the second quarter of the century when many firms were starting. Cooperation among carters was the only solution to the problem of providing reliable and consistent service. Each carter was willing to enter into informal cooperative arrangements with other carters so that each member of the group would provide backup if one member had a problem in servicing his regular schedule of customers.[6]

Extended families facilitated such arrangements. The same could be said for ethnic homogeneity, and there may have been a tendency for ethnic groups with strong intraethnic ties to be more successful in this activity. The low repute of the industry probably also influenced which ethnic groups entered; immigrant groups, with traditions of entrepreneurship, and which were newly arrived in the area when the industry started, were likely to dominate.

The continued ethnic homogeneity in many areas continues to facilitate cooperation, in this case with less benign consequence. Italian domination of the industry in New Jersey, Long Island, and New York has eased the involvement of the Mafia.

The national firms (of which Waste Management and Browning Ferris Industries [BFI] are the largest) emerged in the 1970s, constituting an entirely new phenomenon for a previously completely fragmented industry. Waste Management reported revenues of $6 billion in 1991; BFI reported $3 billion.

Waste Management and BFI, the "Big Two," were the first to emerge. Each followed a similar strategy of acquiring numerous local firms, issuing stock to the owners of the acquired firms and giving them multiyear management contracts.[7] That enabled the nationals to retain their local knowledge, possibly including intimacy with local conspiracies, while at the same time providing the modern corporate services that have made them so efficient (centralized truck buying, regularly scheduled maintenance). Each was founded by entrepreneurial groups that included highly educated managers with extensive experience outside of the solid waste field. The national firms have diversified as well into disposal (where they have been accused of using difficult-to-obtain licenses to control entry and prices in the collection business) and into toxic waste collection and disposal. They have also been aggressive competitors in international markets, successfully bidding for business from Buenos Aires to Riyadh.

The national firms do not operate in either New York City or Long Island, though both represent major markets. They are active in New Jersey. Their absence from New York City and Long Island is proba-

---

[6] Indeed, such arrangements were still common in the late 1970s, even between carters who were not otherwise on good terms.

[7] The acquisition rate was particularly high in their early years. For example, BFI acquired 157 companies between 1968 and 1973.

bly evidence of the effectiveness of the racketeer reputation of the industry there and of the customer allocation agreements.

II. The Violations

Hearings of the McClellan Committee in the late 1950s in Los Angeles and the New York metropolitan area showed that the garbage collection industry in both regions was characterized by highly institutionalized customer allocation agreements policed by the local labor unions.[8]

The two sets of agreements operated in much the same way, though the Los Angeles hearings, in contrast to those in New York, showed no significant involvement of any outside criminal group. The carters, as members of industry associations, agreed not to compete for each others' customers. Once a customer had accepted service from a carter, no other member of the association would provide service to that customer, even if actively solicited by him. A carter found to have taken a customer from another member was expected to provide compensation, either in money or other customers. For example, one Los Angeles carter acquired the contract to service a residential complex that was dissatisfied with the service provided by its previous carter. The monthly revenues were $800 and the new company was required by the association to pay $7,200 to the original firm.

The union served as the primary disciplinary arm for the Los Angeles association. Where a member of the association did not abide by the terms of an "arbitration," the union was requested to deny him access to the disposal facilities; the union complied with such requests.

Essentially the same agreement had emerged in the New York area, but racketeers had played a role in the formation of the local association, and there was a pattern of violence and intimidation associated with the agreement.[9] A member of the Lucchese family of the Mafia, Tony (Ducks) Corallo, intervened on behalf of a relative who owned a carting firm; the union leader agreed not to enforce the terms of the union contract on that firm. The union played an active role in enforcing the customer allocation agreement by picketing customers of firms that broke the agreement. In general the union appeared to be the instrument of Mafiosi, and it was through the union that racketeers extracted their taxes. At least one murder seemed to be related to

[8] Senator John McClellan of Arkansas was chair of the Permanent Subcommittee of Investigation of the Government Operations Committee from 1955 to his death. He led the committee in major investigations of organized crime throughout his tenure. A good summary of these hearings is presented in Hutchison (1970).

[9] The hearings covered Westchester County and Long Island, as well as the city.

the formation of the agreement; like every one of the eight homicides connected to the industry in the greater New York area, it remains unsolved.

One element of the agreement, which survived in agreements a quarter century later, was that the carter's entitlement was to a location rather than a customer. If a store moved to a new location, which had never had a commercial business before, then carters could compete to service the store at its new location. However, the original carter had the right to service any business that moved into the original location, an arrangement that minimizes the difficulty of operating a customer allocation agreement.

The McClellan Committee hearings led to indictment of the principal racketeer (Vincent Squillante) directly involved in the industry, along with the union president (Bernard Adelstein). Squillante disappeared before the trial and is believed to have been murdered; Adelstein's conviction was overturned on appeal. Otherwise the hearings did little more than help establish the bad reputation of the industry.

Shortly after the McClellan Committee hearings, the New Jersey State Assembly held hearings on the state's garbage collection industry. It focused on municipal contracting and found evidence of a bid-rigging agreement, with the union providing enforcement for the agreement. The union local involved was controlled by organized crime figures; the union leader was indicted and disappeared, presumably murdered, shortly before his trial. Landfills owned by carters were also used to enforce the agreement; "renegade" carters were either denied access or charged higher prices.

Ten years later the New Jersey State Commission of Investigation (SCI) carried out a more detailed investigation of the industry. Its 1969 report covered the commercial sector as well as the municipal contract sector. Most carters serving commercial customers belonged to one of a small number of associations, generally organized along county lines. The bylaws of the associations were perfectly explicit on the nature of the competitive relationship among association members. For example, one required the following: "a. At each meeting every member shall provide a list of his stops which he has lost or which became vacant or to which he discontinued service for non-payment of charges or which he has begun to service as a new stop. b. Stops exchanged or transferred shall be under a formula of 10 times the monthly rate. The member entitled to a stop shall have the option of determining whether he shall receive cash or stops in return. c. The trustees shall fix minimum fees for the different types of stops and customers" (New Jersey State Commission of Investigation 1969).

Other associations had equally explicit restrictions on competition among members. A lawyer who handled the affairs of some ten of these groups defended them before the SCI, arguing that their purpose was to police the members. When asked what he meant, he replied: "Well before I came in the matter back in 1956, members were engaged in stealing stops among the other members. I use the word 'stealing' . . . I mean taking, taking stops that belong to other members and doing other things that need straightening out. . . . With reference to whether one member can supply better service at a lesser price, he still has no right to take the stop from a member. . . . The stop is merchandise belonging to the member for the period of time" (New Jersey State Commission of Investigation 1969).

Curiously enough, the courts of New Jersey had upheld the restrictive agreements of the associations. In at least one case an association had taken a member to court because of failure to pay compensation for "stealing" a customer; the court had ruled for the association, arguing that membership had the nature of a contract.

The SCI produced no specific evidence of organized crime involvement but warned that it had reason to suspect that such involvement was likely to occur and that the state should act to prevent this (New Jersey State Commission of Investigation 1969).

More detailed information is available on the operation of the carting industry in the 1970s and early 1980s in New York City, New Jersey, and Long Island. Though there are differences among the three jurisdictions, the patterns of violation are essentially the same. Consequently, I present the New York City case in some detail and then describe the other two only to the extent they differ in important ways or where material was available that throws light on aspects of the industry arrangements that are not well covered by the New York City description.

A. New York City

The commercial solid waste collection market in New York City in 1979 consisted of 300 firms with approximately 800 trucks. The city Department of Sanitation picked up all residential garbage. The largest private firm had about twenty trucks. None of the national firms was present in the market, though a number of commercial customers had invited them to enter the market.

The firms were either sole proprietorships or partnerships. All were fully unionized; the union involved was Local 813 of the Teamsters, which also represented carting employees in the suburban counties. Nearly a quarter century after the McClellan Committee hearings, Bernard Adelstein, then the head of Local 813, had become its business agent; Adelstein's son and nephew had become the president and secretary, respectively.

The total number of firms had declined substantially since 1956, when regulation was introduced and 500 firms were eligible for licensing. The attrition was gradual, usually involving mergers of small firms when one carter retired from the business. It was difficult to establish that there had been no new entrants (since firms might change corporate names), but officials of the licensing agency could not recall any genuine new entrant in two decades.

The vast majority of carters were members of one of three industry associations; one covered the Bronx and Manhattan, one covered Brooklyn, and the other Queens. The regional organization represented a recognition of the reality that New York City did not constitute a single market. Transportation costs are a significant element of the cost of operation of a carter.[10] Most carters operate in a very confined region within one borough.

1. *Customers as Assets.* Public record information in the late 1970s showed that the anticompetitive practices that created public concern in the 1950s, and eventually led to regulation, still persisted. Customers were treated as assets of the carters who serviced them, and they were transferred between carters in open financial transactions that were routinely approved by the Department of Consumer Affairs (DCA), the industry's regulatory agency. The justification offered for the transfers was that the original carter was selling the goodwill that he had developed among his customers. In fact, the circumstances surrounding individual transactions, as well as the high and uniform prices paid, made clear that this was a pretense. The transfers represented nothing more than the confirmation of a customer allocation agreement among the carters. A fairly detailed account is offered of two illustrative transactions as the detail helps provide a flavor of the regulatory and business environment of the industry.

---

[10] An indication of the significance of transportation cost was provided by an analysis of tariffs filed by New Jersey carters in 1984. Tariffs gave marginal costs of about five cents per cubic yard per mile; they were approximately $4 per cubic yard in the carter's prime territory. A customer twenty miles away would be 25 percent more expensive to service.

The first comes from a rare DCA hearing on one of these transfers. In June 1979 Triboro Carting purchased a set of 149 customers, located in northern Manhattan, from another carter named Cancro.[11] That transaction was never given final approval by the DCA, for reasons that need not detain us here. The next six months saw a number of complaints about the quality of service offered by Triboro. The local newspaper complained of uncollected refuse outside businesses, and some customers complained to Triboro and then to the DCA. Triboro, in the DCA hearing, admitted some service difficulties. Its president said that the company had "nothing but aggravation" from the time it took over the route. The problems had two sources. First, Triboro's equipment was damaged by unexplained attackers on a number of occasions; for example, tires were slashed. These incidents led to service interruptions. Second, Triboro took the attitude that customers should adjust to the company's routine rather than the company providing the types of services customers wanted.

In December 1979, on the eve of a DCA hearing concerning the propriety of the financing of the sale of customers by Cancro to Triboro, three of Triboro's trucks were burned. Though the record stated that these fires were the result of arson, there was no discussion of either the motivation or identity of the arsonist. At this stage Triboro asked another firm, Inwood Carting, to assist by lending equipment for service of these 149 customers; Triboro staff manned the Inwood trucks. Shortly afterward, Triboro agreed to sell these customers to Inwood for a total price of $214,000.

Counsel for the DCA contested the sale to Inwood, arguing that there was no goodwill to be transferred. After all, there was evidence of (justified) widespread customer dissatisfaction with Triboro. Further, Triboro had serviced the customers for only a short period of time and had not even bothered to inform the customers that it regarded Inwood as a fine firm, providing high-quality service. Indeed, Inwood billed the customers directly, and all the customers paid, before any formal transfer took place.

At the hearing, the presidents of both Inwood and Triboro were explicit about the nature of the transaction. Inwood's president asserted that the sale of customers gave his firm "the exclusive right to serve"

---

[11] This description is based on briefs, transcripts, and the hearing officer's opinion filed "In the Matter of the Department of Consumer Affairs, Complainant, against Inwood Sanitation Co. and Triboro Carting," complaints 168889 and 168890, New York Department of Consumer Affairs.

those customers. Both companies agreed that this was industry practice in New York. Hence it was this right that was being sold. Nonetheless, the hearing officer found for the carting companies and against the DCA, arguing that the department had not shown that the goodwill of the prior carter (Cancro) did not still exist and could not be transferred.

The second transaction, which provides even more detail and clearer evidence about the nature of deceptive practices in the industry, concerns the dissolution of a major carting company under court order. New York Carting was a firm with approximately twenty trucks in 1978, when it was convicted of attempted commercial bribery and attempted grand larceny. The firm and its chief operating officer pled guilty to the charges, which involved payments to purchasing agents of the firm's customers for overlooking gross overbillings by New York Carting.

The DCA revoked the company's license, intending that the revocation should take effect immediately. New York Carting went to court and successfully applied for a six-month stay to dispose of its assets. Its physical assets consisted of trucks, containers, and some plants, valued at less than $1 million. However the firm was able to realize over $10 million in disposing of its assets.

The difference between the two figures represented the valuation placed on the firm's customers by other carters. The customers were sold in six separate transactions. In one case the dominant component of the transaction was the transfer of a single customer, the UN building complex.[12] The purchaser of the UN contract was willing to pay $17,600 per month for ten years for the right to pick up the UN garbage ($2.1 million total) for the approximately five years remaining on the contract; the contract with the United Nations yielded revenues of about $20,000 per month ($1.2 million in total). At the end of the five years the contract would be put out for public bid again and be awarded to the low-cost bidder. For other customers, the sales price was at roughly forty times the gross monthly billing provided by the customer, or "stop" (the industry's term for customer).

The New York Carting transactions provided even stronger evidence of an industry-wide customer allocation agreement than did the routine sale of customers by an ongoing carting firm. In the latter case, the new firm either had to pay the existing supplier for an agreement not to compete (i.e., to discontinue service to those customers) or had to

---

[12] The transaction involved one other customer with monthly billings less than 10 percent of those of the United Nations.

enter into direct competition for those customers through price and service quality variation. But in the instance of New York Carting there was another option for a carter who wanted to obtain the customer of a particular stop. New York Carting would not be able to provide service after 1979, the DCA having taken away its license. There was no need to buy a restrictive covenant from New York Carting since it could not compete after that date. Yet the stops were being sold at prices at least as high (expressed as a multiple of the monthly revenues) as those reflected in other transactions at the time.

It might be argued that this was proof that the sale of customers was truly a sale of goodwill. After all, in the New York Carting case, the contract did not provide (as they usually did) for a restrictive covenant. However, the court record suggests the implausibility of this claim. It was shown that New York Carting grossly overbilled many of its corporate customers, often paying a purchasing agent to ensure that this was overlooked.[13] If New York Carting had any goodwill to transfer, it was solely with the corrupted purchasing agents; the DCA could scarcely approve the transfer of goodwill based on the payment of bribes.

A more plausible interpretation is that the purchases were justified for the buyers by the fact that it gave them an exclusive right to service the stops. Implicitly, the purchase involved a restrictive covenant on the part of other members of the carting industry, an agreement not to compete if the stops were purchased.

The sale of customers was a fairly routine activity. I reviewed DCA records for two successive twelve-month periods, starting November 20, 1978. In the first there were twenty-four route sales (in which a carter sold all his customers) and twelve stop sales (in which the carter sold only some of his customers). In the second twelve-month period, the figures were twenty and twenty-four.

2. *Prices.* The prices fetched in sales of customers were just as compelling as the circumstances of customer sales, in demonstrating the existence of a customer allocation agreement. These prices also provide the basis for a crude estimate of the extent to which the price of garbage collection was raised above its competitive level; see Section VI for an estimate of this price increase.

The price of stops is conventionally measured as a multiple of

---

[13] The district attorney identified approximately $1,100 per week as distributed each week in cash, presumably mostly to purchasing agents. It was able to identify only three of the recipients.

monthly revenues. At the time of the McClellan Committee hearings the ratio may have been as low as ten; by 1980 it had risen to as high as sixty-three for certain classes of customers. For example, the contract for the sale of the UN stop by New York Carting involved a reduction in the sale price of $63 for every $1 the monthly revenues fell below the level stipulated in the contract. More typically, the multiple was about forty for each customer in denser neighborhoods, where marginal cost of a unit of service (a cubic yard of waste picked up) was likely to be low.

To understand the implications of these prices, consider that the Department of Consumer Affairs, in setting maximum prices for services, estimated a margin of only 10.9 percent profit on total operating costs. Thus a carter receiving $100 monthly revenues from a customer should have been earning only $10.90 per month in profits, an annual return of $131. Yet other carters were willing to pay $4,000 for that customer, suggesting a "price earnings ratio" (p/e) of more than thirty, far higher than the ratio in most corporate acquisitions; such a high p/e is particularly striking in a stagnant market such as that for solid waste collection, where the large number of firms and small barriers to entry would suggest considerable risk.

The comparison is somewhat oversimplified. There are returns available to owners of small businesses that are not available to equity holders in large corporations because they show up in forms other than recorded profits. For example, it is difficult to monitor the claimed expenses of businessmen so as to ensure that truly personal expenses are not charged to the business. For businesses as small as the carting firms in New York City, this may add substantially to the available returns of the owner-managers.

More important, it is also likely that the DCA underestimates the true operating margins of carters for two reasons. First, the carter has considerable discretion in estimating the quantity of waste he is collecting from a particular customer; he may exaggerate that quantity so as to effectively charge above the allowed price. Second, he may not report all of his income, thus reducing both his tax obligation and the revenues that the DCA uses in calculating actual profits.

The first of these phenomena is at the heart of the failure of regulation in this industry. Ostensibly, DCA regulation should have greatly hindered the ability of carters, even with a customer allocation agreement, to exploit their market power over individual customers. The department's maximum price, based on actual financial data, allows only a "fair and reasonable" profit, and few contracts were in open violation of the ceiling.

However, most customers have only a vague knowledge of the amount of waste collected by their carter. It is the carter who usually provides the container in which the waste is placed; indeed, the carter may actually manufacture the container, which requires no more than the equipment of a sheet metal shop. The container may or may not have a label giving its volume and that label may be inaccurate; containers other than simple cubes have volumes that are difficult to estimate by eye, so that the customer needs to make an effort to determine the volume. One prosecutor in another state claimed that a sample of containers were on average 30 percent smaller than claimed (personal communication with anonymous informant 1980). Carters may also pick up containers that are not completely full, thus exaggerating the amount of service provided. Alternatively, they may not completely empty the container when they do pick it up.

New York Carting was convicted because it claimed to be picking up 213 cubic yards per month at the Roger Smith Hotel. A new owner, with a civil engineering background, correctly estimated that the total waste generated was only forty-eight cubic yards. The ensuing investigation showed that this level of overcharge had continued for some years. In 1974, the Brooklyn district attorney's case against fifty-five members of the Kings County (Brooklyn) Trade Waste Association showed that overcharging of 500 percent occurred routinely.

Underreporting of income was also a critical element of the failure of regulation in the 1970s. Carters routinely concealed the existence of cash customers and thus understated their total revenues.[14] Small businesses may themselves be happy to pay in cash. This underreporting also helps explain the high prices paid for customers, since much of the income can be sheltered from taxes. Underreporting undermined the DCA regulatory process since the prices set were based on the difference between expenses (calculated from fully-reported aggregate payments for wages, equipment, disposal, etc., incurred in servicing all customers) and the revenue that would be generated by those prices, charged only to the customers listed.

An anonymous informant who had worked for a major carter in the

---

[14] A consultant working for the industry reported that firms had a second set of books covering their cash customers, which was kept separately from those provided to the DCA.

late 1970s provided specific data on his former employer in 1979.[15] It
had gross billings of $150,000 per month, of which it reported about
$135,000. The remaining $15,000 was deposited in a separate bank
account and not shown in the company books. This was used to make
payments to various officials of customer companies, totaling $3,000
per month. The rest was divided among the three partners in the firm
and was, as far as the informant could tell, scrupulously accounted
for.

The underreporting of income and charging of personal expenses to
the business go far to explain the prices paid for customers. I use
figures from the informant's firm to illustrate. The three partners each
received salaries of $37,500 in 1979, though two of them spent only a
trivial amount of time working there. The working partner charged
$30,000 in personal expenses to the firm; for example, it provided him
with a new Cadillac each year, though the bulk of the car's mileage
was incurred for personal trips. The firm reported a gross profit of
$75,000 to both the Internal Revenue Service and the DCA.

The total entrepreneurial income for the firm then was made up of
four items. Seventy-five thousand dollars was shown as book profit.
Thirty thousand dollars was taken out as unjustified business expenses.
Seventy-five thousand was paid in salaries to partners for no labor
input. Finally, $144,000 was received as unrecorded profits. Total en-
trepreneurial income was $324,000; taxes were paid only on $150,000
(declared profit plus inactive partners' income).

The firm sold for approximately $7.5 million, of which $6.75 million
was payment for customers. At first sight, given the book profits, this
was far too high a price. However, with $174,000 in unrecorded
profits, as well as the $150,000 in taxable income, the price looked
more reasonable. If we assign the 1979 federal corporate tax rate of 40
percent to the untaxed portion of the income, the firm generated the
equivalent of $440,000 of taxable profits. The p/e ratio was then a
reasonable 15.3.

3. *Racketeers.*   Racketeers played a role in the operation of the customer allocation agreement in the late 1970s. Though that role was not
highly visible, it was essential to the continued success of the agreement in the late 1970s.

The McClellan Committee suggested that it was through the union

[15] Some changes have been made in these figures to preserve confidentiality, but the
relevant proportions have been maintained.

that racketeers exerted their influence in the carting industry, both in the city and the suburbs. The union was portrayed as the tool of organized crime members. By the second half of the 1970s, though Bernard Adelstein continued to control Local 813, the situation seemed to have changed. Wage negotiations were conducted aggressively and even led to a moderately lengthy strike in 1978. An informant who worked for a major firm, reputed to be well connected with racketeers, reported that the union leadership was strident in representing workers' interests. Efforts by the firm to fire employees for stealing business (e.g., using the company truck to pick up waste from customers who paid the employee directly) were vigorously contested.

Part of the explanation for this emerged in the investigation of carting activities on Long Island. Adelstein, who served as the crucial link between the racketeers and the union, had managed to attain some independence by playing off interests of two rival Mafia families, the Luccheses and Gambinos. The union leader was more closely associated with the Gambino family than with the Lucchese family, but the Gambinos were only peripherally involved with the carting industry. Consequently, some believed the Gambinos were not willing to push Adelstein to support the Lucchese-run conspiracy but protected him from the Luccheses. Moreover, the Gambino control of Adelstein was not strong, at least in the eyes of Sal Avellino, the Lucchese family member who ran the Long Island industry in the mid-1980s. He and an associate discussed it at one point, with Avellino asserting the following "See, years ago, believe it or not, just between us, years ago he was on our side. . . . And there was a few guys around . . . then how they let, when Paul's (Castellano) son married Tommy's daughter. . . . See, and he went and they more or less drifted over there. They claim him but they don't control him. . . . I'm a firm believer that you can't claim anybody unless you can control him. If you can't say to this guy, stop, and you keep saying no, I'm not going to stop, then I don't have you."[16]

Racketeers played a more direct role in the operation of a "grievance committee," which served to enforce the agreement for at least two of the major associations. According to two former carting company managers (anonymous personal communications with author 1979, 1980), one member of the committee, for over two decades, was a

[16] Hearings of the President's Commission on Organized Crime (1985) (hereafter PCOC Hearings), pp. 680–81.

Mafia member with a long criminal record, including heroin dealing charges.

According to one of the carting executives, the basic criterion for the grievance committee, in determining which of the two carters should service a particular customer, was the date at which each carter first provided service to that site; this was the same rule that the McClellan Committee had found in Los Angeles and the New Jersey State Commission of Investigation had found in its state in the late 1960s. Each carter presented ledger sheets showing when he first had collected garbage there, and the committee ruled accordingly. However, if the racketeer had an interest in the dispute, if it involved some carter with whom he was closely linked (financially or by kinship), then he would probably rule in favor of his client, and the remainder of the committee deferred to him. In most cases he did not have an interest, and the informant reported that the rulings seemed to have been reasonably objective.

The grievance committee was an active body; it met as an adjunct to the association's weekly meeting. Informants claimed that these were the occasions on which carters paid the racketeers, but none provided credible information on the nature or size of those payments.

The grievance committee rule appeared to be simple, allowing little discretion on the part of the committee. It did, however, have to deal with the very American problem of legalistic cheating. The original rule required only the presentation of ledger entries. However, two participants started to cheat systematically by creating false ledger pages, scuffing them up to look old. Eventually, after this had succeeded a number of times, they were caught and the "rules of evidence" were changed, now requiring presentation of external documentation, such as a billing, which was less easily faked.

The critical observation is that the grievance committee seems to have been effective. No one in the industry knew of prolonged disputes between carters, and one informant asserted that he did not know of a single instance of noncompliance.[17] It is difficult to believe that all members of the association accepted that their individual interests were best served by this process. Certainly other cartels, involving decision makers with longer planning horizons, have foundered on the members' impatience with existing market allocations (see Fog 1956). I infer

[17] Occasional incidents of arson or property damage were reported, as in the Cancro-Inwood matter discussed above.

that the presence of the racketeers in the grievance committee facilitated the working of the process. The implied threat of force provided the ultimate incentive to accept the committees' rulings.

B. Long Island

As revealed in the McClellan Committee hearings, the Long Island industry has been plagued by racketeer-associated customer allocation agreements since the mid-1950s. In 1977, as chronicled in newspapers, there was an outbreak of violence as two men attempted to form a union competitive with Local 813 in the carting industry. A wave of arson, resulting in the destruction of twenty-two trucks, ended when the two men were found murdered in a car trunk.

Each of the four decades, from the 1950s to the 1980s, has seen at least one detailed enquiry into the operation of the customer allocation agreement. Towns have complained about the difficulty of getting competitive bids for waste collection contracts. Indeed, one significant difference between the agreements in New York and New Jersey, on the one hand, and Long Island, on the other hand, was that the latter covered municipal contracts as well as commercial customers. The powerful local newspaper (*Newsday*) has given considerable publicity to these matters. But only the mid-1980s investigation by the New York State Organized Crime Task Force (OCTF) (discussed below) resulted in convictions of any of the principal figures in the industry.

1. *The Rebellion.* That 1980s investigation provided detailed information about the operation of the conspiracy, the role of the union, and the involvement of racketeers and is the primary focus here.

The investigation was initiated through the willingness of one of the carters (Robert Kubecka, later murdered, in yet another unsolved homicide) to act as an informant while he tried to break the industry's rules. Kubecka was an outsider of Polish origin in an industry dominated by Italians. He ran a small firm established by his father and attempted to bid away customers from other carters operating in the same small area of Suffolk County. The primary target of Kubecka's "raids" was a larger carting firm, Sail Carting, whose owner, Anthony Vespucci, was planning to retire. An important part of his retirement income was to come from the sale of his business whose major asset was its customers. Vespucci was selling the firm in pieces, each piece consisting of a block of customers and a small amount of equipment. The sales contracts all specified payment over a period of about sixty months, and each was contingent on the purchaser receiving customer revenues of the amount specified in the contract. Loss of customers posed a peculiar threat to Vespucci, since it immediately reduced the capital value of the firm, at a time when he lacked the means to retaliate.[18]

The retaliation against Kubecka's raids was complex, involving the carters. Surprisingly, the union, still led in 1984 by Bernard Adelstein of McClellan Committee fame, was a reluctant ally of the carters. The local agent never picketed Kubecka's customers, despite repeated requests by the other carters. Indeed, an electronic surveillance revealed a striking level of conflict between the carters and the union. The (informal) bargaining committee of the carters, led by the dominant figure in the local industry, Sal Avellino, carefully rehearsed their arguments as to why they could not offer a large increase in wages:

We can't give the store away because there is no store to give away. Things are very bad. The men are all complaining. The bosses are all complaining. You got a few Indians out there, robbing all kinds of work . . . which is not your problem Bernie. That is our problem, an association problem. But in the meantime we got Indians there, losing work. The union can't do nothing to stop them. The union doesn't do nothing to help. We have in Brookhaven, in Islip, in Smithtown firms that are nonunion, so when municipal bids come up they are up there bidding away. This prevailing rate doesn't mean a thing to them.[19]

Nobody abides by it, so when you get a guy that is a union man and he toes the line, he hasn't got a chance to win the bid. He hasn't got a chance. [Taking Adelstein's role]: We go on strike. [Reverting to his own role]: Then I got to say you're not strong enough to make it, to really make a strike go. The strike was only a few days [referring apparently to 1978]. Everybody was ready to go to work. The union people were ready to go to work. You don't have enough people to man the dumps. You didn't have pickets in front of two of the dumps that we had. O.K., we can work with a strike.[20]

[18] The buyers of the customers were less motivated to respond to the retaliation since loss of a customer was mitigated by reduction in the amount owed to Vespucci.

[19] Towns generally require that municipal contractors pay "prevailing wages." If an industry is heavily unionized, the prevailing wage is the union contract figure.

[20] Sentencing memorandum. People v. James Corrigan Jr., County Court of the State of New York, July 1987. This contains over five hundred pages of electronic surveillance.

This certainly conveyed the impression of people preparing to bargain aggressively in the forthcoming negotiations. Avellino laid out the need for such bargaining by showing that the existence of nonunion firms limited the ability of unionized firms to raise the level of wages. He cast aspersions on the union's ability to back up a tough bargaining position with an effective strike, arguing that the 1978 strike was not a success from the union's point of view.

2. *Racketeers.* The role of racketeers was central but difficult to characterize. There was no doubt that they regularly obtained money from carters as a group, though direct payments were a modest $400,000 (see below).[21] However, it was not clear just what services they provided in return for that money. Their involvement is best understood by consideration of Avellino, the central figure connecting the carters and the racketeers.

Avellino had been the owner of a carting company since 1974. He entered the industry in his late thirties, having previously been the owner of a garment manufacturing firm. He had no criminal record, and at the time the OCTF began its investigation it could find no intelligence information suggesting that he was involved in any criminal activity while a garment manufacturer.

He came, however, from a family with extensive criminal involvement. His father was probably a soldier in the Lucchese crime family, in which his uncle was later a capo (middle-level manager, responsible for one branch). His brother was a gambling operator. He himself became a member of the Lucchese family, though it is not known when. It seems implausible that he was not involved in organized crime activities well before 1974.

When Avellino entered the carting industry, he apparently had no particular cachet or connection with the union or other carters. He was subjected to intense union pressure in the mid-1970s. An effort was even made to destroy his property during the 1977 intercarter struggle mentioned above.

At some stage, though, he became a member of the Lucchese family and a prominent figure in the carting industry. The exact sequence is hard to determine, but it seems plausible that the two events were related. He helped organize a new carter's association, the Private Sanitary Industry (PSI), to replace the notorious and faction-ridden Nas-

---

[21] They may also have received other moneys indirectly.

sau-Suffolk Cartmen's Association. He established close relations with other, more experienced and prominent carting company owners. He became the chauffeur and close associate of the Lucchese family leader, Anthony Corallo (he of McClellan Committee fame); he also became close to Corallo's deputy, Salvatore (Tom Mix) Santoro.

Avellino became a dominant figure among the carters. The executive director of the PSI checked with him before making decisions, and other carters deferred to him and expected him to be able to resolve disputes. He took a public role as a spokesman for the carters and was on the board of the PSI. He headed the (unofficial) group that bargained with the union in 1983.

His connections went well beyond the carting industry. For example, he knew some prominent figures in the construction industry on Long Island, and he used those connections to influence the distribution of carting contracts for new construction. He was involved in discussions of efforts to extort money from businesses in the trucking sector of the garment industry.

His involvement in purely criminal activities was also fairly routine. He was active in the management of a gambling business, and he frequently talked with other racketeers about the operation of an illegal casino in New York City.

Avellino had a complex identity. He was clearly a member of the Lucchese family, although he was sometimes not very knowledgeable about its customs, and he actively concerned himself with the politics of the five Mafia families operating in New York City. But he was also an active carting entrepreneur. One of Avellino's major roles appeared to be the delivery of money to the Lucchese and Gambino families. Each quarter, he and a small number of other carters collected monies from a subgroup of the PSI for delivery to the two family heads. The one indication of the amounts involved suggested that more than $50,000 was delivered to each family each quarter.

Avellino was proud of the fact that he increased the amount delivered after he became prominent in the industry. Indeed, he was clearly miffed that his success was not formally acknowledged. In one conversation, he commented on the attitude of the leader to whom he delivered the money: "You want to know the truth, Tommy. He never says a word but they are all doing good. . . . He never asks how much. It's all sealed up. The accounting is inside. All the notes are inside. But you would like, say, 'Gee is there a mistake?' Next time would they say, 'Is there a mistake?' Tommy replied skeptically, 'Take $5 out, see if they find it, Sal.' "[22]

It was often made clear that control of the industry was shared between the Lucchese and Gambino families and that the money must be split evenly between them. A discussion of the possibility of setting up an alternative union (Local 813A) is particularly interesting in this respect. Avellino and his carting associates still proposed to share the profits between the Gambinos and the Luccheses, but the union leader would no longer be entitled to a share.[23] This suggests, though not with certainty, that Adelstein received some money independently of the racketeers. If he did, it must have been through his own agents, for at no stage did Avellino suggest that any carters paid Adelstein directly or that the money he collected included a share for Adelstein.

A striking feature of Avellino's performance was that he persuaded so many of the carters that he was seeking, almost altruistically, arrangements that benefited all. Repeated references were made by others to how much their lot improved after Avellino entered the industry. For example, Avellino reported that Freddy, another carter, "came to my house one Sunday with a brand new Mercedes, the small one, the fifty thousand dollar one, so I walked out, it was a Sunday morning and I said, 'Congratulations, beautiful, beautiful.' He says, 'I just wanted you to see it, cause this is thanks to you and to PSI that I bought this car.' "[24]

In another conversation, Avellino made clear that he understood the value of playing fair in the application of the property rights rules:

> Ya see, out here Frank in Nassau, Suffolk County . . . we don't shake anybody down, we don't steal anybody's work, we don't steal it to sell it back to them like they do every place else, in five or six years . . . whenever I got a stop back for a guy because somebody took it, never was a price put on it, because if it was his to begin with and he was part of the club and he was payin' every three months, then he got it back for nothin' because that was supposed to be the idea. . . . So I never let them think that we were interested or that I was interested in just taking money from them.[25]

[22] PCOC Hearings (1985), p. 691.
[23] See conversation quoted on pp. 686–687 of PCOC Hearings (1985).
[24] Sentencing memorandum (see n. 20 above).
[25] PCOC Hearings (1985), p. 666.

It is clear that the agreement disproportionately favored a relatively small number of carters who received a larger share of new business. But it is also likely that all the members of the PSI, many of whom probably had little contact with Avellino, also benefited from the increased security that Avellino's honest application of dishonest rules provided.

None of the racketeers with whom Avellino conversed showed much independent knowledge of the industry. They occasionally gave advice to Avellino about how he should deal with specific problems, but only when he brought up those problems. For example, Corallo and Avellino discussed the desirability of filings, rather than nuts and bolts, being put into the engines of rebels' trucks. Corallo also told Avellino that, in light of the possibility that the industry was under investigation, strong action against rebels should be delayed: "Once it's over, you get him; you don't make waves, throw gasoline on the fire. That's the gist of it."[26]

Members of the Gambino and Lucchese families may have benefited from their influence in the Long Island carting industry in other ways as well as directly. For example, there were possible ties through the insurance industry, but nothing conclusive was found.

C. New Jersey

I provide only a little information on the New Jersey industry because, despite a long involvement in study of it, I learned less about the details of the operation of the customer allocation agreement there than in the other two areas.

In particular, the evidence concerning racketeer involvement was weakest here. A lengthy investigation by the New Jersey attorney general in the late 1970s showed the existence of a customer allocation agreement. However, though three homicides could plausibly be related to this agreement, the racketeer participation was generally hazy. Carmine Franco, the most significant of the carters, was alleged to be closely related to various racketeers, but they entered into the drama only in narrow and opportunistic ways.[27]

For example, after the killing of an aggressive carter who had refused to follow the rules, two racketeers and three carters met to decide on how the deceased carter's customers should be allocated. One racketeer

[26] See n. 25 above.
[27] I testified in 1986 in a BPU proceeding in which the state sought to strip Carmine Franco and his brother of their license to operate a garbage collection company.

was closely related to the carter's widow, while the other represented the interests of the principal competitor. The meeting resulted in a decision to reallocate customers according to a status quo associated with an arbitrary date in the middle of the period of the dispute.

Most striking was lack of any evidence that Local 945 had retained any role in the operation of the agreement. It certainly had been involved in the 1960s, as evidenced by the New Jersey State Commission of Investigation (1969). But, despite continued evidence of racketeering in the local, the state's lengthy investigation failed to find any indication that the carters were able to use the union for enforcement purposes.

III. Racketeering Assets and Cartel Strategies

If the previous section's description is correct, then the carting industry around New York has been characterized by enduring customer allocation agreements. These are highly unusual because they represent economic conspiracies that have lasted for decades despite the involvement of very large numbers of participants; each has had at least 100 members. After something less than an exhaustive search, I have been unable to find any report of similarly durable cartel agreements, let alone one involving hundreds of participants.

A distinctive feature of the conspiracies that have marked the garbage collection industry in the greater New York area is the involvement of racketeers. As already hinted, a central argument of this essay is that the racketeers' role has been critical to the maintenance of these agreements. The following pages analyze the problem of creating effective cartels and then consider the assets that racketeers bring to such cartels.

By "racketeers" I mean persons who are members of a large criminal group with a continuing identity known to others and who use that membership and identity to extort others involved in legitimate or illegitimate business.[28] Mafia members and their close associates are potential racketeers, but not every one of their income-generating activities constitutes racketeering. A Mafia member who engages in book-

[28] This is consistent with Webster's definition of "racket": "a usually illegitimate enterprise or activity that is made workable by coercion, bribery or intimidation . . . a system of obtaining money or other advantage illegally, fraudulently or undeservedly, usually with the outward consent of the victims." The same dictionary provides a useful and distinctive definition of "racketeer": "one who extorts money or advantage by threats of violence or by blackmail or by threatened or actual unlawful interference with business of employment" (*Webster's Third New International Dictionary*).

making is a bookmaker; when he receives payments from other book-
makers in order to protect them either from himself or from other
criminals, then he is engaged in racketeering.[29]

A. Designing Conspiracies

The economic conspiracies we are considering are nothing more or
less than cartels. They must face up to most of the problems encountered by illicit cartels generally. Customer allocation agreements are
peculiarly attractive for a cartel. Such an arrangement is only possible
in a few industries, including garbage collection. For a number of
reasons discussed below, the garbage industry in New York and its
environs is peculiarly vulnerable to the operation of a racketeer-
enforced cartel.

The problem for cartels, particularly those with large numbers, is
to design agreements that can be maintained over time. Three aspects
of agreements are relevant: the rules to be followed by members, the
means for detection of rule violators, and the sanctions to be imposed
against violators. Weakness in any of these three is likely to lead to
repeated defections and breakdown of the cartel.

There are at least three dimensions to the rules that affect cartel
members' willingness to remain in the association. First, the rules must
produce results that, over time, are perceived as equitable. Certainly
no cartel member must perceive himself to be worse off in the cartel
than he was prior to its creation. More important, the percentage increase in profits must not be very skewed toward a small number of
members.[30] Second, the agreement must be compatible with continued
entrepreneurial autonomy. Loss of autonomy, as might arise if the
cartel decided (correctly) that production facilities must be centralized
to maximize joint profits, transforms the later bargaining relationship
between members. Those members who have lost production facilities
are now dependent on the willingness of the others to honor the original commitment. Here the illegality of the agreement is important
since no contract enforceable by a court can be written.

Third, there is likely to be a strong inclination to avoid rules that
require "side payments" among members. Payments from one member
to another can provide valuable evidence for a prosecutor. More gener-

---

[29] Reuter (1983) argues that the primary role of organized crime in illegal markets is
precisely racketeering rather than direct provision of the illegal good or service.

[30] Fog (1956) reports some evidence of this for a sample of Danish cartels.

ally, illegal agreements are likely to seek to minimize the number of transactions and contacts necessary for their effective execution.

The second important issue is the speed and cost of detecting violations. The longer it takes to detect a violation, the greater the return to violation and the lower the expected lifetime of the cartel (Stigler 1964). Similarly, the profitability of the cartel will be lowered by high costs of monitoring. Price agreements, where there are a small number of large customers, may be particularly volatile since they fail on both accounts. Secret rebates can go undetected for a long time, while detection costs, through monitoring of internal documents of sellers and buyers, may be high.

The final consideration is the nature of available sanctions. Members will doubt a cartel's potential stability if continued violation of the rules cannot be punished without ending the cartel. The possibility of selective and cheap sanctions will increase stability. Price agreements may be difficult to enforce; the problem is to find means for members to offer discounts to the offender's customers without offering them to all customers.

Cartels have a limited number of rules available to them for carrying out their aim of extracting the available monopoly profits. The primary alternatives are price fixing, output quotas (designed to limit total output and thus raise price), territorial allocations, and customer allocations. The feasibility and desirability of each is dependent on characteristics of both demand and supply in the given market. For example, price fixing is difficult where the good or service involved is custom-made; that was a problem for the famous electrical conspiracy of the 1950s in dealing with government purchases of major machinery that had to be tailored to the specifications of the purchaser.[31] Indeed, there are few settings in which pure price-fixing agreements have proven enforceable over long periods of time. The efforts by the railroads prior to the passage of the Interstate Commerce Commission Act in 1887 illustrates the problems where an industry has high fixed costs and few customers (Kolko 1965). Stocking and Watkins (1946) point to the problems during the 1930s when, because of the National Recovery Act, such agreements were arguably legal. In each case some members of the agreement started offering secret rebates to increase their market share. This led to the collapse of the agreements.

Output quotas are another important alternative. Stocking and Wat-

---

[31] See Herling (1962) for a detailed account of this conspiracy.

kins (1951), in an analysis of two major American quota agreements (covering salt production and container production), and Wilson (1962) (examining a number of British agreements in the 1950s) found that they required extensive and intrusive inspection for their maintenance; these are not attractive for an illegal cartel. Adding a small amount of capacity, particularly where this can be done through using existing capital more intensively, is difficult to detect.

Territorial allocation allows for easy detection of violations. However, it also allows for easy detection of the agreement by antitrust authorities. Moreover, its formation may require substantial dislocation of existing customer-supplier relationships, with consequent loss of goodwill.

Customer allocation dominates the other cartel rules, where it is feasible, a matter I take up shortly. Violations are easily detected within a short period of time and selective sanctions are readily applied that do not threaten the operation of the agreement involving the other members. Detection occurs almost automatically because each customer is allocated to a particular firm. If a cartel member provides service to the customer of another member, that member will be aware of the loss of the business of that customer. Identifying the violator is likely to be a simple matter for those goods and services in markets where a customer allocation is feasible. Selective sanctions can be applied by aggressive solicitation of the violator's customers.

The rule is also equitable, simple to understand and easy to apply. It gives to each participant what he thinks of as his already, namely, his existing customers. It requires no active monitoring to ensure compliance. Nor does it require active transfer of information or other cooperation that leaves paper trails for investigators. Members can charge different prices and provide different quality of products, though there may be limits on the variation depending on the ease of comparison by customers.

A customer allocation rule still leaves one problem unsolved: how to allocate new customers. Without territoriality, there is no obvious allocation formula. Customers might be allocated on the basis of existing market shares; a firm with 10 percent of the market gets one out of ten new customers. However that requires an exchange of information about output levels in a situation where participants want to minimize the demands for active cooperation. Another alternative (suggested by this case study) is that there is competition for new customers, but then they become subject to the basic rule.

Under what conditions is a customer allocation agreement feasible? The essential condition appears to be immobility of customers, that is, the necessity of having the supplier come to the customer. This permits a supplier to determine whether the loss of a customer is the result of the customer ceasing to purchase the good or service or the result of a shift to another firm. It also permits him to determine, through surveillance, which competitor now is servicing that customer. That, of course, is made easier where service provision is conspicuous, frequent, and regular.

The condition of fixed-location customers is a very restrictive one. It essentially eliminates the retail sector; customers are, in modern times, highly mobile. Moreover, there are so many that the cost of detection will be a high proportion of the profits from any single customer. Refusal of service (as is required when a customer solicits service from other than his current supplier) is more difficult where the customer has placed himself in a position to buy the good or service by entering the supplier's store. The only part of the retail trades where a customer allocation agreement appears feasible is the small segment consisting of services or goods supplied directly to the household. Home delivery of milk is one example, though the elasticity of demand (given the density of retail outlets for milk and the availability of refrigeration) limits the profitability of such an agreement.[32]

Solid waste collection meets the criteria for customer allocation very well. Customers are indeed immobile.[33] It is difficult to substitute for the service, so that if a customer requests discontinuance of garbage collection, it is highly likely that he is obtaining the service from another firm.[34] Since the waste must be collected at least once a week by a large labeled truck, it is particularly simple to identify the violator.

B. Racketeer Role

Even where conditions facilitate a customer allocation agreement, agreements with many parties have a tendency to break down because there is always a short-run incentive for an individual to break the

[32] Antitrust violations in the milk delivery industry have been found at the wholesale level. See Chambers (1981).

[33] An exception is the collection of waste from construction sites; the site operates for only a few weeks or months. In Long Island and New Jersey (certainly) and New York (probably), this sector of the business was not subject to the customer allocation agreement.

[34] Though customers can self-haul, probably at considerably higher expense.

cartel rules. Racketeers bring certain assets to the operation of these agreements.

One asset is simply the initiating spirit and energy. Not all entrepreneurs have the same willingness to enter into illegal arrangements. Racketeers, whose primary skills relate to criminal activities, are presumably more willing and capable than businessmen to initiate these arrangements. Further, entrepreneurs may be more willing to attend meetings for the purpose of launching illegal agreements if the invitation is issued by a threatening figure.

More important, racketeers offer the prospect that the conspiracy will work, simply because they provide credible enforcement. Cartels with many participants appear generally to have short lives because there is always an incentive for a member to leave the agreement and take advantage of the restrictions imposed on the remaining members (Scherer 1970, chap. 6). Potential conspirators are presumably aware of this and may be reluctant to enter into an arrangement that is probably short-lived and also illegal. Racketeers, by promising to take illegal but effective actions against any member who violates the rules of the agreement, provide potential members with credible assurance that it is likely to be of lasting benefit.

Racketeers may use their control of corrupt unions for the enforcement effort. That seemed to be the import of the McClellan Committee findings about labor racketeering (U.S. Senate 1957). The union is able to dress up unattractive cartel enforcement as the more acceptable activity of protecting unionists' rights.

But the racketeer involvement has another benefit, once it becomes known. It reduces the willingness of customers to protest the high prices charged under the agreement or to solicit competing bids from other carters, tempting violation. Note that the customers in the commercial sector of the carting industry include large corporations competent at understanding and exercising their rights. The unspoken threat, perhaps occasionally articulated in a vague way, that aggressive action might be punished by Mafia interventions, smooths customer relations for the carters. Indeed, the New Jersey State Commission of Investigation (1989) noted that one carter told a reporter that a story about racketeer involvement in the industry would only help his business.

Finally, the racketeer involvement also provides a reputational barrier to entry. Entrants must be concerned that they will be the objects of retaliation by racketeers. Their trucks and plants may be destroyed and their customers threatened or subjected to violence. This was what the Brooklyn district attorney's office found when it started a carting firm in 1972; most customers approached by the firm said that they were concerned about the risks of giving up their current carter (Reuter 1981).

Racketeer involvement provides a second kind of barrier to entry. Any firm that succeeds in a racketeer-controlled market is at risk of coming under suspicion of racketeer involvement itself. A national firm, attempting to overcome the somewhat unsavory reputation of the garbage collection industry generally, is likely to pause at the prospect of adding to its problems by acquiring the additional taint; successful entry might turn out to be just as costly as unsuccessful.

What are the preconditions, then, for racketeers to enter the industry? I am unwilling to draw any general conclusions on the basis of a case study, but it seems reasonable to identify three factors that have facilitated racketeer involvement in the carting industry in New York:

1. *Low Educational Status and Ethnic Propinquity with the Mafia.* The entrepreneurs who head the privately owned carting companies in the three areas are generally not highly educated. They may be no more prone to law-breaking than more highly educated managers, but they may well be more willing to work with racketeers than those managers. That they share ethnic ties with the Mafia also eases the relationship.

2. *Large Numbers.* An agreement among a few parties requires less initiating energy and less active maintenance. An agreement with many dozens of participants is likely to require external force both for initiation and maintenance.

3. *Little Technological Innovation and Low-skilled Labor Force.* The union may no longer be critical to the operation of the agreement, but it was clearly involved in its initiation; less educated workers have shown less resistance to racketeer involvement in their unions. Major innovation would strain the operation of an agreement since it would permit innovators significant advantage over other participants in the cartel and thus give them strong incentive to break its rules.

IV. Investigation

The tendency of this industry to allocate customers and the involvement of racketeers has led to numerous investigations by authorities at every level of government. Ignoring purely administrative procedures by agencies such as the DCA or the City Investigations Commission, it is possible to identify at least fifteen separate investigations of criminal behavior in the solid waste industry in New York City and its New York suburbs between 1956 and 1984. Some were initiated by specific complaints, others by law enforcement concern with racketeering. Some produced convictions, others nothing more than newspaper articles. A great variety of investigative and legal tactics were used. At least two of the investigations were based on undercover operations, while others focused on tax evasions as the point of legal vulnerability. They may have been unsuccessful, but law enforcement efforts have lacked neither variety nor number. The following section describes three of the more ambitious recent investigations.

A. Brooklyn, 1974

The Brooklyn district attorney's (D.A.) investigation, started in 1972, nicely illustrates the limitations of investigation. Customers had generally refused to testify before grand juries, believing that they ran significant risk of retaliation and that police could not provide protection over the long haul. Given this problem, the D.A. began an undercover investigation, purchasing a truck for $4,000 and obtaining a license from the DCA. A number of police officers were assigned to solicit customers and work on the truck: "Many of the merchants . . . were very surprised to find a private carting firm offering competitive rates. . . . A few merchants actually retained the services of the undercover company, and our covert operation was in business."[35]

The investigation uncovered most of what was expected. Some customers who tried to switch to the undercover firm were threatened, and in at least one case the customer's store was vandalized following the threat. Out of 2,000 approached, only nineteen customers actually signed up. The undercover firm was unable to join the Brooklyn Trade Waste Association. It seems that other carters were, correctly, suspicious that this new firm was controlled by the police. Surveillance of the headquarters of the association showed that organized crime figures were in attendance at a private meeting each week, following the association dinner. Evidence was found that these racketeers settled disputes and received regular payments from the officers of the association.

The result was an indictment of fifty-five of the carting firms and nine other persons (racketeers and association officials) for "restraint of trade"; interestingly, no union officials were indicted. Firms were

[35] "Supporting Affidavit" for wiretap application by District Attorney Eugene Gold of Kings Country, June 22, 1973, p. 2.

found to have threatened customers and to have overcharged many of them with fraudulent bills. Most of the defendants pled guilty; those that did not were able to have the indictment quashed on a technicality. The judge ordered the dissolution of the Brooklyn Trade Waste Association. The Department of Consumer Affairs issued temporary license renewals to the indicted carters but then gave them permanent renewals and a fine of $500 per truck. The court imposed light fines on those who pled guilty.

The DCA response was clearly inadequate, viewed either as a punishment or a deterrent. A fine of $500 per truck represented less than 1 percent of the extortionate revenue that the district attorney credibly alleged was being generated annually. The renewal of licenses and failure to determine whether prices had changed or that customers were less constrained in their choice surely signaled to the carters that they faced only minor costs in the continuation of the customer allocation agreement.

B. New Jersey, 1981

The New Jersey attorney general launched a major investigation of the carting industry in 1978. The investigation lasted over three years and produced a series of indictments in 1981, largely dependent on the testimony of Harold Kaufman, an informant who had worked for Bernard Adelstein at Local 813 and then for Charles Macaluso, the aggressive founder of Statewide Environmental Contractors, a New Jersey carting firm.[36] As noted above, though the relevant union local (Teamsters Local 945) was subject to intense scrutiny (and has a long record of racketeering and corruption that led to a court-appointed trustee in the mid-1980s), it seemed to play no role in the operation of the customer allocation agreement.

The indictments alleged a customer allocation agreement and the involvement of three racketeers. The latter, who were serving long sentences for other crimes, were dismissed from the indictments by the trial court; moreover, the allegations showed them to have a quite marginal role, relating to just one transaction. The vast majority of the carters pled guilty to the charges (a BFI affiliate being the most important exception; it was acquitted after two trials). Only three of the

---

[36] Charles Macaluso was the son of the founder of New York Carting and brother of the president of that company, who was convicted of commercial bribery in New York City.

principals were given jail time, and then with work release. The rest received sanctions involving probation, fines, and community service.

The Board of Public Utilities sought to deprive the principal figures (Carmine and Salvatore Franco) of their licenses to collect waste. The BPU proceedings unfolded over a five-year period, with what, to a nonlawyer, seemed almost Byzantine twists. The state attorney general had accepted pleas to a charge of conspiracy in restraint of trade. The statute by which the BPU regulated the carting industry specified only monopoly as a ground for license removal, though a later BPU regulation had included restraint of trade; the BPU felt that it should proceed under the authority of the statute rather than its own regulation. The state spent over $1 million in the legal proceedings and eventually prevailed, depriving the Francos of their license. However, it was widely believed that the brothers continued to operate their business, using the names of other firms. The BPU, stung by criticism of the legal bills and the slowness of proceedings, largely abandoned its interest in the regulation of the solid waste collection business.

C. Long Island, 1984

In 1983 the New York Organized Crime Task Force began an eighteen-month investigation of the Long Island carting industry, triggered by Robert Kubecka's willingness to act as an informant while trying to buck the existing agreement. Numerous wiretaps were installed; Avellino's Jaguar was bugged, so as to permit surveillance of his conversations with Corallo, the head of the Lucchese family. The wiretaps yielded a wealth of detail on the operation of the efforts to punish Kubecka's attempts to take customers from Sail Carting and others.

After eighteen months of investigation, the OCTF brought a series of indictments against the principal figures in November 1984. Those indicted included Tony (Ducks) Corallo and his underboss Salvatore (Tom Mix) Santoro; Salvatore Avellino, Corallo's chauffeur and principal racketeering representative in the Long Island garbage industry; James Corrigan, director of the Private Sanitation Industry; four local officials; one state official; and eleven other carters, together with their companies.

The indictments covered a wide variety of offenses. The local officials were indicted for agreeing to influence the Huntington town council to increase rates for residential collection. The state official, head of the regional branch of the Department of Motor Vehicles, was indicted for providing Corrigan with information that confirmed his suspicion that he was under state investigation. But the principal indictments concerned the property rights agreement and efforts to discipline the rebel carter.

Another two years passed in litigation concerning the technical aspects of the investigation. The principal focus of this litigation was electronic surveillance—for example, did the OCTF have authority for wiretaps in certain locations, was adequate effort made to minimize the extent of such surveillance, and did the transcripts accurately reflect the content of the wiretaps? Given the large number of defendants (who retained approximately thirty lawyers), these were inevitably complex proceedings.

Some defendants were dismissed on technicalities. For example, it turned out that two of the carters were immune from prosecution because they had testified before a Nassau County grand jury.

At the end of all this, most of the defendants, including the ringleader, Avellino, pled guilty to the charges. The pleas did not include any agreement with OCTF prosecutors on sentencing recommendations to the court. The prosecutors did provide some signals about the relative status of the defendants; three ringleaders were required to plead guilty to a D felony, while the others pleaded to a lesser E felony.

The judge gave all those who pleaded almost identical nonpenal sentences: five years' probation plus some community service. Avellino was required to provide 840 hours of garbage collection; some of those hours could be worked by an employee if he worked with Avellino.

Without denying the complexity of determining the appropriate sentence for a criminal offense, the penalties imposed here certainly raise serious questions for public policy. If we view such sentences as setting the "price" of the crime, then they are clearly too low; this price is far below any reasonable estimate of the return to the participants.

My very rough estimate of the total annual income accrued by the carters was about $14 million.[37] The total value of the penalty imposed on the industry by the judge, measured in terms of lost freedom and legal costs, was clearly a great deal less than that. Unless those involved were extraordinarily risk averse, the penalty was highly unlikely to change their calculation as to the net returns from continuation of the customer allocation agreement.

Matters may actually be even worse than this suggests. The investi-

[37] See Reuter 1987 (sec. 2) for the basis of these estimates.

gation produced a great deal of publicity about the involvement of racketeers in this industry and about the network of political favors generated by the current carters. Neither potential entrants nor customers were likely to derive any comfort from this information even if it only confirmed their prior beliefs. Together with the light sentences imposed on the principals, this publicity may well have increased the barriers to entry into the industry and the passivity of customers.[38]

Indeed, prosecutors face an awkward dilemma. For the more aggressively they attack the industry, the more notorious it becomes. Every investigation, with its concomitant headlines in the newspapers (for even the staid *New York Times* continues to give considerable prominence to allegations of racketeering in this industry), adds to the bad name of the industry and further deters honest businessmen from considering entry. The barrier to entry that protects the conspiracy may be augmented by each investigation and prosecution.

But what if an investigation actually led to the elimination of the agreement? Surely in that case prosecution would induce entry. But the experiences of New York and New Jersey prosecutors suggest the implausibility of getting effective sanctions. The three cases above showed extraordinary price gouging (Brooklyn), involvement with organized crime (Brooklyn and Long Island), and suppression of competition by a variety of means (all three). None of this was adequate to persuade courts to impose significant sentences. Efforts to obtain injunctive relief, such as restructuring of the industry, were readily tied up in legal proceedings.

The head of the Organized Crime Task Force, Ronald Goldstock, reasonably concluded that only basic restructuring of the industry would reduce the extent of racketeer involvement; prosecution and conventional regulation were not enough. His efforts to generate interest on Long Island in this matter were unsuccessful.[39]

V. Regulation

The reputation of the industry for repeated conspiracy and racketeer involvement has led, in addition to repeated investigations, to the im-

[38] A slight piece of evidence for this may be found in the later effort by the town of Babylon, in Nassau County, to obtain bids for garbage collection. The town actively sought bids from firms (new as well as old) for a long-term contract to pick up waste from the entire community. The total annual value of the contract was at least $5 million. No companies other than those currently operating there entered a bid.

[39] I should admit my own involvement in this effort. The final section of my study on the Long Island industry (Reuter 1987, sec. 4) outlined a reform program, and I made visits to local legislators and editorial writers on behalf of the scheme.

position of regulation in New York City and New Jersey. Though regulation appears to have had little impact on the targeted behavior, this essay gives some attention to that regulation because the failure is instructive of the difficulty faced in trying to root out the problem of conspiracy.

A. New York City

In 1956, Mayor Wagner appointed a special committee to review the collection of solid waste from commercial establishments following "complaints of abuses in the private cartmen's industry and charges of the existence of a monopoly [sic]" (New York Times 1956). The committee made two major recommendations. The first was that the city should discontinue free sanitation department collection of waste from commercial establishments in residential blocks, mostly small stores; this added 52,000 new customers to the 70,000 already served by the carters. At the same time it recommended that the industry should be regulated, with a price ceiling and written contracts between customer and carter, filed with the city. These remain the basic elements of the regulatory system today.

The Department of Consumer Affairs is the regulatory agency. It requires each carter to obtain a license. The licensing covers all officers and stockholders, who must be fingerprinted at the DCA offices.[40] The Commissioner of Consumer Affairs can deny a license on rather vague grounds of "bad character." In fact, this has been interpreted very strictly; only persons with felony convictions related to the garbage collection business have been denied licenses. In 1980, a long-time member of the relevant part of the DCA could not remember a license denial by any commissioner after the initial implementation in 1956 (anonymous personal communication with author 1980). Even the fifty-five Brooklyn carters who pled guilty to price gouging misdemeanors in 1974 received only minor fines and were permitted to retain their licenses (Bird 1974).

The second component of the regulatory system is the setting of maximum rates. From time to time, the carters petition the commissioner for an increase in the maximum rate they may charge customers per cubic yard. The petition is based on claims of increased costs, typically after the union contract has been negotiated or the city has

---

[40] In the 1970s this presented a barrier to licensing of publicly traded companies. Regulations in the 1980s limited the fingerprinting requirement to major stockholders.

raised disposal costs. The commissioner is required to set a rate that allows a "fair and reasonable return" to licensees. Absent any other statutory guideline, the department has adopted the approach of the Interstate Commerce Commission in its regulation of trucking firms prior to 1980, namely, allowing a fixed percentage mark-up on total operating costs (Moore 1978).

The third regulatory element is the filing of contract cards for each customer. The card records the price per unit and the total amount and frequency of collection (e.g., two cubic yards, three times per week, at $5 per cubic yard). The department asks, but does not require, that the customer as well as the carter sign the card; though the card constitutes a contract, it is terminable at will by the customer.

The Trade Waste Bureau of the DCA has a small staff responsible for inspection and audit. Much of the activity is concerned with the accuracy of the contract cards. Auditors inspect the various ledgers of the carters in an annual random sample of carters. The most common offense is the identification of customers in business ledgers for whom no cards have been filed with the DCA. The department may administer a $25 fine for each violation; it usually levies a smaller average fine for a large number of such infractions detected in a single audit. With only five inspectors and three auditors in 1979, the department could do little more serious monitoring of its 300 regulated firms.

The DCA also requires carters to file for approval of every acquisition or divestiture of assets. The sale of customers to another carter is one such action that must be approved. Few such transactions are disapproved. Indeed, it is hard to determine what would constitute possible grounds for disapproval, except for misrepresentation of actual facts in the contract. When the department does question a transaction, it is usually because of doubt that the persons listed as the purchasers are really the principals (i.e., the department is concerned that they are "fronts" for racketeers).

B. New Jersey

New Jersey imposed regulation following the 1969 State Commission of Investigation report, and it was intended to prevent price gouging by carters. An irony is that the SCI report focused mostly on bid rigging in the municipal contract market, which is not the primary object of the regulation.

The regulatory regime in New Jersey in the 1980s was much more elaborate than that set up by New York City. Carters were not only licensed by the Board of Public Utilities but also were required to have individually approved rate schedules (giving prices for many different kinds of service). The rules governing the determination of those schedules constituted almost a parody of the public utility framework.

Each firm must submit data necessary to establish prices that permit the carter to earn the "allowed rate of return" on invested capital, using the methods developed for regulation of electric and communication utilities. The fact that these firms are typically only one-thousandth the size of those other utilities, have a negligible capital base, and have costs dominated by wages and fuel rather than capital costs, did not affect the BPU; "one regulatory rule fits all" seemed to be the motto. In fairness, the legislature, in giving the BPU responsibility for regulating the carting industry, gave it no direction as to how that regulation was to be implemented; the BPU understandably chose to use its existing tools, however inappropriate. But rate of return applications for a firm with only $300,000 in revenues and a capital base of $50,000 strains the framework; the cost of capital may be only 3 percent of total operating costs.

A carter violates BPU regulations if he charges below his filed tariff; this was intended to guard against predatory pricing, a sinister practice not given much credence in the economic literature.

The initial tariffs filed in 1970 were not subject to rate of return regulation; they were intended simply to reflect actual prices. Observers believe that many carters filed tariffs far higher than they were actually charging, so as to minimize the need to make application later, when rate of return regulations would be applied. As a consequence, few carters applied for price increases in the following decade. Nor did the BPU receive many complaints from customers alleging charges over filed tariffs. That probably reflected ignorance on the part of customers about the carters' obligations. An unpublished BPU staff survey of a small sample of commercial customers found that most of them, during the period 1975–80, had been required to pay higher prices at some stage. None of the customers indicated checking with the BPU to determine whether the listed tariffs for their carter had been raised. In fact, almost none of the carters had filed for increases during that period.

I reviewed three of the few rate hearings of the first decade. Three observations emerged. First, the BPU made no effort to verify the financial statements of the carters, at least with respect to revenue, despite a belief by the staff that most carters understated their revenues by a substantial margin. Second, decision criteria were elusive; most carters got less than they sought, but the method of calculation was hard to determine. Third, the cost of application, given its highly formalistic nature, was significant for small carters, who had to hire a lawyer and an accountant.

In the 1970s the BPU was essentially reactive in its dealings with the carters; its inspectors only responded to complaints. They were as likely to penalize a carter for charging below tariff as for charging above tariff. Indeed, where there was an "outbreak of competition" in an area, one of the tactics of an affected carter was to bring a complaint against a competitor for tariff violation.

One case provides a nice illustration of the farcical nature of the regulatory process. A customer complained when his carter raised his price. The customer applied to the BPU, alleging an overcharge. The BPU found that, in fact, the new rate was still below the filed tariff. The carter promptly responded by charging his filed tariff and seemed to be genuinely surprised to learn that the filed tariff was not a ceiling but the level he was required to charge.

Though there have been no instances of dramatic overcharges, as found in New York City in the New York Carting and Brooklyn Trade Waste Association cases discussed above, it seems likely that customers were generally overcharged. Customers did not know the carters' tariffs or even, in 1980, know that there was regulation of this market. Even if they were aware, they were likely to be uncertain of how much waste they generated. I reviewed a sample of bills presented by carters; not a single bill provided information that would enable either the customer or a BPU inspector to determine whether the carter was in compliance with his filed tariff.

As in New York, the regulators must approve all acquisition of assets, including the purchase of customers. In the period to 1981 no such sale had ever been disapproved, and, again as in New York, it was unclear what grounds could have been offered for such a disapproval. One ground was that the transfer of customers would reduce the competitiveness of a local market. This was ritualistically dealt with by showing the total number of customers was small in comparison with the total in a county or some broadly defined geographic area; antitrust market analysis it was not.

Customer sales were less frequent than in New York City; in one eighteen-month period the BPU approved thirty-one transfers; there were 900 licensees. Prices for customers fell between fifteen and eighteen times monthly revenue, noticeably less than in New York. The ostensible motivation for the sales of customers, since the BPU required that some statement of purpose be filed, was either the age of the selling carter (e.g., retirement or ill health) or the desire for increased specialization (e.g., not servicing a particular area any longer or only wanting a particular type of customer). Curiously, the BPU did not allow the purchase price of customers as a capital cost.

The BPU, like the New York DCA, also had the right to deny licenses to persons not of good character. And like the DCA it had interpreted this very narrowly. Even a criminal conviction of the chief operating officer and of the firm itself was insufficient to deprive the chief executive officer of his license. The only denial of license before 1981 involved an applicant who had been convicted of criminal charges in the garbage business in another state.

In 1983 the state legislature passed Assembly Bill 901, barring the licensing of firms and key individuals with criminal records, habits, or associations; it was argued that this would promote competition in an industry that had just seen massive indictments for anticompetitive agreements. Litigation delayed implementation of Assembly Bill 901 for two years. The coverage of the bill, in terms of the number of companies and individuals needing to be investigated, then turned out to be enormous. The attorney general in 1988 (cited in New Jersey State Commission of Investigation 1989) estimated that there might be 4,000 corporate entities and 13,000 individuals subject to the terms of the bill. Even with twenty-one state police detectives, the licensing scrutiny process had not reached even half the eligibles, using a narrow definition.

In understanding the behavior of the BPU at this time, it is important to note that the garbage collection industry constituted, by any measure, a very small part of its responsibilities. Certainly the total revenues of the state's carting industry were less than those of a single major electricity generating company. The solid waste bureau within the BPU employed a total of twenty staff, compared to 500 in the agency as a whole. The commissioners took little interest in the industry until the mid-1980s, when they responded to the conviction of twenty-four carters in 1983 on criminal antitrust charges by trying to remove licenses and impose penalties.

C. Conclusion

Regulation in both New York City and New Jersey has done very little to control the behavior that generated the demand for regulation

in the first place, namely, the tendency to conspiracy. In neither jurisdiction has it even dealt with the symptoms, namely, the treatment of
customers as assets, let alone with the underlying cause. The regulatory apparatus has been highly bureaucratic and formalistic. If anything, by openly permitting the market in customers, the regulators
have condoned the primary symbol of the customer allocation agreement. Regulatory barriers to entry and competition have not been
great, but they certainly have not helped induce price and quality
competition. The new regulations for monitoring of the fitness of individuals and corporations licensed in New Jersey promised to become
another monumental bureaucratic program with no useful consequence.

VI. Consequences

What was the result of all this collusion in New Jersey, Long Island,
and New York City? Perhaps the most significant was that the cost
of garbage collection for commercial establishments was significantly
increased, although we can only infer this indirectly.

There may be substantial discrepancies between the actual per-unit
prices and those apparently paid. As already suggested, carters can
cheat customers in at least four ways described in Section I. Anecdotes
from the three areas suggest that all four methods have been used,
although the anecdotes are certainly not overwhelming in number.

The result of such cheating is that data on the amounts paid by
customers to their carters cannot be converted into unit prices, since
there are no independent data on the quantity of waste being collected,
and the cost of trying to obtain such independent data would be pro-
hibitive. Hence, we can only use an indirect analysis, based on the
prices paid by carters when buying and selling customers, to infer how
much the customer allocation agreement raised service prices.

The justification for these transfers of customers is the claim that
the carter has developed goodwill, a transferable asset. However, it is
apparent from various investigations described above, together with
such sources as the *Newsday* survey of Long Island in 1978, that the
quality of service is not generally high.

Moreover, it would be surprising if high-quality service were provided, since the existence of the customer allocation agreement reduces
the incentive for offering service of higher quality than necessary to
prevent aggressive search behavior by customers. The carters have an
interest in ensuring that customers are not so unhappy that they frequently seek alternative suppliers; complaints by large corporations

about the existence of a customer allocation agreement are likely to be triggered if they are dissatisfied with the quality of service and find themselves unable to obtain competitive bids from other carters. Even more than for the traditional monopolist, the optimal reward for an illicit cartel is a "quiet life," to use the famous phrase of Hicks (1935).

This means that the cartel wants to ensure that none of its members offered very low-quality service, which could have endangered them all. But the cartel may also seek to prevent any member from offering noticeably better service than the others, since that might make other customers dissatisfied and induce them to test the strength of the customer allocation agreement.

We have only one direct observation on this kind of behavior. A member of the Private Sanitary Industry, serving residential customers on Long Island, consistently provided low-quality service. This generated numerous complaints to public officials. One of those officials, an ally of the PSI leadership, passed on the complaints to the PSI. The association leaders were concerned about the threat posed by the complaints and forced the carter to resign from the PSI.

The excess costs of garbage collection arising from the existence of the customer allocation agreement can be estimated; I use Long Island in the mid-1980s for illustrative purposes. As stated above, commercial customers were sold for forty to forty-five times the monthly revenues they provided the carter. To make a conservative estimate, I use the lower figure.

In a competitive market, what would the multiple be if the carters were providing high-quality service? In the New York/New Jersey study (Reuter, Rubinstein, and Wynn 1982) it was suggested that a multiple of ten was appropriate as an upper bound, based on the figure that apparently was used in the early days of the customer allocation agreement in New York City. It is also close to the figure that apparently prevailed in the residential market on Long Island in the early 1970s (as reflected in some company documents), when a relatively weak customer allocation agreement was in operation. It is likely, then, to be a generous estimate of the baseline multiple.

The differential in the two multiples is thirty. This provides the basis for a rough estimation of the rents being extracted by the carters from customers. We can calculate the increase in the capitalized value of the customers resulting from the allocation agreement. Since each carter can either sell the customers to another carter and invest the proceeds in equity or bonds or continue to service the customers, those who stay in the business must earn at least as much from doing so as they would from the other option.

Assume that the rate of return on relatively safe investments is r percent per month. Consider a customer yielding revenues of $\$p$ per month. Let $\$(m)$ be the price paid by a carter for a customer yielding $\$1$ per month (i.e., the multiple). The cartel price equals the competitive price plus the rents the carter must earn on the increase in the capitalized value of customers arising from the customer allocation agreement:

$$p\# = p + r([m\#] \times [p\#] - m \times p),$$

where #'s refer to values with a customer allocation agreement, and those without that sign are the values that would prevail in a competitive market.

Assuming that in 1984 $[m] = 10$, $r = 0.01$ (an annual interest rate of 12 percent), and $[m]\# = 40$, we obtain $p\#/p = 1.5$. That is, the price under the customer allocation agreement was 50 percent higher than that which would have prevailed in a competitive market.

This is probably a conservative estimate. It assumes that the operating costs of carters were the same with customer allocation as with competition. In fact, the customer allocation agreement may have reduced incentives to minimize costs. That would have the effect of further raising the difference between the cartel and competitive prices. The only factor that might make the initial estimate an overestimate is the possibility that a significant proportion of profits were unreported for tax purposes, which would have lowered the rate of return that carters needed to earn on the excess capitalized value of the customers.[41]

The estimate of a 50 percent increase applies only to the commercial sector. In the residential sector, the multiple was between twenty and twenty-five. Using the same formula and $m\# = 22.5$, we obtain $p\#/p = 1.15$: prices in the residential sector were 15 percent higher than they would have been in the absence of a customer allocation agreement.

The lower multiples in the residential sector, observed in both Long Island and New Jersey, are readily explained. The overcharging of

---

[41] Income concealment is not a cartel function. Carters may conceal cash customers with or without a conspiracy.

residents is both more visible and borne more directly than that of stores and factories. Residents in different towns can readily compare how much they pay and have a sense of whether they are overcharged since the amount of waste being generated by the average household is fairly uniform across similar communities. Moreover, households cannot pass on the higher costs as can commercial customers. If each restaurant in New York City has to pay a 50 percent surcharge for its waste collection, it is a uniform tax, albeit collected by a nongovernmental authority, and disadvantages none of them, an insight that Schelling (1967) brought to the analysis of organized crime extortion generally. Even where a business is in competition with businesses in other parts of the country (as for manufacturing plants), where similar extortion is not found in garbage collection, the overcharge is on such a small share of total operating costs that it makes only a modest difference.

Finally, note that the residential sector is likely to be more politically aggressive than the commercial sector at the local level. Indeed, numerous towns on Long Island have regulated residential "scavenger" rates while none have attempted to regulate commercial rates. Towns also have the option, if the overcharges become too egregious, of taking on garbage collection directly; this acts to reduce the optimal level of extortion for the carters.

The customer allocation agreements thus appear to permit overcharging that generates overcharge revenues; how are they distributed among carters, union officials and members, and racketeers? For this we need estimates of total revenues, which can only be constructed rather awkwardly since there is no centralized registry that provides an estimate of even the total number of trucks in Long Island, let alone the revenues generated. Estimating total industry revenues and the share of those revenues that can be allocated to excess profits is important because it would enable us to determine the share going to racketeers. The absolute annual amount seems to have been about $400,000, shared equally between the Gambino and Lucchese families.

I estimate that the industry had a total of 500 trucks, taking the 300 registered in Suffolk County to represent half the total for the two counties and allowing for overlap of one-third between the counties. I also assume that they were divided equally between commercial and residential markets. Finally, assume, using New York City and New Jersey figures, that the average commercial truck generated a total of $125,000 in revenues in 1986. Commercial collection revenues in 1984 then totaled $31.25 million, of which $10.4 million was assigned to the customer allocation agreement. Residential trucks generally earned less, say $100,000. If prices were 15 percent higher than they would have been with competition, the $25 million in revenues generated by residential collection included $3.2 million in excess profits.

This yields a total of $13.6 million in returns to the customer allocation agreement in 1984. It should be clear that this is a very rough estimate, particularly since the base estimate of total revenues is built on so many assumptions. But the true figure is not likely to be less than $5 million, suggesting that the prime beneficiaries of the agreement were the carters themselves, rather than the racketeers, receiving only $400,000 (at least directly).

The other potential beneficiary was the union, including both members and officials. The existence of the customer allocation agreement permitted the union to make higher wage demands, just as Teamsters were able to obtain high wages and benefits under the national master agreement when the interstate trucking industry was subject to Interstate Commerce Commission regulation (Moore 1978). The discussion among the carters in preparing for preliminary negotiations with the union in 1983 suggests that they believed the union did bargain aggressively, despite the ties between its leadership and the Gambinos.

Union officials benefited from both the higher wages and benefits, which provided a more substantial base for their own salaries and benefits, and from other consequences of the agreement. The local union organizer certainly received monies for not enforcing the union wage scale at some companies. Presumably, he also received benefits from enforcement actions on behalf of the conspiring carters, though no direct evidence of that was available.

Thus it seems that the primary beneficiaries of collusion, in economic terms, have been the carters. Though racketeers have extracted profits from their involvement in the industry, the bulk of the moneys go to the carters themselves, as evidenced by the high prices they are willing to pay for the right to serve customers.

VII. Conclusions

This essay has described the garbage collection business in the New York metropolitan region in the period to about 1985. From more limited evidence it appears that the industry continues to be characterized by customer allocation agreements. This section presents that evidence, examines evidence on the generality of the phenomenon of customer allocation and racketeer involvement in this industry in the rest of the nation, and offers some general conclusions about racketeering in legitimate industries.

A. The New York Area Industry in Recent Years

Despite the spate of successful prosecutions in the 1980s described above, the evidence strongly suggests that the tendency to allocate customers continues. Nor, despite almost universal criticism of the regulatory methods adopted by New York City and New Jersey, has there been any significant change in regulatory approaches.

In 1987 New York Mayor Koch announced an effort by the city to set up a city-run competitor for the private carters, initially servicing just the Chinatown area in Manhattan.[42] The New York Times carried various stories over the next year chronicling difficulties in obtaining the data necessary to implement the scheme. After a while the scheme seems just to have dissolved; certainly it has never been implemented.

Shortly after the mayor's announcement, the Wall Street Journal (Penn 1988, p. 54) carried an article repeating the now time-honored complaints: carters evade price regulation by overstating the quantity of garbage being picked up; aggressive competitors face the threat of physical punishment; customers have no choice of service provider. Even the major electrical utility, Con Edison, angered by its carter's effort to raise its price after one year of a two-year contract, was unable to persuade another carter to offer bids.

Three years later the New York Times (Gold 1991, p. A17) reported another effort by the city to increase competition, this time by persuading the national firms to enter the city's market. As an inducement, the city offered to buy back the routes if the new entrants were intimidated by the existing carters; the city would then operate the routes itself. The Department of Consumer Affairs said, once again, that "carters violate the rules of economics by not competitively bidding for business" (Gold 1991, p. A17). The United Nations, still in the hands of the firm that had purchased the contract from New York Carting, had given up putting the contract out for bid.

On Long Island, notwithstanding the state's successful prosecution of the Private Sanitary Industry and most of its leading members, the

---

[42] The mayor drew somewhat on the plan developed by the author for restructuring the industry on Long Island (Reuter 1987, sec. 4). The plan required that the government operate as a competitor in the market so that customers would be willing to switch to a lower-priced firm and other outside carters would also enter the market.

customer allocation agreement continued to operate. In 1989 the federal government brought a civil Racketeer Influenced and Corrupt Organizations lawsuit against those convicted in the state's earlier case, seeking full divestiture. Thirty-two years after Bernard Adelstein had been named as a principal in the McClellan hearings, the federal government was once again seeking his removal from control of Teamster's Local 813.

The New Jersey State Commission of Investigation, whose 1969 investigation had led to regulation of the industry, published a twenty-year update in 1989 and pointed to continuing evidence of customer allocation agreements. The only improvement seemed to be in the related municipal contract system where the report found a dramatic decline in the percentage of towns receiving single bids for their contracts.

Racketeer involvement was assumed to have continued in all three areas. No fresh evidence was offered for this claim.

B. Other Areas

There is spotty evidence of customer allocation agreements outside of New York and New Jersey. For example, the state of Illinois alleged in 1971 that the local Chicago association (the Chicago and Suburban Refuse Disposal Corporation) had formal rules allocating customers. As summarized by the *Wall Street Journal* (Bailey 1991, p. 2) the suit, which was settled by a $50,000 payment to the state (without admitting wrongdoing), alleged that members "would not solicit each other's customers; if a customer of one hauler sought a bid from another hauler, the second hauler would either refuse to bid or quote a higher price; if a hauler nevertheless ended up with another hauler's customer, something of equal value—money or comparable account—would be paid to even the score; and bidding for all government contracts would be rigged ahead of time."

Allegations of racketeer involvement have been made against the industry in western Florida in the 1970s. In the 1960s the U.S. Department of Justice brought charges against the local carting association in Philadelphia that included use of violence in the furtherance of restraint of trade (Hay and Kelly 1974).

The two major national firms have a dismayingly long record of convictions for restrictive practices. The BFI has been included in government criminal antitrust suits in New Jersey (resulting in acquittal by a jury); Georgia (where the suit was settled without admission of the charges); and Florida and Ohio, where affiliates of the companies were convicted of customer allocation. Waste Management also has been convicted of price fixing charges in Wisconsin and California and pled no contest to charges in Florida and Georgia. Just as dismayingly, a private class-action suit alleging price fixing in numerous local markets resulted in a private settlement, with the defendants paying $50 million to settle the suit (Bailey 1991, p. 2).

Despite these problems, the nationals have been seen as aggressive competitors in some markets. The emergence of competition in the New Jersey municipal contract market is believed to be the result of active bidding by the nationals, following their settlement of a civil suit brought by the state against the Municipal Contractors Association.

More recently, the U.S. Department of Justice has tried to induce entry by the nationals into the New York City market. The department took over two large carting firms in 1990 when their owners were convicted of illegal dumping. It sought to have the firm's customers serviced by a new entrant to the business and was reported by the *New York Times* (Gold 1991) to have either BFI or Laidlaw, a Canadian-based hauler, take over the service responsibilities.

It is difficult to determine, then, just how generally the industry exhibits the phenomenon of either customer allocation or racketeer involvement. In most areas there are neither Mafia families nor any other comparable racketeering group. For our purposes it would be most interesting to obtain data on service prices and on the market for customers among carters. A 1980 effort to obtain such data was unsuccessful (Reuter 1981, app. B) since the carters refused to provide answers to questions on either topic.

Fragments of evidence suggest that some markets are quite competitive. For example, in the antitrust suit cited in footnote 4, testimony showed that in Houston new firms had grown rapidly by aggressive solicitation of customers and price cutting. It may be that in newer cities, particularly those with rapidly expanding markets and populations, the flow of new customers is such that old customer allocation agreements can do little to impede entry into a market with many unallocated customers.

C. Conclusions: Racketeering and Customer Allocation

The greater New York garbage collection industry is not the only one in which racketeers have a long established role. Among those that are prominently and accurately labeled this way are the stevedoring industry on the East Coast (U.S. Senate 1981), the casino industry in Nevada (Skolnick 1978), and garment manufacturing in the Northeast (President's Commission on Organized Crime 1986).

However, the nature of the racketeer involvement varies in these different industries. For example, stevedoring firms have been subject to extortion by racketeers through unions, while the Nevada casinos were used as means for laundering money or for evading regulation by those same racketeers. Only in the garment trucking sector do they operate in ways that resemble a customer allocation agreement. In none of these industries does it appear that the businesses themselves are beneficiaries of the racketeering.

But one characteristic that all these industries share is the durability of the presence of racketeers. For example, credible allegations of their involvement in the waterfront go back at least to the 1950s (Jensen 1974). Another characteristic is that all these industries have been subject to numerous investigations aimed at rooting out the racketeers. Only in the Nevada industry, where their presence was historically opportunistic (racketeers being the only capitalists willing to provide large-scale finance for a pariah industry), not based in the structure of the industry or its finance, has their presence clearly declined.

The problem of racketeer involvement in the New York carting industry seems also to be one that is unlikely to yield to conventional solutions of either prosecution or regulation. The reputational barrier to entry is a powerful one, which has served to keep the nationals out. With customers cowed and conspiracy richly rewarded, there is little to disturb the existing arrangements. Even the declining power of the Mafia is likely to affect this industry only slowly; organizational reputation is a long-lived asset. It is that reputation that permits the rarest of phenomena—stable, long-lived, and large number cartel arrangements. Given the difficulty of dealing with the problem, it is fortunate that the circumstances for its creation seem to be highly localized and idiosyncratic.

REFERENCES

Bailey, Jeff. 1991. "Garbage Firms Antitrust Woes Pile Up." *Wall Street Journal* (September 10), p. 2.

Bird, David. 1974. "City Will Take Indicted Carters' Routes." *New York Times* (July 22), p. 1.

Chambers, Marcia. 1981. "Two Panels Indict Seventeen Milk Dealers in Price-fixing." *New York Times* (November 10), sec. 2, p. 1.

Fog, Bjorke. 1956 "How Are Cartel Prices Determined?" *Journal of Industrial Economics* 15:16–23.

Gold, Allen R. 1991. "U.S. Acts to End Monopolies in New York Trash Hauling." *New York Times*, national ed. (February 6), p. A17.

Hay, George, and Daniel Kelly. 1974. "An Empirical Survey of Price-fixing Conspiracies." *Journal of Law and Economics* 17:13–38.

Herling, John. 1962. *The Great Price Conspiracy: The Story of Anti-trust Violations in the Electrical Industry*. Washington, D.C.: Luce.

Hicks, John. 1935. "Annual Survey of Economic Theory: The Theory of Monopoly." *Econometrica* 3:1–20.

Hutchison, John. 1970. *The Imperfect Union*. New York: E. P. Dutton.

Jensen, Vernon. 1974. *Strife on the Waterfront: The Port of New York since 1945*. Ithaca, N.Y.: Cornell University Press.

Kolko, Gabriel. 1965. *Railroads and Regulation: 1877–1916*. Princeton, N.J.: Princeton University Press.

Moore, Thomas G. 1978. "The Beneficiaries of Trucking Regulation." *Journal of Law and Economics* 21:327–43.

New Jersey State Commission of Investigation. 1969. *In the Matter of the Investigation of Waste Disposal and the Garbage Industry in New Jersey*. Trenton: New Jersey State Commission of Investigation.

———. 1989. *Solid Waste Regulation*. Trenton: New Jersey State Commission of Investigation.

New York Times. 1956 (February 8). "Economies Urged in Refuse Service," p. 35.

Penn, Stanley. 1988. "NYC Will Confront Mafia in Chinatown by Bidding to Haul Garbage of Some Businesses." *Wall Street Journal* (April 25), p. 54.

President's Commission on Organized Crime. 1985. *Hearings: Organized Crime and Labor-Management Racketeering in the United States*. Washington, D.C.: U.S. Government Printing Office.

———. 1986. THE EDGE: *Organized Crime, Business and Labor Unions*. Washington, D.C.: U.S. Government Printing Office.

Reuter, Peter. 1981. "Racketeering in Legitimate Industries: An Economic Analysis." Unpublished manuscript. New York: Center for Research on Institutions and Social Policy.

———. 1983. *Disorganized Crime: The Economics of the Visible Hand*. Cambridge, Mass.: MIT Press.

———. 1987. *Racketeering in Legitimate Industries: A Study in the Economics of Intimidation*. Santa Monica, Calif.: RAND.

Reuter, Peter, Jonathan Rubinstein, and Simon Wynn. 1982. *Racketeering in Legitimate Industries: Two Case Studies*. Executive summary. Washington, D.C.: National Institute of Justice.

Schelling, Thomas. 1967. "Economic Analysis of Organized Crime." President's Commission on Law Enforcement and Administration of Justice.

Task Force Report: Organized Crime. Washington, D.C.: U.S. Government Printing Office.

Scherer, Frederick M. 1970. *Industrial Market Structure and Economic Performance.* Chicago: Rand-McNally.

Skolnick, Jerome. 1978. *House of Cards.* Boston: Little, Brown.

———. 1978. "Scale, Market Structure and the Cost of Refuse Collection." *Review of Economics and Statistics* 59:428–38.

Stevens, Barbara. 1978. "Scale, Market Structure and the Cost of Refuse Collection." *Review of Economics and Statistics* 59:428–38.

———. 1991. "Privatization of Solid Waste Management." Unpublished manuscript. Westport, Conn.: Ecodata.

Stigler, George. 1964. "A Theory of Oligopoly." *Journal of Political Economy* 72:44–61.

Stocking, G., and M. Watkins. 1946. *Cartels in Action.* New York: Twentieth Century Fund.

———. 1951. *Monopoly and Free Enterprise.* New York: Twentieth Century Fund.

U.S. Senate. 1957. Select Committee on Improper Activities in the Labor Management Field (McClellan Committee). Hearings, pt. 17. Washington, D.C.: U.S. Government Printing Office.

———. 1981. "Waterfront Corruption." Hearings before the Permanent Subcommittee on Investigations of the Committee on Governmental Affairs, 97th Congress.

Wilson, Thomas. 1962. "Restrictive Practices." In *Competition, Cartels and Their Regulation*, edited by John Perry. Amsterdam: North-Holland.

Henry N. Pontell and Kitty Calavita

The Savings and Loan Industry

ABSTRACT

Crime and fraud were central factors in the savings and loan crisis.
Insider abuse was in large part a product of the organizational
environment within which thrifts operated in the 1980s. Thrift
deregulation in the early 1980s, in conjunction with federal insurance
on thrift deposits, produced a "criminogenic environment" in which
opportunities for fraud were extensive and risks were minimal.
Various common patterns of fraud—"illegal risk taking," "collective
embezzlement," and "covering-up"—can be attributed to the economic
and regulatory structure of the deregulated savings and loan industry.

Fraud in savings and loan (S&L) institutions may constitute the most
costly set of white-collar crimes in history. In 1989, official estimates
of the bailout costs for insolvent thrifts were placed at $200 billion
over the next decade and ranged from $300 billion to $473 billion by
the year 2021 (U.S. Congress, House Committee on Ways and Means
1989, p. 20; U.S. Congress, Senate Committee on Banking, Housing,
and Urban Affairs 1989, p. 9). The General Accounting Office (GAO),
revising an earlier, more conservative estimated, claimed that it "will
now cost at least $325 billion and could cost as much as $500 billion
over the next 30 to 40 years" (Johnston 1990). The GAO further noted
that the new figure was "subject to significant change" depending on
the general economic health of the country. Edwin Gray, former chair

Henry N. Pontell and Kitty Calavita are professor and associate professor of criminology, law, and society at the University of California, Irvine. The research reported here
was supported under award 90-IJ-CX-0059 from the National Institute of Justice. Points
of view in this document are the authors' and do not necessarily represent the official
position of the U.S. Department of Justice.

of the Federal Home Loan Bank Board, estimated the eventual cost of the debacle will exceed one trillion dollars (Gray 1991). Another recent estimate is that the final figure will approximate 1.4 trillion dollars (Hill 1990, p. 24). Since its inception in August 1989, the Resolution Trust Corporation (RTC), which was formed by federal legislation to dispose of seized S&L assets, had "resolved" (closed, sold, or merged with another institution) 583 insolvent thrifts through November 1991 and had managed over $181 billion in thrift assets (Resolution Trust Corporation 1992).

There is abundant evidence that willful criminality was involved in significant numbers of these insolvencies. Government reports suggest that criminal activity was a central factor in 70–80 percent of thrift failures (U.S. Congress, House Committee on Government Operations 1988, p. 51; U.S. General Accounting Office 1989a). A Resolution Trust Corporation report estimated that about 51 percent of insolvent thrifts controlled by RTC had suspected criminal misconduct referred to the FBI and that "fraud and potentially criminal conduct by insiders contributed to the failure of about 41 percent of RTC thrifts" (Resolution Trust Corporation 1990a, p. 9). In 1990, RTC investigatory official James R. Dudine testified before Congress on the extent of misconduct in failed S&Ls. He reported that 138 of the 392 thrifts that by then had come under RTC conservatorship had had criminal misconduct referred to the FBI, that insider abuse and misconduct contributed significantly to the failure in about 50 percent of failed thrifts, and that in about 15 percent of the insolvencies, possible fraudulent transactions involved the participation of other financial institutions (Dudine 1990).

Congressional hearings reveal a backlog of extremely complex criminal cases that point to the potential inability of federal enforcement agencies to respond effectively to "the crisis." In April 1990, there were 1,298 "inactive cases" in Department of Justice files, each involving over $100,000, which then-current guidelines classified as "significant." Despite the seriousness of these "significant cases," backlogs grew as there were not enough FBI agents or U.S. Attorneys to keep up with the rapid pace of criminal referrals (Rosenblatt 1990a). One senior FBI official noted in an interview in 1990 that he did not expect referrals to level off for at least 4–5 years.[1] In 1990, Congress allocated additional resources to the Department of Justice to process S&L fraud

---

[1] Attribution of views or comments of unnamed individuals are based on field notes and interview records from interviews we conducted with individuals as part of our research on the S&L crisis.

cases. In recognition of the unprecedented volume of such cases, other federal agencies, most notably the Secret Service, joined the investigative effort. Records from the Office of Thrift Supervision (OTS), since 1989 the supervisory and enforcement agency for thrifts, indicate that it made 7,799 criminal referrals to the Department of Justice from 1989 through June 1990 alone (Resolution Trust Corporation 1990a, p. 9).

There is little doubt that deliberate crime is an integral part of the S&L crisis and contributes significantly to the losses that will accrue to generations of taxpayers. Of course, the amount of thrift crime officially uncovered and prosecuted depends in part on the response of regulators and law enforcement officials. Unlike most common crimes that are easily recognizable, and in which extensive investigations are not usually necessary before criminal cases can be brought, thrift industry crimes are often well hidden by intricate "paper trails" and require extensive documentation before the case can even be brought to a prosecutor. As Katz (1979) has noted in this regard, the investigative and prosecutorial functions in white-collar crimes are often one and the same. Thus, a central determinant of the "extent of white-collar crime" is the capacity and willingness of enforcers and other state officials to define it as such.

This essay examines the origins of the thrift crisis, focusing on the impact of deregulation and the federal deposit insurance system, which together provided significant opportunities for profit and minimal risks for fraud. In addition, we trace the essential forms of thrift crime, suggesting that each is derived from the organizational environment and regulatory structure that characterized the thrift industry in the mid-1980s, as well as the distinctive subcultures and networks operating in particular regions of the country. Finally, we examine government responses to this epidemic of financial fraud, delineating prevailing investigative strategies, civil and criminal procedural alternatives, and preliminary sanctioning patterns. We conclude with a brief discussion of the potential for a second round of fraud, and related taxpayer expenses, as the government manages and sells—often to individuals who were formerly affiliated with the moribund thrift industry—the billions of dollars of assets it has seized from insolvent thrifts.

I. Underpinnings of the Crisis

The federally insured savings and loan system was put into place in the 1930s, primarily to encourage the construction and sale of new homes during the Depression and to protect these savings institutions from the kind of disaster that followed the 1929 panic. The Federal Home Loan Bank Act of 1932 established the Federal Home Loan Bank Board (FHLBB), designed to provide a credit system to ensure the availability of mortgage money for home financing and to oversee federally chartered savings and loan institutions. Two years later, the National Housing Act created the Federal Savings and Loan Insurance Corporation (FSLIC) to insure deposits in savings and loan institutions.

Until the broad reforms enacted by the Financial Institutions Reform, Recovery, and Enforcement Act of 1989 (FIRREA), the FHLBB was the primary regulatory agency responsible for federally chartered savings and loans. An independent agency with a chair and two members appointed by the president, the FHLBB oversaw twelve regional home loan banks that served as a conduit to the individual savings and loans that constituted the industry. These regional district banks provided a pool of funds for their member institutions at below market rates, in order to disburse loans and cover withdrawals. In 1985, the district banks were assigned the task of examining and supervising the savings and loans within their regional jurisdiction. Thus, although the central FHLBB was officially responsible for promulgating and enforcing regulations, agents of the district banks oversaw the thrifts' operations and had the authority to initiate corrective measures and to notify the FHLBB of suspected misconduct. This dual role of the district banks and the FHLBB both to promote *and* to regulate the savings and loan industry contributed to their curiously complacent response to emerging indications of fraud in the industry.

In return for the protection provided by federal deposit insurance provided by the FSLIC, thrifts were tightly regulated. Until 1974, all federally chartered savings and loans were by law "mutual" institutions, owned by the depositors, who, instead of receiving interest on deposits, received dividends based on the profits of the association. These mutual associations were limited to making home loans, as they had been created and were protected by federal insurance as a way to encourage home ownership. Furthermore, thrifts were limited geographically, being confined to the issuance of home loans within fifty miles of the home office. In 1966, the Financial Institutions Supervisory Act redefined the nature of the "dividends" paid to depositors. Recognizing that these "dividends" were essentially interest on deposits, Regulation Q set a limit on the interest rate thrifts could pay, establishing a ceiling slightly higher than that allowed banks, in recognition of the home ownership function served by thrifts. In 1974, new federal regulations began to allow thrifts to sell stock, gradually moving them from mutually owned to shareholder-held institutions. During the same period, there was a loosening of geographical restrictions. Nonetheless, these minor changes did not significantly alter the protection/regulation formula that had worked for over thirty years.

Economic conditions of the 1970s substantially undermined the health of the industry and ultimately contributed to the dismantling of the traditional boundaries within which they had operated. Perhaps most important, high interest rates and slow growth squeezed the industry at both ends. Locked into low-interest mortgages from previous eras, prohibited by Regulation Q from paying more than 5.5 percent interest on new deposits, and with inflation reaching 13.3 percent by 1979, the industry suffered steep losses. As inflation outpaced the meager 5.5 percent return on thrift deposits, savings and loans found it increasingly difficult to attract new funds. Compounding their problems, the development of money market mutual funds by Wall Street allowed middle-income investors to buy shares in large denomination securities at high money-market rates, which triggered "disintermediation," or massive withdrawals of deposits from savings and loans.

In 1979, Paul Volcker, then head of the Federal Reserve Board, tightened the money supply in an effort to relieve the inflationary spiral, sending interest rates up to their highest levels in this century, contributing to a serious recession. Confronted with rising defaults and foreclosures as the recession deepened, and increasing competition from new high-yield investments with the hike in interest rates, savings and loans seemed doomed to extinction. The industry's net worth fell from $16.7 billion in 1972 to a *negative* net worth of $17.5 billion in 1980, with 85 percent of the country's savings and loans losing money (Pizzo, Fricker, and Muolo 1989, p. 11).

A. Deregulation: Setting the Stage for Disaster

Along with these economic forces, a new ideological era had begun. While policymakers had been considering loosening the restraints on savings and loans since the early 1970s, it was not until the deregulatory fervor of the early Reagan administration that this approach gained widespread political acceptance as a solution to the rapidly escalating savings and loan crisis. Referring to the new deregulatory mentality and the conviction and enthusiasm with which deregulation was pursued, a senior thrift regulator said in an interview, "I always describe it as a freight train. I mean it was just the direction and everybody got on board." In a few strokes, the policymakers dismantled most of the regulatory infrastructure that had kept the thrift industry together for four decades (Mayer 1990). These deregulators were convinced that the free enterprise system works best if left alone, unhampered by perhaps well-meaning but ultimately counterproductive government regulations. The problems of the savings and loan industry seemed to confirm the notion that government regulations imposed an unfair handicap in the competitive process. The answer was to return the industry to what were perceived to be the self-regulating mechanisms of the free market.

In 1980, the Depository Institutions Deregulation and Monetary Control Act (DIDMCA) made four major changes. First, it created the Depository Institutions Deregulation Committee, whose task it was to phase out limits on deposit interest rates by 1986. Second, the law authorized federally chartered thrifts to make commercial real estate loans and consumer loans and to purchase corporate debt instruments. Third, it abolished all remaining geographic limits. Finally, it authorized the issuance of credit cards. But, the move to the "free market" model was both incomplete and accompanied by a decisive move in the *opposite* direction. At the same time that the new law unleashed savings and loans to compete for new money, it *bolstered* the federal protection accorded these "private enterprise" institutions, increasing FSLIC insurance from a maximum of $40,000 to $100,000 per deposit. The increase came during a late-night session of the Senate and House Conference Committee. The Senate bill would have raised federal insurance to $50,000 per deposit; the House bill made no mention of any increase. During negotiations, conference committee members went off the record, moving from the conference room to a back chamber. When they returned, a provision had been added to the conference bill raising deposit insurance to $100,000 per account. The U.S. League of Savings Institutions—the powerful S&L lobby—apparently pushed for the change, withholding its support for the bill until the increase was assured. Deposit insurance only four years earlier had been limited to $25,000, and since the average deposit was only $6,000, this large increase seemed to some to be aimed more at saving the institutions, rather than at protecting individual depositors (Eichler 1989; Mayer 1990; Waldman 1990).

Industry losses continued to mount, as the 1980 reform triggered an even more pronounced "negative rate spread." Thrifts did attract more new money at higher interest rates, but the discrepancy between these high rates and the low rates at which they had earlier invested in long-term, fixed-rate mortgages widened. The most notable effect of the 1980 deregulation was to precipitate larger losses on more money. However, congressional enthusiasm for deregulation did not wane. Convinced that the "free market" was the cure for the S&L doldrums, Congress enacted further deregulation to "improve (S&L's) ability to generate current earnings to sustain the growth capital needed for future operations" (U.S. Congress, Senate 1982, p. 87). The Garn-St. Germain Depository Institutions Act of 1982 accelerated the phase-out of the ceiling on interest rates initiated in the 1980 reform. Probably more important, it dramatically expanded the investment powers of savings and loans, moving them farther away from their traditional role as providers of home mortgages. They were now authorized to increase consumer loans up to a total of 30 percent of their assets; make commercial, corporate, or business loans; and invest in nonresidential real estate worth up to 40 percent of their total assets. Furthermore, the Garn-St. Germain Act allowed thrifts to provide 100 percent financing, requiring no down-payment from the borrower, in an apparent effort to attract new business to the desperate industry.

Industry regulators joined in the deregulation, eliminating a 5 percent limit on brokered deposits in 1980, giving thrifts access to unprecedented amounts of cash. Brokered deposits were placed by middlemen who aggregated individual investments as "jumbo" certificates of deposit (CDs). Since the maximum insured deposit was $100,000, these brokered deposits were packaged as $100,000 CDs, on which the investors could command high interest rates. So attractive was this system to all concerned—brokers who made hefty commissions, individual investors who received high interest for their money, and thrift operators who now had almost unlimited access to these funds—that between 1982 and 1984 brokered deposits as a percentage of total thrift assets increased 400 percent (U.S. General Accounting Office 1985, p. 7). By January 1984, federally insured thrifts had access to $34 billion in brokered deposits (Pizzo, Fricker, and Muolo 1989, pp. 79–80). Some of the most troubled institutions had become virtually dependent on brokered deposits, with Charles Keating's Lincoln Savings and Loan, for example, getting 50 percent of its deposits in this form (Waldman 1990, p. 31).

In 1982, regulators opened the door for a single entrepreneur to own and operate a federally insured savings and loan, dropping a requirement established in 1974 that thrifts have at least 400 stockholders, with no one owning more than 25 percent of the stock. Furthermore, single investors could now start thrifts with noncash assets, such as land or real estate, as backing. While some initial cash investment was still necessary for start-up costs, regulators regarded real estate and other assets as "capital" for the purposes of chartering and licensing new thrifts. Presumably hoping that the move would attract innovative entrepreneurs who would salvage the industry, the deregulators seemed unaware of the disastrous potential of virtually unlimited charters in the vulnerable industry. A senior thrift regulator in an interview described the cumulative impact of the deregulation: "The government created tremendous opportunity in 1982 for anybody that wanted to engage in any kind of criminal activity or just get rich quick."

Losses continued to plague the industry. In 1982, FSLIC spent over $2.4 billion to close or merge insolvent savings and loans, and by 1986 the federal insurance agency was itself insolvent (U.S. Congress, House Committee on Banking, Finance, and Urban Affairs 1989, p. 286). With the number of insolvent thrifts climbing steadily, FSLIC, knowing that it had insufficient funds to cope with the disaster, slowed the pace of closures, allowing technically insolvent institutions to stay open. Not surprisingly, the "zombie" thrifts continued to hemorrhage losses. In the first half of 1988, the thrift industry lost an unprecedented $7.5 billion (Eichler 1989, p. 119).[2]

Martin Mayer, former member of the President's Commission on Housing under the Reagan administration, describes these deregulatory years: "What happened to create the disgusting and expensive spectacle of a diseased industry was that the government, confronted with a difficult problem, found a false solution that made the problem worse. This false solution then acquired a supportive constituency that remained vigorous and effective for almost five years after everybody with the slightest expertise in the subject knew that terrible things were happening *everywhere*. Some of the supporters were true believers, some were simply lazy, and most were making money—*lots* of money—from the government's mistake" (Mayer 1990, p. 27).

B. Transformation of the Industry

The classic Frank Capra movie, *It's a Wonderful Life*, aptly portrayed—albeit in Hollywood's exaggerated style—the savings and loan

[2] Some have pointed out that the 1986 Tax Reform Act, disallowing the "passive loss" deductions authorized in 1981, removed the tax-shelter potential of real estate investments, thereby undermining the value of thrift assets and sending the real estate

industry prior to the "stagflation" of the 1970s and subsequent deregulation. George Bailey, played by Jimmy Stewart, struggles to keep his "building and loan" afloat despite a Depression Era "run," by appealing to the idea that his neighbors' money was not in the building where they deposited it, but in each others' homes, and that they were in effect lending that money to each other, to be paid back with interest. Thrifts traditionally made loans on single-family homes in the local market, and thrift executives lived by the comfortable "3-6-3" rule, which was to pay 3 percent on deposits, lend money at 6 percent interest, and be on the golf course by 3 o'clock in the afternoon. This simple scenario, which guaranteed stable—if modest—profits, changed dramatically during the 1970s due to high inflation and a more competitive financial market that took funds out of thrifts. In the 1980s, deregulation remade the industry and in the process ultimately destroyed it.

As President Reagan signed the deregulatory Garn-St. Germain Act in the White House Rose Garden on October 15, 1982, he declared with characteristic confidence, "All in all, I think we hit the jackpot." The original legislation was written by one of his appointees, Dick Pratt, chair of the FHLBB between 1981 and 1983 (Mayer 1990). Savings and loans, now free from government reins, changed dramatically from their traditional organizational roots. Single owners with entrepreneurial intentions, and sometimes no banking experience, bought troubled thrifts at bargain prices. Large brokered deposits swelled the size of many thrifts, with Texas S&Ls growing 500–1,000 percent a year.

The deregulation of savings and loans' investment powers had unleashed an escalating competitive process in which brokered deposits were a key ingredient. Overnight, ailing savings and loans could obtain huge amounts of cash to stave off their impending insolvency. But brokered deposits had a downside. The more these institutions used brokered deposits, the more they depended on them, and the more they were willing to, and had to, pay to get them. As brokerage firms shopped across the country for the best return on their money, thrifts had to offer ever-higher interest rates to attract them. Furthermore, the most desperate institutions needed these deposits most and paid the highest interest rates. In a contortion of the theory of the survival

market into a downward spiral. While this undoubtedly contributed to the S&L crisis, both the epidemic of fraud and thrifts' solvency problems had commenced well before the 1986 tax reform. Indeed, by 1986, FSLIC itself was insolvent.

of the fittest to which the free-market deregulators subscribed, in this environment it was the weakest thrifts that grew the fastest.

With their newfound wealth, thrift operators were free—indeed were *impelled* by their dependence on high-interest brokered deposits—to make risky investments in junk bonds, stocks, commercial real estate projects, anything that had the potential to reap windfall profits. And, the magic was that every deposit up to $100,000 was federally insured, and therefore these "high-risk" investments, were, from the depositors' and bankers' perspective, essentially "risk-free." A staff member of the House Banking Committee summed up the nature of the vast opportunities and minimal risks that the combination of deregulation and federal insurance opened up. After deregulation, he said in an interview, "Thrifts could do bloody anything. . . . And it was all federally insured. It's almost like when you are walking along and you see a $10 bill on the sidewalk and you know it's not yours . . . but it's so easy to pick it up and stuff it in your pocket and no one knows." Some of the transactions were legitimate—if foolhardy—attempts to raise capital in an environment that effectively stacked the deck against traditional lending practices. Others were outright scams involving insiders, borrowers, Wall Street brokers, and developers. The organizational environment was altered by the deregulation of the 1980s, transforming the industry virtually overnight, precipitating its demise, and opening up opportunities both to those seeking windfall profits from high-risk investments and to those who used the industry as their personal "money machine."

II. Opportunities for Law-breaking and Regional Subcultures

Significant regional variation exists in the magnitude of thrift fraud and prevailing patterns of illegal activity. In part, these differences are the result of regional variations in the structure of the thrift industry, decentralized regulatory structures, and local market conditions. In addition, it appears that distinctive regional subcultures and networks influenced the scope of fraud and the style and preferred schemes of fraudulent thrift operators across the country.

Of the 357 failed banks and thrifts under FBI investigation by 1988, over one-third were located in Texas and California, with Texas alone accounting for eighty-five cases (FBI report on "White-Collar Crime," in U.S. Congress, House Committee on Banking, Finance and Urban

Affairs 1990, p. 166). In 1989, the General Accounting Office examined twenty-six of the most costly failed thrifts in the United States, accounting for 60 percent of total FSLIC losses at that time. Of these twenty-six worst cases, ten were Texas thrifts and eight were in California (U.S. General Accounting Office 1989a).

This pattern is consistent with the regional development of deregulation. The federal system of thrift regulation was accompanied by a sometimes overlapping state system. State-chartered, as opposed to federally chartered, thrifts were regulated by state agencies and governed by their regulations but could be insured by FSLIC as long as they paid the insurance premiums, which most did. Federally chartered thrifts were *required* to have FSLIC insurance, while for state-chartered thrifts the insurance was optional. Considering the advantages deposit insurance provided a thrift, the 1/12 of 1 percent of an institution's deposits for the FSLIC premium in 1984 was a bargain. By 1987, of the 2,000 federally chartered thrifts and 2,600 state institutions, only 600 of the latter were not members of FSLIC. Furthermore, unlike traditional insurance policies, FSLIC premiums were not tied to risks. Kane (1989, pp. 6–7) explains the ironic result, "FSLIC insurance can simultaneously be unreasonably expensive for a conservatively run firm and unreasonably cheap for an aggressively run enterprise that has little of its own capital at risk."

This dual system had disastrous consequences within the context of deregulation. Since funding for the state regulatory agencies was derived largely from its member institutions, state agencies that were perceived by thrift operators as more restrictive or enforcement-oriented than those of other states or the federal government risked losing their funding as thrifts sought out more lenient jurisdictions.

Texas was one of the first states to deregulate and, by the time of the federal deregulation drive, already was more lax than even the deregulated national system. In fact, until 1984, the Texas Savings and Loan Commission was barred by law from turning down any application for a thrift charter as long as the applicant met the relatively meager capital and other bureaucratic requirements (Pilzer and Deitz 1989, pp. 168–69). With Texas thrifts free to make almost any kind of investment, and virtually anyone with funds welcome to enter the business, they experienced unprecedented growth. William Black, former deputy director of FSLIC, reported to Congress that the forty worst Texas failures (known as the infamous "Texas 40") experienced growth rates between 1983 and 1986 that were over five times the national average (testimony of William Black, in U.S. Congress, House Committee on Banking, Finance, and Urban Affairs 1990, p. 213).

The phenomenal growth in Texas thrifts was largely the result of risky "direct investments" in acquisition, development, and construction (ADC) loans. Acquisition, development, and construction loans were notorious in the industry as the highest-risk investments, since loans are made to developers before a project is undertaken and often involve 100 percent financing. While 100 percent financing for development projects was not uncommon in the banking industry by the 1970s, the risk was compounded for Texas thrifts by an almost total absence of underwriting. In part, the operative assumption was that Texas commercial real estate would continue its steady and dramatic increase in value. In addition, however, thrift executives made short-term profits *regardless* of the long-term viability of their lending practices. Points and fees were paid up-front, and the steadily increasing "profits" recorded as the thrift expanded its volume of business many times over meant generous bonuses and dividends for thrift management. Equally important, the new owners who entered the Texas thrift industry in the early 1980s were often developers themselves, attracted to the thrift industry as "money machines" for their own construction projects and those of their friends and affiliates. The Governor's Task Force on the Savings and Loan Industry in Texas revealed in 1988 that seven of the eleven most troubled Texas thrifts had been purchased by developers between 1982 and 1983 (Governor's Task Force, in U.S. Congress, House Committee on Banking, Finance, and Urban Affairs 1990, p. 241). According to a 1987 report of the Texas Savings and Loan League Special Issues Commission, "Entrepreneurs with backgrounds in real estate development either own or owned 20 of the 24 most deeply insolvent thrifts in Texas" (quoted in ibid., p. 181).

The personal and financial networks among and between the thrift industry in Texas and the development and construction industries, together with the substantial up-front profits to be made, produced a devil-may-care attitude. Indeed, many thrift operators dispensed millions of dollars in high-risk ADC loans with little concern for the actual viability of the projects. William Black, at the time a senior thrift regulator in San Francisco, testified to Congress that, in Texas in the mid-1980s, "It was not unusual to find massive ADC loans made before an application was even received" (testimony of William Black in ibid., p. 179). The mentality behind such practices was expressed bluntly by Tyrell Barker, owner and CEO of State Savings and Loan, who told developers in Dallas, "You bring the dirt, I bring the money. We split 50-50" (quoted in Pizzo, Fricker, and Muolo 1989, p. 191).[3]

"Ol' boy networks" dominated the Texas thrift scene. Arthur Leiser, for thirty-five years an examiner with the Texas Savings and Loan Department, kept a diary and noted the interconnections among thrift insiders, developers, brokers, and a variety of borrowers. One network he describes included seventy-four participants (U.S. Congress, House Committee on Banking, Finance, and Urban Affairs 1990, pp. 815–25). Leiser's flow charts and diagrams are virtually indecipherable in their complexity. It is revealing, however, that all the most costly thrift failures in Texas were represented in these networks. Other investigators have focused their Texas network analysis on a number of "high-flyers" who repeatedly surface as participants in the costliest failures (see, e.g., Adams 1990, p. 270).

These networks were critical in the perpetration of the complex transactions that successful thrift fraud depended on. But, they were also central to staving off the closure of thrifts and keeping regulators at bay. A particularly useful strategy in this regard, demonstrating not only the importance of the networks but the conspiratorial mentality that permeated them, involved Texas thrift operators exchanging their bad assets to get them off the books and artificially enhance their financial picture. When examiners were expected, S&L operators sold bad loans to other thrifts in the network, with the understanding that they would buy bad loans from obliging thrifts in the future. These transactions, referred to cynically by the participants as trading "dead cows for dead horses," kept "zombie" institutions open long after their actual insolvency and multiplied the final cost of government bailouts. In one notorious case, nineteen of the largest thrifts in Texas sent representatives to a secret meeting in Houston in 1985 to trade "dead cows and horses" for the explicit purpose of confounding regulators (Pizzo, Fricker, and Muolo 1989, pp. 209–10).

The evolution of the thrift debacle in California followed a somewhat different course, although ultimately the same patterns of fraud were replicated. When the federal system of thrift supervision was deregulated in 1980 and 1982, California still had one of the most carefully regulated systems in the country. Beginning in 1975, the California Department of Savings and Loan had been staffed by no-nonsense

---

[3] Tyrell Barker has pleaded guilty to misapplication of bank funds.

regulators who imposed strict rules and tolerated little deviation. The California thrift industry complained bitterly, and when federal regulations were relaxed in 1980, they switched en masse to federal charters (U.S. Congress, House Committee on Government Operations 1987, pp. 12–13). With the exodus of thrifts from its jurisdiction, the California agency lost over half of its funding and more than half its staff. In July 1978, it had 172 full-time examiners; by 1983, the number of examiners had shrunk to fifty-five (U.S. Congress, House Committee on Government Operations 1988, p. 62). California policymakers learned the hard way that if the state's Department of Savings and Loan was to survive (and if California politicians were to continue to have access to the industry's generous campaign contributions), they had to loosen the restrictions on the industry. In 1983, the Nolan Bill passed with only one dissenting vote, making it possible for California thrifts to invest in virtually any venture and allowing them to put 100 percent of their deposits in risky commercial real estate.

Suddenly, the California Savings and Loan Commission was inundated with hundreds of applications for new S&L charters from entrepreneurs around the country. Los Angeles consultants and law firms spread the word, offering seminars on how to start an S&L. One prominent firm appropriately titled its seminar, "Why Does It Seem Everyone Is Buying or Starting a California S&L?" (quoted in Pizzo, Fricker, and Muolo 1989, p. 21). In his first six months as savings and loan commissioner in 1983, Lawrence Taggart issued sixty new charters, approving virtually all applications. Attracted to Commissioner Taggart's permissive policies and laissez-faire approach in the face of growth rates that sometimes surpassed 1,000 percent annually, a new breed of thrift entrepreneurs flocked to California's newly deregulated industry. The "list of colorful characters" (Pizzo, Fricker, and Muolo 1989, p. 23) included Southern California dentist Duayne Christensen, who opened North America Savings and Loan in Santa Ana, California, in 1983 as a way to fund his real estate ventures. Teaming up with real estate agent Janet McKinzie, the two used North America as their personal slush fund until it was closed down in 1988, at a loss of $209 million to taxpayers. Regulators cleaning up after North America's demise tell of extravagant birthday parties with Sammy Davis, Jr., providing the entertainment, hundreds of thousands of dollars spent at Neiman-Marcus, $500 gold paper clips, Jaguars, and Rolls-Royces.

Such stories were repeated around the state. In Pomona, carpet salesman John Molinaro, and Donald Mangano, owner of a construction company, bought their own thrift in 1984, using it to finance condominium projects built by Mangano's firm and outfitted with Molinaro's carpets. When Ramona Savings failed less than two years later, succumbing to risky loans and excessive compensation schemes, it cost FSLIC $70 million. Summarizing the epidemic of thrift failures in California and the role of the new breed of financial entrepreneurs, William Crawford, Taggart's successor as commissioner of the California Department of Savings and Loan, explained in 1987, "We built thick vaults; we have cameras; we have time clocks on the vaults; we have dual control—all these controls were to protect against someone stealing the cash. Well, you can steal far more money, and take it out the back door. *The best way to rob a bank is to own one*" (quoted in U.S. Congress, House Committee on Government Operations 1988, p. 34; emphasis in the original).

While clearly a number of unscrupulous entrepreneurs were attracted to thrifts in the 1980s, the point here is not simply to highlight individualistic explanations or focus on greed as the central causal explanation for the thrift industry's collapse. Instead, what is clear from the pattern of thrift fraud is that a criminogenic environment was created from the profit squeeze of the 1970s and the subsequent deregulatory policies of the 1980s, policies that were even more liberal in a few critical states. Indicative of the role that lax state regulations played in the demise of Texas and California thrifts, the majority of insolvencies and related criminal investigations involved state-chartered, not federally chartered, institutions (testimony of William Black, in U.S. Congress, Committee on Banking, Finance, and Urban Affairs 1990, p. 191). Roy Green, former president of the FHLB in Dallas, estimates that 95 percent of the most troubled thrifts in Texas were state-chartered (cited in Governor's Task Force, in U.S. Congress, House Committee on Banking, Finance, and Urban Affairs 1990, p. 231).

III. Patterns of Violations

The Federal Home Loan Bank Board (quoted in U.S. General Accounting Office 1989*b*, p. 22) has defined fraud as it relates to the savings and loan industry:

> Individuals in a position of trust in the institution or closely
> affiliated with it have, in general terms, breached their fiduciary
> duties; traded on inside information; usurped opportunities or

profits; engaged in self-dealing; or otherwise used the institution for personal advantage. Specific examples of insider abuse include loans to insiders in excess of that allowed by regulation; high risk speculative ventures; payment of exorbitant dividends at times when the institution is at or near insolvency; payment from institution funds for personal vacations, automobiles, clothing, and art; payment of unwarranted commissions and fees to companies owned by the shareholder; payment of "consulting fees" to insiders or their companies; use of insiders' companies for association business; and putting friends and relatives on the payroll of the institutions.

Using this broad definition, a GAO study of twenty-six of the most costly thrift failures found that every one of the thrifts in its sample was a victim of fraud and abuse in some form. Evidence presented by the FHLBB to the GAO indicates that fraud was by no means confined to the twenty-six thrifts selected. In fact, the FHLBB referred over six thousand cases for criminal investigation in 1987, and another five thousand were referred during 1988, up significantly from 1985 and 1986—434 and 1,979, respectively (U.S. General Accounting Office 1989a, p. 11).

Some of the more common pervasive weaknesses at the twenty-six failed thrifts investigated by the GAO included "inadequate board supervision and dominance by one or more individuals"; "transactions not made in thrifts' best interest"; "inadequate underwriting of loan administration"; "appraisal deficiencies"; "noncompliance with loan terms"; "excessive compensation and expenditures"; "high risk ADC (Acquisition, Development and Construction) transactions"; "loans to borrowers exceed legal limits"; "inadequate record keeping"; and "transactions recorded in a deceptive manner" (U.S. General Accounting Office 1989a, pp. 13–24).

The GAO (1989a) cites one thrift that paid a chairman of its board a $500,000 bonus the same year the thrift lost almost $23 million, an expenditure that, according to thrift regulators, violated the federal regulation against "excessive compensation." At another thrift, regulators told management that a bonus of over $800,000 (one-third of the institution's earnings) paid to one officer was a waste of assets; the management paid the individual in question $350,000 to relinquish his right to future bonuses, and increased his salary from $100,000 to $250,000. The GAO also found that extravagant expenditures were made to officers and their families, for private planes, homes, and expensive parties. In one case, a majority stockholder used $2 million of thrift funds to buy a beach house and spent another $500,000 for household expenses, all of which were non-business-related.

The hidden and complex nature of bank fraud is described in detail by Alt and Siglin, who use the term broadly to include frauds against "all depository institutions, including banks, thrifts and credit unions" (1990, p. 1). According to Alt and Siglin, the term can include three different levels of misconduct: an arrangement that violates the criminal law; any deliberate violation of thrift regulations, such as loan-to-one-borrower restrictions; or transactions that are not in themselves illegal, but which are used as a cover for, or accompaniment to, illegal transactions (1990, pp. 1–2). In most cases, conduct that constitutes criminal bank fraud will also qualify for a civil bank fraud suit by victims, such as shareholders or the government.

A report issued by the U.S. Congress, Senate Committee on Banking, Housing, and Urban Affairs (1989, p. 9), summarized Department of Justice findings relating to the magnitude and varieties of thrift fraud:

> According to the United States Department of Justice, the most prevalent forms of fraud and insider abuse included nominee loans, double pledging of collateral, reciprocal loan arrangements, land flips, embezzlement, and check kiting. In addition, witnesses have told the Committee of extravagant parties, exorbitant spending on frivolous corporate aircraft, lavish office suites, and numerous other squanderings of federally-insured deposit monies. "At the very least," related David W. Gleeson, president of Lincoln Asset Management Company, "there was an enormous failure of individuals to exercise their fiduciary responsibilities as managers, directors, auditors, appraisers, and lawyers . . . The extent of irresponsible and questionable transactions was so pervasive, and reckless lending policies, wildly aggressive appraisals, and ludicrous deals were so widespread, that each new round of transactions enticed the perpetrators on to larger, more complex, and more (creative) deals with an ever-increasing disregard for sound economics and market demand."

A. Savings and Loan Industry Crime: Insiders

While the list of potential frauds open to thrift operators and related outsiders is a long one, the misconduct can be classified into three analytically distinct categories of white-collar crime. These are "unlawful risk taking," "collective embezzlement," and "covering up" (Calavita and Pontell 1990). The categories often overlap in actual cases, both because one individual may commit several types of fraud and because the same business transaction may involve more than one type.

1. *Unlawful Risk Taking.* In its study of twenty-six of the most costly savings and loan insolvencies, the General Accounting Office concluded, "All of the 26 failed thrifts made non-traditional, higher-risk investments and in doing so . . . violated laws and regulations and engaged in unsafe practices" (U.S. General Accounting Office 1989*b*, p. 17). While deregulation made it legal for thrifts to invest in "nontraditional, higher-risk" activities, regulations and laws were often broken in the process. For example, investment activities were frequently extended beyond permissible levels of risk—for instance, by concentrating investment in one area, such as ADC loans. These high-risk levels were often accompanied by inadequate marketability studies and poor supervision of loan disbursement, both of which constitute violations of regulatory standards.

The factors that triggered this unlawful risk taking are similar in some ways to those described in classic white-collar crime studies. Sutherland (1949), Geis (1967), Farberman (1975), and Hagan (1985), for example, note the importance of competition, the desire to maximize profit, and related corporate subcultures as major determinants of corporate crime. Studies of white-collar crime generally follow Sutherland's (1949) lead in locating corporate crime within the context of an economic environment that rewards profit making as the top priority. In his overview and synthesis of white-collar crime theory, Coleman (1987, p. 427) points out that the "demand for profit is one of the most important economic influences on the opportunity structure for organizational crime." Geis's (1967) study of the infamous electrical company price-fixing conspiracy reveals the central role played by the corporate emphasis on profit maximization and the related corporate subculture conducive to, or at least tolerant of, illegal behavior in the interest of advancing profits. Similarly, Farberman (1975) argues that the necessity to maximize profits within the context of intense competition has produced a "criminogenic market structure" in the automobile industry.

Analyses of Medicaid fraud (Pontell, Jesilow, and Geis 1982, 1984*a*, 1984*b*) have documented how conflicts between government regulation and the norms of the medical profession result in an environment where fraud is likely to occur. Bureaucratic red tape, low payment schedules, and state regulations limiting the autonomous nature of medical practice provide structural conditions that breed resentment among doctors and allow them to rationalize or justify behavior that constitutes lawbreaking. In his explanation of violations in the thrift industry, the refrain of a Houston developer and savings and loan consultant illustrates the impact of such corporate norms and the economic forces from which they derived: "If you didn't do it, you weren't just stupid—you weren't behaving as a prudent businessman, which is the ground rule. You owed it to your partners, to your stockholders, to maximize profits. Everybody else was doing it" (quoted in Lang 1989, p. 21).

In addition, the opportunity structure is often cited as a facilitating factor in the commission of corporate crime. Some analyses emphasize the ease with which corporate crime can be committed, rather than focusing on the profit motive per se in the generation of such crime (Wheeler and Rothman 1982). The electrical company conspiracy of the 1940s and 1950s that involved price-fixing in government contract bids provides an excellent example (Geis 1967). In that case, the small number of very large corporations and their domination of the industry provided an ideal opportunity structure and facilitated the criminal conspiracy among the nation's largest electrical manufacturing companies.

The unlawful risk taking in the savings and loan industry, however, is distinct in a number of ways from such traditional corporate crimes. While "successful" corporate crime traditionally results in increased profits and long-term liquidity for the company, unlawful risk taking in the thrift industry is a gamble with very bad odds. Unlike more traditional corporate and white-collar crimes in the industrial sector, these financial crimes often result in the bankruptcy of the institution.

One of the most critical ingredients found by the GAO study of twenty-six failed thrifts was the extensive use of ADC transactions, often with related parties (U.S. General Accounting Office 1989a). A high degree of risk was assumed by the institution in these transactions, with the thrift providing most, if not all, of the necessary funds. To compensate for this high degree of risk, the thrift was to receive a portion of the profits generated from the completed projects, which is why these transactions are sometimes referred to as "direct investments." This arrangement, in turn, relieved developers from any personal liability to repay the funds. If the developer defaulted, the thrift had only the property as an asset. The thrift's return on its investment, however, was dependent on the original project being completed and subsequently turning a profit.

Deregulatory policies in the early 1980s gave legal authority to thrifts to pursue such deals. However, many did so in an inappropriate, unsafe, and often illegal manner. The GAO has documented that a combination of poor underwriting, the large proportion of thrift assets involved, and excessive geographic concentrations of transactions spelled disaster for the industry. In one case, a thrift lent $40 million to one borrower to build condominiums and a shopping center. No feasibility study was conducted, violating the regulation requiring investigations of borrowers' creditworthiness and project viability prior to dispensing loans. Examiners claimed that, had such an investigation been done, it would have shown that the proposed site was overdeveloped and the borrower already heavily in debt. The transaction cost the thrift over $10 million when the developer declared bankruptcy (U.S. General Accounting Office 1989*b*, p. 32).

Unlawful risk taking was in some cases the result of otherwise legitimate entrepreneurs attempting to reverse the imminent insolvency of their institutions. The U.S. Congress, House Committee on Government Operations (1988, p. 34), concluded that "normally honest bankers (including thrift insiders) . . . resorted to fraud or unsafe and unsound practices in efforts to save a battered institution. In those cases an incentive existed to turn an unhealthy financial institution around by garnering more deposits and then making even more speculative investments, hoping to 'make it big.'" The commissioner of the California Department of Savings and Loan described the pressure to engage in fraud in the competitive environment dominated by brokered deposits: "If you have got a lot of money, high-cost money pushing you, and you have to make profits, you have to put it out awful fast" (U.S. Congress, House Committee on Government Operations 1987, p. 13). Federal Home Loan Bank Board Chair M. Danny Wall described the bind of thrift operators on a "slippery slope of a failing institution trying to save probably their institution first and trying to save themselves and their career" (U.S. Congress, House Committee on Government Operations 1988, p. 46). The words of an unidentified witness best summed up the formula that produced an epidemic of unlawful risk-taking in the thrift industry: "If you put temptation and the opportunity, and the need in the same place, you are asking for trouble" (U.S. Congress, House Committee on Government Operations 1987, p. 9).

2. *Collective Embezzlement.* "Collective embezzlement," also referred to here as "looting," refers to the siphoning off of funds from a savings and loan institution for personal gain, at the expense of the institution itself and with the implicit or explicit sanction of its management. This "robbing of one's own bank" is currently estimated to be the single most costly category of crime in the thrift industry, having precipitated a significant number of the largest insolvencies to date (U.S. Congress, House Committee on Government Operations 1988, p. 41; U.S. General Accounting Office 1989*b*, p. 19). The GAO concluded that, of the thrifts it studied, "almost all of the 26 failed thrifts made transactions that were not in the thrift's best interest. Rather, the transactions often personally benefited directors, officers, and other related parties" (U.S. General Accounting Office 1989*b*, p. 19).

Embezzlement is by no means an isolated or uncommon form of white-collar crime. The advent of computers and their proliferation in business makes access to "other people's money" easier than ever. Not surprisingly, the toll from such crime is considerable. Conklin (1977) notes that, between 1950 and 1971, at least one hundred banks were made insolvent as a result of embezzlement. Moreover, in the mid-1970s commercial banks lost almost five times as much money to embezzlers as they did to armed robbers (Conklin 1977, p. 7).

The traditional embezzler is usually seen as a lower-level employee working alone to steal from a large organization. In discussing various forms of white-collar lawbreaking, Sutherland noted that "the ordinary case of embezzlement is a crime by a single individual in a subordinate position against a strong corporation" (1983, p. 231). Similarly, Cressey (1953), in his landmark study, *Other People's Money*, examined the motivations of the lone embezzler. The *collective* embezzlement referred to here, however, differs in important ways from this traditional pattern.

Sherman's (1978) study of corruption in police departments distinguishes between deviance *by* an organization and deviance *in* an organization. Deviance in an organization is composed of those acts that directly harm the attainment of an organizational goal, such as making a profit. In contrast, deviance by an organization involves "collective rule breaking" that helps achieve organizational goals. Traditional embezzlement is clearly an example of deviance *in* an organization, insofar as it is perpetrated by an individual stealing from the institution and thereby jeopardizing its organizational goals. Collective embezzlement, however, not only is deviance *in* an organization—in the sense that the misconduct harms the viability of the institution—but also constitutes deviance *by* the organization. Not only are the perpetrators themselves in management positions, but the very goals of the institution are precisely to provide a money machine for its owners and other insiders. The formal goals of the organization thus constitute a "front" for the real goals of management, who not infrequently purchased the institution in order to loot it. The S&L could be discarded after serving its purpose. It is a prime example of what Wheeler and Rothman (1982, p. 1406) have called "the organization as weapon": "the organization . . . is for white-collar criminals what the gun or knife is for the common criminal—a tool to obtain money from victims." The principal difference between Wheeler and Rothman's profile of the organization as weapon, and the case of collective embezzlement presented here, is that the latter is an organizational crime *against* the organization's own best interests. That is, the organization is both weapon *and* victim.[4]

Numerous examples of this form of thrift crime can be found in media and journalistic accounts, as well as government investigations of the S&L crisis (U.S. Congress, House Committee on Government Operations 1988; Pizzo, Fricker, and Muolo 1989; U.S. General Accounting Office 1989b). One of the most infamous cases of collective embezzlement involved Janet McKinzie and North America Savings and Loan. The indictment against McKinzie and five business associates charged that the failed thrift had operated as a fraudulent enterprise since its inception in 1983.[5]

Regulators claimed that McKinzie and her partners had looted more than $16 million from depositors in a systematic scheme to use the institution as a front for bogus real estate transactions. The defendants then used part of the fraudulent earnings to make the thrift appear to have adequate capital long after it was insolvent. The remainder of the money was siphoned off to purchase expensive homes in Newport Beach, Rolls-Royces, and other luxuries. The fifteen-month FBI investigation concluded that the failed thrift represented the worst case of

---

[4] Wheeler and Rothman (1982, p. 1405) note the distinction between embezzlement and corporate crime in previous work, pointing out that "either the individual gains at the organization's expense, as in embezzlement, or the organization profits regardless of individual advantage, as in price-fixing." They argue that this separation ignores cases where both organization and individual may benefit, as when an individual's career is advanced by crime perpetrated on behalf of the organization. What they neglect to note, however, is the possibility of organizational crime in which the organization is a weapon for perpetrating crime against *itself*.

[5] The case was the first on the West Coast to use racketeering laws (RICO) to bring charges against thrift executives.

insider fraud uncovered in California and could be directly traced to the fraudulent activities of the institution's top management (Murphy 1989).

One scam perpetrated by McKinzie and her partner Duayne Christensen involved the creation of a series of phony real estate escrows, into which $11 million in thrift funds were deposited and then diverted to Christensen and McKinzie. Another scheme involved $5.6 million that was lost through the creation of false billings for fictitious construction costs to the thrift for two real estate projects. The money was diverted to a company owned by McKinzie (Murphy 1989).

The major difference between these cases of collective embezzlement and the more traditional forms of corporate crime is that it involves the *intentional "looting" of the resources of the organization itself*. And it differs from traditional embezzlement in that it usually involves a *network* of individuals, it is committed by the institution's own executive officers, and it eventually leads to the total demise of the organization itself.

3. *Covering-up*.   A considerable proportion of the criminal charges leveled against fraudulent savings and loan institutions involve attempts to cover up or hide both the thrift's insolvency and the fraud that contributed to that insolvency. "Covering-up" is usually accomplished through manipulation of S&L books and records. This form of fraud may be the most pervasive and widespread criminal activity of thrift operators. Of the alleged 179 violations of criminal law reported in the twenty-six failed thrifts studied by the GAO, forty-two were for covering-up, constituting the single largest category (U.S. General Accounting Office 1989*b*, p. 51). The same study found that *every one* of the thrifts had been cited by regulatory examiners for "deficiencies in accounting" (p. 40). Covering-up has been employed to a variety of ends by S&L operators. First, it is used to produce a misleading picture of the institution's state of health or, more specifically, to misrepresent the thrift's amount of capital reserves, as well as its capital-to-assets ratio. Second, deals may be arranged that include covering-up as part of the scheme itself. For example, in cases of risky insider or "reciprocal" loans, a reserve account may be created to pay off the first few months (or years) of a development loan to make it look current, whether or not the project has failed or was phony in the first place. Third, covering-up may be used after the fact to disguise illegal investment activity. In other words, previously honest bankers, responding to the competitive pressures of the 1980s and the deregu-

lated thrift environment, may have stepped over the line into unlawful risk taking or other unlawful attempts to save their ailing institutions; covering-up then became an essential part of the fraud, as they attempted simultaneously to rescue their institutions and their own reputations.

Regulators (in responding to the crisis in the thrift industry in the early 1980s) may have sent the wrong message to thrift operators in 1981 when "regulatory accounting procedures" (RAP) were instituted. The new procedures allowed thrifts to sell off their below-market-rate loans and spread out their losses over many years, thereby enhancing their image of financial health. The new RAP techniques provided a "gray area" within which deceptive bookkeeping in the interest of artificially improving the balance sheet was considered normal.

B. Outsiders

Savings and loan fraud was not confined to insiders. Thrift officers were often joined in the largest scams with "outsiders" from various occupations and professional groups. "The Keating Five," which included five U.S. senators who were formally investigated for their role in influencing regulators on behalf of Charles Keating's now defunct Lincoln Savings and Loan of Irvine, California, is but one example of the participation of high-ranking politicians in the crisis. Lewis (1989) describes how Wall Street brokerage firms enriched themselves through fraud against their clients, many of them thrifts that had invested in stock market schemes and related securities and junk bond deals. Finally, real estate developers and deposit brokers have been named as coconspirators in numerous cases of thrift fraud.

Industry regulators and FBI investigators have reported in interviews that appraisers, lawyers, and accountants whose well-paid services made many of the S&L frauds possible were among the most egregious offenders. Perhaps most important was the role of accountants, whose audits and scrutiny of savings and loan records allowed many scam transactions to go unnoticed, while disguising the state of the financial institution's health. Although not usually in violation of the criminal law, some of the largest accounting firms in the country are now involved in civil suits, as they are being sued by government regulators for their negligence in reporting potential malfeasance. Professional accounting firms were highly paid for their services, creating the temptation to turn a blind eye when evidence of wrongdoing surfaced. In one study conducted by the General Accounting Office, of eleven failed thrifts in Texas, six involved such laxity on the part of auditors that investigators referred them to professional and regulatory agencies for formal action (U.S. General Accounting Office 1989c). Among the firms referred were Arthur Young and Company; Ernst and Whinney; and Deloitte, Haskins, and Sells, three of the largest accounting firms in the United States. Arthur Young and Company audited the books of Don Dixon's Vernon Savings and Loan just months before it was seized by federal regulators, who discovered that 90 percent of the thrift's loans were in default. The same firm gave a stamp of approval to Western Savings and Loan, which was led to insolvency through a number of fraudulent land-flip transactions. William Black, a top government regulator, charged that "the CPA firm's Dallas office offered the 'K-Mart blue-light special' to thrifts that shopped for friendly auditors" (Waldman 1990, p. 49).

Lawyers constitute another group of professionals involved in the demise of S&Ls. Lawsuits have been initiated against lawyers and their firms for negligently advising thrift officials in making risky loans that violated federal regulations. One Philadelphia firm, Blank, Rome, Comisky and McCauley, settled a major suit in August 1988, by agreeing to pay FSLIC $50 million for its part in the collapse of Sunrise Savings and Loan in Fort Lauderdale, Florida. The thrift's top management was convicted of conspiracy in 1989, at which time the prosecutor dubbed a partner and associate at the thrift's law firm "unindicted coconspirators" for their part in putting together the bogus loan transactions (Waldman 1990, pp. 49–50). The law firm was charged with negligence and aiding and abetting Sunrise management in the violation of state and federal laws.

Appraisers were central players in the epidemic of fraud as well. As assessors of property values, appraisers are essential to the real estate and banking systems. In many states where the thrift industry was particularly hard hit, such as Texas, the appraisal business is entirely unregulated. Like many other professionals involved in the thrift crisis, appraisers are susceptible to designing their results to meet clients' wishes, as they are particularly dependent on repeat business and referrals. Thrift regulators report in interviews that inaccurate and inflated appraisals have been found in the wreckage of failed thrifts throughout the country.

Accountants, lawyers, and appraisers interested in retaining lucrative contracts with S&Ls in the 1980s inevitably were confronted with the tension between safe banking procedures, statutes and regulations, and professional standards on one hand, and the demands of their clients on the other. Periodically the line was crossed, as these "outsiders" violated not only professional codes of conduct but, in some cases, statutory obligations. Much as the criminogenic environment of the S&Ls triggered insider abuse and fraud, the very structure of the relationship between insiders and professionals on the outside assured that some segment of those outsiders would become accomplices to the fraud.

Some of the outsiders who took advantage of the newly deregulated thrift industry had direct and indirect connections to traditional organized crime. Pizzo, Fricker, and Muolo (1989), for example, document the activities of Mario Renda, a money broker from New York, whose moving of union pension funds around the country caused numerous thrift failures. Renda's "hot" money often required that the thrift make nonrecourse loans to Renda's affiliates, who then frequently defaulted on the "drag away loans." Pizzo, Fricker, and Muolo present evidence that Renda was actually laundering money for the New York organized crime families through his brokered deposits. Herman Beebe has similarly been labeled a "Typhoid Mary" of thrifts, moving from one institution to another, leaving a string of insolvent thrifts in his wake. Pizzo, Fricker, and Muolo (1989, p. 20) call Beebe "a veritable godfather of thrifts and banks," so generous was he in their financing. A secret report to the comptroller of the currency in 1985 estimated that over one hundred thrifts and banks across the country were directly or indirectly controlled by Beebe in the form of networks of ownership, corporate shells, and partnerships or personal connections (cited in Pizzo, Fricker, and Muolo 1989, p. 230).

IV. Government Regulation and Law Enforcement

Until 1989, the primary thrift regulatory agency was the Federal Home Loan Bank Board, together with its twelve regional banks. It is now widely recognized that the dual function of the FHLBB as both promoter and regulator of the thrift industry institutionalized the "captive agency" syndrome (Lowi 1969; Levi 1984; Snider 1991) and limited its potential as an effective watchdog (U.S General Accounting Office 1989a). Budget restrictions exacerbated the problem, precluding adequate training, competitive salaries for examiners, and timely inspections. According to a Congressional report: "Prior to July, 1985, OMB (Office of Management and Budget) seriously disregarded the safety and soundness of the S&L industry by refusing to provide to the

FHLBB sufficient numbers of examiners to detect misconduct and regulatory violations. Therefore, OMB has indirectly contributed to numerous thrift failures and larger FSLIC losses than would have otherwise occurred" (U.S. Congress, House Committee on Government Operations 1988, p. 15).

In July 1985, Ed Gray, chair of the FHLBB, successfully removed the supervisory budget of the bank board from OMB jurisdiction by transferring all investigatory authority from the central office to the quasi-independent regional home loan banks. The effect was immediate, as regulators' modest salaries increased and the number of examination and supervisory staff almost doubled, from 757 in June 1985 to 1,424 by October 1987 (U.S. Congress, House Committee on Government Operations 1988, p. 15).

The frequency of examinations rose slightly as a result of these increases, but a lax approach to enforcement persisted. According to the House Committee on Government Operations, the thrift regulatory agency shirked its responsibility to exercise effective oversight and enforcement through its "graduated response" strategy, which typically followed this pattern: "An agency uncovers abuse and issues a directive or letter; the abuse continues and becomes worse, and the agency then issues a MOU (Memorandum of Understanding) or a supervisory agreement; and then, as the situation worsens, the agency issues one or more supervisory directives, and possibly a C&D (Cease and Desist) order or removal (of management), but by then the institution is failing" (U.S. Congress, House Committee on Government Operations 1988, p.16).

"Formal administrative actions" (a cease and desist order, removal of management, or civil penalties) were used only as a last resort. Similar to discovery proceedings in civil cases, "formal examinations" preceding such actions often require the issuance of subpoenas for testimony or documents. The proceedings are conducted under oath, and any official of the agency may preside at the hearing. If formal actions are deemed necessary, a "notice of charges" may be filed; if a settlement is still not reached, the case may go before an administrative law judge who makes a recommendation regarding agency action. The agency may accept, reject, or modify this recommendation, and its final order is subject to judicial review. In most cases, a settlement is reached before the formal administrative proceeding runs its full course.

In the late 1980s, both the House Committee on Government Operations and GAO reported a general lack of such formal actions against even the most serious offenders. One study (U.S. General Accounting Office 1989b) examined 424 "Significant Supervisory Cases," that is, thrifts that had serious internal control problems and were in danger of insolvency. It found that regulators had taken formal actions in fewer than 50 percent, and in most of these cases the formal actions were taken after the thrift was already insolvent. Another report (U.S. General Accounting Office 1989d, p. 4) concluded that "numerous safety and soundness problems" had been documented by examiners in twenty-six of the nation's most costly insolvencies over the course of five years or more. Despite the examiners' notes that these thrifts required "urgent and decisive corrective measures," in most cases nothing was done before it was too late (General Accounting Office 1989d, p. 4). The U.S. Congress, House Committee on Government Operations (1988, pp. 75–77), reported that formal enforcement actions, which they had argued in a 1984 report were already too rare to constitute a deterrent, declined even further after 1986.

The Financial Institutions Reform, Recovery, and Enforcement Act of 1989 reorganized the thrift regulatory system, transferring supervisory and enforcement authority from the FHLBB to a number of new and existing agencies. Primary among these are the Federal Deposit Insurance Corporation (FDIC; which previously had had oversight authority only over commercial banks), the Office of Thrift Supervision, and the Resolution Trust Corporation. The FDIC has general regulatory authority over what remains of the savings and loan industry and provides deposit insurance, thereby placing banking and thrift regulation in the same agency. The examination and enforcement functions of the regulatory apparatus are located in the newly created OTS. The RTC, the huge government "corporation" created to manage and dispose of seized thrift assets—discussed in more detail below—also plays an important enforcement role. A large proportion of the civil and criminal cases mounted by the federal government against thrift operators originate in evidence uncovered by the RTC in the course of their "autopsies" of insolvent institutions.

This multiple-agency structure helps resolve the dual-functions problem that had hamstrung the FHLBB. Nonetheless, a number of limitations continue to restrict the potential effectiveness of thrift regulation. While the centralization of bank and thrift regulation in the FDIC streamlines the regulatory machinery, it is unclear whether FDIC, which for years has been closely identified with the banking industry, will adopt a rigorous approach to regulation. There is substantial evidence that, in the 1980s, the FDIC was by far the most lenient of the financial institutions regulators. In their investigation of the FDIC, the FHLBB, and the NCUA (the National Credit Union Administration), the House Committee on Government Operations found that the FDIC was the *least* likely to conduct timely examinations, hire and retain experienced staff, and impose formal enforcement actions, despite a large number of bank failures and insider abuse and misconduct (U.S. Congress, House Committee on Government Operations 1988, pp. 9–17).

It is too early to tell whether the FDIC will reverse its historically lax approach. Regardless of the regulatory philosophy adopted, however, a catch-22 complicates bank and thrift regulation. Hints as to the nature of this catch-22 are scattered throughout government reports and congressional hearings. In 1987, the U.S. Attorney for the Southern District of Texas testified before the U.S. Congress, House Committee on Government Operations, Subcommittee on Commerce, Consumer, and Monetary Affairs (1987, p. 126), "The public's faith in the security and integrity of their banking institutions is considered so vital to the continued viability of the banking system that Congress has promulgated laws to prevent people from even starting rumors about a bank's solvency or insolvency." The following year, the U.S. Congress, House Committee on Government Operations (1988, p. 17), reported, "Although every other Federal regulatory agency discloses final enforcement actions, the banking agencies continue to refuse to routinely disclose the existence or a summary of final civil enforcement orders." The reason given for this reluctance to reveal evidence of misconduct or imminent insolvency was that it might damage public confidence in the institution, worsening its condition.

Dependent on public confidence in the viability and integrity of financial institutions, regulators in the 1980s took a wait-and-see stance that, according to the U.S. Congress, House Committee on Government Operations (1988, p. 17), contributed substantially to the epidemic of thrift misconduct. This catch-22—based as it is on the nature of the banking system and the central ingredient of trust in financial institutions—continues to present a formidable challenge to thrift regulators.

Compounding these difficulties, current economic conditions, particularly the stagnant real estate market and declining investment activity, have renewed the pressure on bank and thrift regulators to loosen restrictions on lending, to exercise leniency in the recording of bad real estate loans, and to ease up on capital requirements. Treasury Secretary Nicholas Brady applauded the new, less aggressive guidelines adopted by regulators in response to the lingering recession, saying that "improving credit availability is necessary to sustaining economic recovery" (Rosenblatt 1991, p. D1). Savings and loan regulators must now walk a fine line between discouraging investment activity and tolerating dangerous levels of risk and potential insolvency.

A significant body of literature has recently developed that explores the potential of self-regulation in industries where law enforcement approaches have failed or where government regulation is prohibitively expensive, disruptive, or both (Hopkins 1978; Braithwaite 1985; Shapiro 1985). A number of researchers have investigated the possibility of "informal social control" mechanisms such as negative publicity campaigns against offending businesses and cooperative strategies emphasizing voluntary compliance and internal systems of self-regulation (Stone 1975; Bardach and Kagan 1982; Braithwaite and Fisse 1983; Scholz 1984a, 1984b). These scholars point out that the rigid law-enforcement, "criminalization" approach to regulation has failed in part because it establishes an adversarial relationship and thereby fosters resistance—rather than cooperation—from industry management. Braithwaite (1985, 1988) proposes instead a staggered approach to regulation in which internal controls and cooperative strategies are tried first, with punitive, law-enforcement strategies being used only as a last resort.

In light of the historical deficiencies and continuing dilemmas surrounding thrift regulation, it might be argued that such measures should be considered. However, there are a number of potential problems with a self-regulatory approach to thrift supervision. First is the issue of whether self-regulation is intrinsically limited as a way to prevent or deter corporate misconduct. Some scholars argue along these lines that only the high cost and social stigma associated with aggressive enforcement and criminal penalties will induce industry compliance (Watkins 1977; Hawkins 1984; Levi 1984).

Second, and more important here, the fraud perpetrated in the thrift industry in the 1980s, unlike traditional corporate crime, was often the product of deliberate strategies to loot the institution. Appeals to institutional interests, including the business's reputation and long-term profitability, which may conceivably work in an environment in which corporate actors are committed to institutional survival, are largely irrelevant to the prevention of such collective embezzlement. Nor, it seems, would additional layers of internal control prevent this form of thrift fraud. As investigators sift through the paper trail of insolvent institutions, they discover evidence of vast networks of co-conspirators attracted to the instant wealth available in the thrift industry. Comprised of lawyers, appraisers, accountants, and brokers, as well as thrift insiders and occasionally even government regulators, these networks have been described as "go-along, get-along, get-rich-too crews" (Pizzo, Fricker, and Muolo 1989). Given the nature of these crimes and historical precedent, it is predictable that, in a significant number of cases, the addition of internal control personnel would achieve little more than extend the network of fraud to include them.

Despite these drawbacks to institutional self-control as a way to limit S&L fraud, it may be that the concentration of ownership in a few hands was in part responsible for the magnitude and extent of thrift fraud. In other words, while formal internal control mechanisms may not have prevented fraud, insider abuse might have been limited had regulations not permitted a concentrated ownership structure. A San Francisco regulator with the Office of Thrift Supervision has recently completed a study demonstrating that fraud and insider abuse in California, Arizona, and Nevada in the 1980s were statistically related to the concentration of thrift ownership. In the 230 federally insured thrifts in these states operating between 1984 and 1988, fraud by insiders was both much more frequent and more costly among thrifts owned by a few individuals than among thrifts where ownership was widely distributed (Deardorff 1991). Thus, while formal systems of internal control may not curtail insider fraud, requiring a more diffuse ownership structure may significantly limit the opportunity to use the institution for personal gain.

A. Processing Thrift Fraud

Suspected thrift fraud may be reported by a wide range of parties, including employees or officers of the thrift, independent auditors, borrowers, and FDIC, OTS, or RTC personnel. Depending on such factors as the amount of money potentially involved, the extent of the evidence, whether the alleged perpetrator is a thrift insider, and available resources, the matter is handled administratively through the formal and informal enforcement actions described above, or is slated for civil or criminal action.

1. *Civil Litigation.* As a receiver of failed institutions, the federal

government, primarily through the FDIC and RTC, can become involved in civil fraud litigation. When the RTC seizes a thrift, it receives certain assets of the institution—usually real estate—and investigates the possibility of filing legal claims against former officers, directors, and outsiders. Government authorities generally do not know at the outset the precise value of legal claims and assets, necessitating an examination by investigators and attorneys. These examinations focus on the validity of a potential legal claim, the chances of actual recovery, and whether the size of the recovery is sufficient to warrant a costly and time-consuming civil suit. Because litigation costs in complex financial cases may be substantial, the potential defendants must have either significant assets or substantial insurance coverage in order for the case to move forward.

Within the RTC, the "professional liability section" of the legal division is responsible for litigating such cases. These lawsuits may target directors and officers, attorneys, accountants, commodity and securities brokers, and appraisers. The lawyers of this division work with RTC investigators and outside "fee counsel" to pursue civil recoveries for the RTC. As of July 1990, the RTC was involved in eighty-four civil lawsuits involving forty-eight thrifts, and many more such cases were anticipated (Resolution Trust Corporation 1990*b*).[6]

The amount of civil litigation arising from bank and thrift failures in recent years is significant and is likely to increase in the future. The extent to which it increases depends on the amount of recoverable assets and the ability of enforcement agents to locate and uncover them. Preliminary RTC reports indicate that professionals may be liable for malpractice in about 20 percent of failed thrifts. Professional liability claims are important, as they provide a potential source of recoverable funds through professional liability insurance. It should be pointed out, however, that the amounts recovered will be relatively small compared to the overall losses incurred from thrift failures.

2. *Criminal Prosecution.*   The criminal justice system becomes involved in thrift fraud cases when a financial institution or a regulator refers a potential criminal violation to the Department of Justice. Once a criminal referral is made, the FBI or, more recently (as of January 1991), the Secret Service in the Department of the Treasury, investigates to determine if criminal charges can be brought. FBI and Secret Service investigators usually work with a U.S. Attorney's Office in

[6] While the RTC is responsible for the bulk of these civil lawsuits, it must often coordinate with other agencies, including the Justice Department, OTS, and the Securities and Exchange Commission for collecting civil recoveries.

the early stages, both to determine if the investigation should proceed and to set expectations regarding what evidence will be needed in order to prosecute successfully.[7]

Prosecutions are handled by U.S. Attorneys' Offices in the various federal districts. Minor cases involving relatively small sums of money may be referred to local district attorneys for prosecution at the state level. The decision whether to prosecute is complex and can reflect numerous factors including current workloads and resources, the importance of the case relative to others, recoverable assets, the perceived need to punish the defendant for wrongdoing, and potential deterrent effects, both specific and general.

Prosecutorial "task forces" provide a useful enforcement tool in many areas of the country, bringing together a variety of agency experts to work on particularly complex financial fraud cases (see Geller and Morris 1992). These task forces usually combine the resources of the U.S. Attorney's Office; the Criminal, Tax, and Civil Divisions of the Justice Department; the FBI; IRS; FDIC; OTS; RTC; and other agencies. The first major task force, formed in August 1987, was the Dallas Bank Fraud Task Force, which has served as a model for those that have since been established throughout the country. With the director of the Regional Fraud Section of the Justice Department assisting in the coordinative effort, it has been involved in some of the most notorious thrift fraud cases, including Vernon Savings and Loan and Sunbelt (also known by investigators as "Gunbelt") Savings Association. Through 1990, the Dallas Bank Fraud Task Force had charged ninety-five individuals, of whom seventy-one had been convicted (U.S. Attorney, Northern District of Texas 1991).

B. Legislative Reforms

The Financial Institutions Reform, Recovery, and Enforcement Act of 1989 was the Bush administration's bailout plan for the nation's troubled thrift industry. It was approved by Congress within six months and went into effect in August 1989. The bill raised $50 billion over three years through the sale of bonds to be paid back over forty years in order to finance the federal seizure of hundreds of insolvent savings and loan institutions and to provide funds to cover insured deposits. Since bonds are financing the effort, at least half of the total bailout cost will consist of interest payments on these bonds. In the

---

[7] The Justice Department and the Secret Service have also recently become active in civil enforcement. In cooperation with regulatory agencies, efforts are under way to maximize the recovery of assets, at the least cost to government.

last year, the estimated cost of the bailout has increased again and was estimated to be well over the $500 billion predicted by the General Accounting Office in August 1990. This means that the original $50 billion authorized under the 1989 law will provide only a small percentage of the final cost.

The act repealed many of the deregulatory measures instituted in the early 1980s. The reform requires an S&L to hold at least 70 percent of its assets in home mortgages or mortgage-related securities in order to retain its "qualified thrift lender" status, which enables it to obtain below-market-rate advances from the Federal Home Loan Bank Board and to take tax deductions for loan loss reserves. It prohibits thrifts from purchasing junk bonds with insured deposits and requires that they sell whatever junk bonds they already hold by 1994. In an effort to prevent the concentration of thrift loans to a handful of thrift affiliates, FIRREA limits loans to one borrower to 15 percent of the thrift's capital. Importantly, ADC loans must now be booked as *investments*, which precludes the payment of fees and bonuses to thrift insiders. Finally, the law raised thrift capital standards to those of banks and, for the first time, tied capital requirements to the investment risks of their portfolios.

Recognizing the structural impediments to effective regulation in the past, Congress reorganized the regulatory agencies that oversee thrifts, abolishing the FHLBB and FSLIC. Deposits are now insured by a division of the Federal Deposit Insurance Corporation, which had previously insured only commercial banks, while oversight responsibilities are located in the Office of Thrift Supervision. The most unwieldy and politically vulnerable piece of the regulatory apparatus created by FIRREA is the Resolution Trust Corporation. The RTC has been assigned the unenviable task of managing and disposing of billions of dollars of failed thrift assets.

Finally, FIRREA provides new tools for law enforcement. One of the most important is a civil forfeiture provision for thrift-related offenses. This new measure makes it possible for enforcement agents to seize defendants' assets prior to conviction in an effort to salvage funds before they are transferred offshore, consumed, or otherwise "disappear." The law also provides for increased penalties for financial institution crimes committed on or after August 9, 1989 (from five years to twenty years per offense), and extends the statute of limitations on such crimes from five to ten years. While not affecting the many offenses committed prior to 1984, the new statute of limitations constitutes official recognition of the large workloads of investigators and the unprecedented backlog of financial fraud cases. At the same time, FIRREA provided substantial increases in FBI agents and prosecutors to work on these cases and authorized $75 million annually for three years to enhance the Justice Department's efforts to prosecute financial fraud.

A second major federal statutory change, the Comprehensive Thrift and Bank Fraud Prosecution and Taxpayer Recovery Act of 1990 strengthened some of the provisions in FIRREA and added new ones. Unlike FIRREA, which focused primarily on reforming the regulatory apparatus, this 1990 law concentrated almost entirely on law-enforcement efforts and enhancing sanctions against thrift fraud. It increased penalties for concealing assets from government agencies, obstructing their functions and placing assets beyond their reach, as well as obstructing examination of a financial institution. The law also increased maximum statutory penalties from twenty to thirty years imprisonment for a range of violations, including false entries or reports, bribery, embezzlement, mail and wire fraud, and intentional misapplication of thrift funds, reserving the most severe sanctions for "financial crime kingpins." In apparent recognition of the error of the "open doors" of the deregulatory period, the new legislation imposed greater restrictions on the granting of thrift charters.

Finally, the act authorized the creation of a Financial Institutions Fraud Unit within the Office of the Deputy Attorney General, to be headed by a special counsel for a period of five years. A presidential appointee, this special counsel supervises and coordinates investigations and prosecutions of financial institution crimes and manages civil enforcement and resource issues for the processing of such crimes.

V. Law in Action: Detecting and Processing Violators

Detecting and prosecuting S&L fraud constitutes one of the most challenging tasks in the history of American law enforcement. The nature of the crimes, and the complex financial transactions within which they are usually embedded, makes it extraordinarily difficult to detect such acts in the first place and then to uncover adequate evidence to prosecute them successfully. The magnitude of the workloads resulting from this epidemic of financial fraud ensures that a substantial number will fall through the cracks.

A. *Interagency Coordination*

Established in 1984, in Washington, D.C., the federal "Bank Fraud Working Group" was designed to assist in coordinating efforts among different agencies involved in dealing with financial institution fraud and abuse. It is composed of representatives from the Fraud Section of the Department of Justice, the Federal Bureau of Investigation, the Federal Deposit Insurance Corporation, the Office of the Comptroller of the Currency, the Federal Reserve Board, the Office of Thrift Supervision (formerly the Federal Home Loan Bank Board), the Resolution Trust Corporation, the Internal Revenue Service, the Department of the Treasury, and the Secret Service. The Working Group has been responsible for reforms in the criminal referral system and has coordinated and enhanced training programs for regulators and investigators. In addition, it has successfully supported legislative reforms to improve the coordination and exchange of information among regulatory agencies.

More than twenty "local working groups" around the country supplement the federal effort (Dudine 1990). Strategically placed in Dallas, Miami, Los Angeles, Houston, and other cities with heavy concentrations of thrift fraud, these local working groups assist in the timely investigation of particularly complex cases.

B. Obstacles to Coordination

Despite these ongoing efforts at interagency coordination, a number of hurdles remain. Perhaps the largest organizational obstacle concerns parallel civil and criminal proceedings, as they relate to the different functions of regulatory and enforcement agencies. Regulatory agencies, such as the RTC and FDIC, although necessarily concerned with enforcement, investigations, and criminal referrals, are not responsible for criminal investigations or proceedings. Their primary responsibility subsequent to an insolvency lies with the recovery of assets and the achievement of civil remedies. Thus, conflict may surface if a defendant is named in both civil and criminal proceedings. If the defendant is first convicted of a crime directly related to what is being sought in the civil case, the civil case may be lost if it seeks to recoup funds through professional liability insurance since most such insurance policies are nullified if a crime is involved. This conflict may not only affect the timing of parallel cases but may also affect the timely referral of a case for criminal prosecution. Furthermore, partly as a result of this conflict, and the different priorities of regulatory—as opposed to law enforcement—agencies, communication gaps periodically arise. While a number of enforcement officials during interviews have reported improvements, the sharing of information among agencies has been problematic (the RTC and OTS are required to share information with the FBI, but not vice versa) and has periodically hampered effective prosecution, both civil and criminal.

C. Prosecution and Sentencing

A report issued by the U.S. Department of Justice (1991) documented enforcement activities for "major" savings and loan prosecutions. Major cases are defined as those that satisfy any one of the following conditions: the amount of fraud was $100,000 or more; the defendant was an officer, director, or owner (including shareholder); the schemes involved multiple borrowers in the same institution; and "other major factors." Using this broad definition, the report presents the following results for the period from October 1, 1988, to May 31, 1991: 764 defendants had been charged in cases involving thrifts with losses of $7.7 billion; ninety-five of these defendants were board chairmen, chief operating officers, or presidents, and 131 were directors or other officers; 550 defendants (93 percent of those tried) were convicted, and forty-two were acquitted (twenty-one of these involved a single case in Florida); sixty-nine of those convicted were board chairmen, chief operating officers, or presidents, and 103 were directors or other officers; 326 defendants (79 percent) of the 412 defendants who were sentenced received prison sentences; and fines of $8,091,000 were imposed and restitution of $270,703,000 was ordered.

While these data give a general description of the results of law enforcement efforts, they of course cannot provide an accurate account of the full extent of fraud in the S&L crisis, nor can they be relied on to identify the key roles played by different occupational groups and organizations in committing fraud. In the absence of other information regarding the nature of criminal referrals, investigative strategies, and resources, and the ease with which criminal intent can be diffused by ordinary occupational and organizational routines, such official processing data are largely "ceremonial" in nature. That is, they function to legitimate the activities of the organization reporting them and are thus "production figures." As Meyer and Rowan (1977, p. 351) have noted: "Ceremonial criteria of worth and ceremoniously derived production functions are useful to organizations with internal participants, stockholders, the public, and the state as with IRS or the SEC. They demonstrate socially the fitness of an organization."

These data thus reveal at least as much about organizational activities as they do about patterns of financial crime. For example, of the 764 defendants reported, fewer than a third (226) were directly affiliated with a thrift, and most were apparently borrowers. This may mean that more borrowers than insiders commit fraud against thrifts (after all, there are more borrowers than thrift officials in the general population), *or* it may simply mean that fraud by borrowers and other outsiders is easier to detect and prosecute since the institution itself is more likely to report it and provide evidence. Despite such limitations of official data, at a minimum, the reported figures speak to the sheer volume of financial fraud prosecutions, the widespread participation of insiders in the looting of their institutions, and the high percentage of convictions despite the formidable obstacles to successful prosecution.

VI. Conclusion

The financial losses incurred in the savings and loan crisis are due in no small part to deliberate criminal activity. The combination of deregulation, increased government insurance for deposits, and the absence of effective oversight mechanisms provided an environment in which misconduct proliferated (Needleman and Needleman 1979). This environment was criminogenic in that it provided ample incentives and opportunities for fraud at minimal risk. Given the nature of this criminogenic environment, it was perhaps inevitable that thrift fraud and insider abuse proliferated in the 1980s. Participants in this epidemic of fraud included both those who deliberately entered the thrift industry in order to loot it and legitimate thrift operators who found themselves on the "slippery slope" of insolvency, unlawful risk taking, and cover-up.

Government bailout efforts remain complicated by the uncertainty that still characterizes the industry and the larger economy. In 1990, thrifts lost a record $19.2 billion, surprising authorities who thought the industry had already reached its low point (Rosenblatt 1990*b*). Officials in the Office of Thrift Supervision believe that the profit margin of the industry remains "totally inadequate," suggesting that the final cost of the thrift debacle will continue to rise (Rosenblatt 1990*b*).

Government efforts to recoup losses through the sale of billions of dollars of assets from seized thrifts deserves careful scrutiny, as the disposal of these assets could trigger another round of fraud. Award-winning journalist Stephen Pizzo, in a nationally televised interview, predicted that the same criminals who looted thrifts into insolvency would use some of their ill-gained bounty to buy up the assets at bargain-basement prices. Noting the limited capacity of the government to monitor the unwieldy bailout process and the likelihood that some assets would be sold to those implicated in the first round of fraud, one senior regulator lamented in an interview that there will inevitably be a "couple of major embarrassments."

As policymakers attempt to bail out the thrift industry, it is important to examine the causes and dynamics of the crimes that played such a major role in its demise. Such an examination is central to our understanding of white-collar crime in the late twentieth century. Financial fraud of the kind described here is of course not new. What is new is its magnitude and scope, at a time when the economic structure of the United States, and to a lesser extent other Western democracies, is increasingly focused on financial transactions rather than the manufacturing enterprises of the Industrial Era. As the incidents of financial crime (including insider trading, junk bond scams, insurance fraud, and securities violations, as well as thrift and banking fraud) are revealed with increasing frequency, and money management replaces production as the locus of profit making, it is critical to investigate the similarities and differences between this form of white-collar crime and more traditional forms. We have argued here, for example, that "illegal risk taking" and "collective embezzlement" are distinct from much of the corporate crime discussed in previous literature and that these distinctions derive largely from the organizational environment within which thrifts operated and the nature of the financial enterprise itself. Further research, focused on the thrift and banking industries as well as other comparable financial institutions, is vital to advancing our theoretical understanding of the dynamics of white-collar crime in the postindustrial period.

As the government undertakes the most expensive industry bailout in history, and policymakers consider extensive reforms to invigorate the ailing banking system, a clear understanding of the thrift crisis is central to enlightened decision making. This essay represents an effort to provide the analytical infrastructure on which effective policymaking depends.

In particular, three principles must be rigorously upheld if a recurrence of the savings and loan debacle is to be avoided. First, the chartering and licensing of new financial institutions must be strictly supervised. Not only must the number of thrifts be kept in line with market demand in order to avoid the reckless competition of the 1980s, but applicants for thrift charters must be carefully scrutinized for character as well as capital. Related to this, diffuse ownership and control structures must be encouraged if the kind of collective embezzlement and other insider abuse described here is to be curtailed. Second—and more important—given the virtually unique investment *protection* that federal insurance provides, investment *risk* must be tightly regulated, and in any case risk must always be tied to capital requirements, with higher-risk institutions required to retain larger cushions of capital. It was the criminogenic combination of extensive, high-risk investment opportunities (and concomitant opportunities for fraud) with deposit insurance ensuring a steady stream of new deposits that set the stage for the thrift crisis. Deposit insurance is an important stabilizing mechanism and functioned effectively in the decades prior to deregulation to instill depositor confidence and stave off bank runs. However, this protective mechanism must be accompanied by strict limitations on certain forms of investment—such as junk bonds, concentration of loans to one borrower, ADC loans, and the like—which are "high risk" not only in terms of their investment return but in terms of their potential to encourage and conceal fraud. Finally, oversight of these financial institutions must be rigorous. It is the function of thrifts and banks to manage other people's money in the form of deposits; they do so with relatively little of their own capital at stake, within the context of federal insurance on deposits and, therefore, must endure little customer scrutiny. Opportunities and pressures to commit fraud are endemic to this organizational environment. If these opportunities are to be offset by the risk of detection and prosecution, serious regulatory oversight—in the form of regular inspections and severe penalties for violations—is imperative.

While this analysis specifically addresses the S&L crisis, lessons learned from that crisis can be extended to other financial institutions—such as credit unions, banks, insurance companies, and pension funds—which are entrusted with investing other people's money within a relatively "risk-free" environment. As Congress turns its attention to those other areas, it is urgent that their organizational structures, particularly the components of those structures that encourage and facilitate fraud, be understood.

REFERENCES

Adams, James Ring. 1990. *The Big Fix: Inside the S&L Scandal*. New York: Wiley.
Alt, Konrad, and Kristen Siglin. 1990. Memorandum on bank and thrift fraud to Senate Banking Committee members and staff, U.S. Congress, July 25.

Bardach, Eugene, and Robert A. Kagan. 1982. *Going by the Book: The Problem of Regulatory Unreasonableness.* Philadelphia: Temple University Press.

Braithwaite, John. 1985. "White-Collar Crime." In *Annual Review of Sociology,* edited by Ralph Turner. Palo Alto, Calif.: Annual Reviews.

———. 1988. "Toward a Benign Big Gun Theory of Regulatory Power." Canberra: Australian National University, Australian Institute of Criminology.

Braithwaite, John, and Brent Fisse. 1983. "Asbestos and Health: A Case of Informal Social Control." *Australian–New Zealand Journal of Criminology* 16:67–80.

Calavita, Kitty, and Henry N. Pontell. 1990. " 'Heads I Win, Tails You Lose': Deregulation, Crime and Crisis in the Savings and Loan Industry." *Crime and Delinquency* 36:309–41.

Coleman, James William. 1987. "Toward an Integrated Theory of White-Collar Crime." *American Journal of Sociology* 93:406–39.

Conklin, John E. 1977. *Illegal, but Not Criminal: Business Crime in America.* New York: Spectrum.

Cressey, Donald. 1953. *Other People's Money: A Study of the Social Psychology of Embezzlement.* Glencoe, Ill.: Free Press.

Deardorff, Charles A. 1991. "The Relationships between the Incidence and Cost of Abuse and Fraud by Insiders and the Concentration of Thrift Ownership." Unpublished manuscript. San Francisco: Regional Office of the Office of Thrift Supervision.

Dudine, James R. 1990. "The Extent of Misconduct in Insolvent Thrift Associations." Testimony before the Commerce, Consumer, and Monetary Affairs Subcommittee of the House Committee on Government Operations, U.S. Congress, March 15.

Eichler, Ned. 1989. *The Thrift Debacle.* Berkeley and Los Angeles: University of California Press.

Farberman, Harvey A. 1975. "A Criminogenic Market Structure: The Automobile Industry." *Sociological Quarterly* 16:438–57.

Geis, Gilbert. 1967. "The Heavy Electrical Equipment Antitrust Cases of 1961." In *Criminal Behavior Systems: A Typology,* edited by Marshall B. Clinard and Richard Quinney. New York: Holt, Rinehart & Winston.

Geller, William, and Norval Morris. 1992. "Relations between Federal and Local Police." In *Modern Policing,* edited by Michael Tonry and Norval Morris. Vol. 15 of *Crime and Justice: A Review of Research,* edited by Michael Tonry. Chicago: University of Chicago Press.

Gray, Edwin. 1991. Personal communication with author, March 25.

Hagan, John. 1985. *Modern Criminology: Crime, Criminal Behavior, and Its Control.* New York: McGraw-Hill.

Hawkins, Keith. 1984. *Environment and Enforcement.* Oxford: Clarendon.

Hill, G. Christian. 1990. "A Never Ending Story: An Introduction to the S&L Symposium." *Stanford Law and Policy Review* 2(Spring):21–24.

Hopkins, Andrew. 1978. *Crime, Law, and Business: The Sociological Sources of Australian Monopoly Law.* Canberra: Australian National University, Australian Institute of Criminology.

Johnston, Oswald. 1990. "GAO Says S&L Cost Could Rise to $500 Billion." *Los Angeles Times* (April 7), p. 1.

Kane, Edward J. 1989. *The S&L Insurance Mess: How Did It Happen?* Washington, D.C.: Urban Institute Press.

Katz, Jack. 1979. "Legality and Equality: Plea Bargaining in the Prosecution of White-Collar and Common Crimes." *Law and Society Review* 13:431–59.

Lang, Curtis J. 1989. "Blue Sky and Big Bucks." *Southern Exposure* 17(1):20–25.

Levi, Michael. 1984. "Giving Creditors the Business: The Criminal Law in Action." *International Journal of the Sociology of Law* 12:321–33.

Lewis, Michael. 1989. *Liar's Poker*. New York: Penguin.

Lowi, Theodore J. 1969. *End of Liberalism*. New York: W. W. Norton.

Mayer, Martin. 1990. *The Greatest Bank Robbery Ever: The Collapse of the Savings and Loan Industry*. New York: Charles Scribner's Sons.

Meyer, John W., and Brian Rowan. 1977. "Institutionalized Organizations: Formal Structure as Myth and Ceremony." *American Journal of Sociology* 83:340–63.

Murphy, Kim. 1989. "6 Are Indicted in O.C. Thrift Case." *Los Angeles Times* (April 12), p. 1.

Needleman, Martin, and Carolyn Needleman. 1979. "Organizational Crime: Two Models of Criminogenesis." *Sociological Quarterly* 20:517–39.

Pilzer, Paul Zane, and Robert Deitz. 1989. *Other People's Money: The Inside Story of the S&L Mess*. New York: Simon & Schuster.

Pizzo, Stephen, Mary Fricker, and Paul Muolo. 1989. *Inside Job: The Looting of America's Savings and Loans*. New York: McGraw-Hill.

Pontell, Henry N., Paul D. Jesilow, and Gilbert Geis. 1982. "Policing Physicians: Practitioner Fraud and Abuse in a Government Benefit Program." *Social Problems* 30(October):117–25.

———. 1984a. "Practitioner Fraud and Abuse in Medical Benefit Programs: Government Regulation and Professional White-Collar Crime." *Law and Policy* 6(October):405–24.

———. 1984b. "Practitioner Fraud and Abuse in Government Medical Benefit Programs." Final report and executive summary of grant 82-1J-CX-0035 to the U.S. Department of Justice, National Institute of Justice.

Resolution Trust Corporation. 1990a. "Report on Investigations to Date: Office of Investigations, Resolutions, and Operations Division." December 31. Washington, D.C.: Resolution Trust Corporation.

———. 1990b. "Report on Fraud Abuse and Malpractice in RTC-controlled Thrift Associations." Statement of James R. Dudine to the Oversight Board, July 18. Washington, D.C.: Resolution Trust Corporation.

———. 1992. *RTC Review* vol. 3, no. 1 (January).

Rosenblatt, Robert A. 1990a. "1,000 Bank, S&L Fraud Cases Go Uninvestigated, Lawmaker Says." *Los Angeles Times* (March 15), p. D1.

———. 1990b. "S&Ls Suffer $19.2-Billion Loss for Worst Year Ever." *Los Angeles Times* (March 27), p. 1.

———. 1991. "Bank Agencies Act to Alleviate the Credit Crunch." *Los Angeles Times* (November 8), p. D1.

Scholz, John T. 1984a. "Cooperation, Deterrence, and the Ecology of Regulatory Enforcement." *Law and Society Review* 18:179–224.

————. 1984*b*. "Voluntary Compliance and Regulatory Enforcement." *Law and Policy* 6:385–404.

Shapiro, Susan. 1985. "The Road Not Taken: The Elusive Path to Criminal Prosecution for White Collar Offenders." *Law and Society Review* 19:179–217.

Sherman, Lawrence. 1978. *Scandal and Reform*. Berkeley: University of California Press.

Snider, Laureen. 1991. "The Regulatory Dance: Understanding Reform Processes in Corporate Crime." *International Journal of the Sociology of Law* 19:209–36.

Stone, Christopher. 1975. *Where the Law Ends: The Social Control of Corporate Behavior*. New York: Harper & Row.

Sutherland, Edwin. 1949. *White Collar Crime*. New York: Dryden.

————. 1983. *White Collar Crime: The Uncut Version*. New Haven, Conn.: Yale University Press.

U.S. Attorney. Northern District of Texas. 1991. "Fraud in Financial Institutions II: January 1, 1985–December 31, 1990." Report. Washington, D.C.: U.S. Department of Justice.

U.S. Congress. House Committee on Banking, Finance, and Urban Affairs. 1990. *Effectiveness of Law Enforcement against Financial Crime*. Hearings before the committee, April 11. Washington, D.C.: U.S. Government Printing Office.

————. Subcommittee on Financial Institutions Supervision, Regulation, and Insurance. 1989. *Financial Institution Reform, Recovery, and Enforcement Act of 1989* (H.R. 1278). Hearings before the subcommittee, March 8, 9, and 14. Washington, D.C.: U.S. Government Printing Office.

U.S. Congress. House Committee on Government Operations. 1988. *Combatting Fraud, Abuse and Misconduct in the Nation's Financial Institutions: Current Federal Reports Are Inadequate*. Seventy-second report by the Committee on Government Operations, October 13. Washington, D.C.: U.S. Government Printing Office.

————. Subcommittee on Commerce, Consumer, and Monetary Affairs. 1987. *Fraud and Abuse by Insiders, Borrowers, and Appraisers in the California Thrift Industry*. Hearings before the subcommittee, June 13. Washington, D.C.: U.S. Government Printing Office.

U.S. Congress. House Committee on Ways and Means. 1989. *Budget Implications and Current Tax Rules Relating to Troubled Savings and Loan Institutions*. Hearings before the committee, February 22 and March 2 and 15. Washington, D.C.: U.S. Government Printing Office.

U.S. Congress. Senate Committee on Banking, Housing, and Urban Affairs. 1989. *Problems of the Federal Savings and Loan Insurance Corporation (FSLIC)*. Hearings before the committee, part 3, March 3 and 7–10. Washington, D.C.: U.S. Government Printing Office.

U.S. Congress. Senate. 1982. *Senate Conference Report*. 97th Cong., 2d sess. S. Rept. 641. Washington, D.C.: U.S. Government Printing Office.

U.S. Department of Justice. Office of the Attorney General. 1991. "Attacking Financial Institution Fraud: A Report to the Congress of the United States." Report submitted to Congress, May.

U.S. General Accounting Office. 1985. "Thrift Industry Restructuring the

Net Worth Certificate Program." Report submitted to Congress. GAO/66D-85-79. Washington, D.C.: U.S. Government Printing Office.

———. 1989a. "Failed Thrifts: Internal Control Weaknesses Create an Environment Conducive to Fraud, Insider Abuse and Related Unsafe Practices." Statement of Frederick D. Wolf, assistant comptroller general, before the Subcommittee on Criminal Justice of the House Committee on the Judiciary, March 22, 1989. GAO/T-AFMD-89-4. Washington, D.C.: U.S. Government Printing Office.

———. 1989b. "Thrift Failures. Costly Failures Resulted from Regulatory Violations and Unsafe Practices." Report submitted to Congress, June 1989. GAO/AFMD-89-62. Washington, D.C.: U.S. Government Printing Office.

———. 1989c. "CPA Audit Quality: Failures of CPA Audits to Identify and Report Significant Savings and Loan Problems." Report to the chairman, House Committee on Banking, Finance and Urban Affairs. GAO/AFMD-89-45. Washington, D.C.: U.S. Government Printing Office.

———. 1989d. "Troubled Thrifts: Bank Board Use of Enforcement Actions." Briefing report submitted to the Honorable Henry B. Gonzales, chairman, House Committee on Banking, Finance, and Urban Affairs. GAO/66D-89-68BR. Washington, D.C.: U.S. Government Printing Office.

Waldman, Michael. 1990. *Who Robbed America? A Citizen's Guide to the S&L Scandal*. New York: Random House.

Watkins, John C. 1977. "White-Collar Crime, Legal Sanctions, and Social Control." *Crime and Delinquency* 23:290–303.

Wheeler, Stanton, and Mitchell Lewis Rothman. 1982. "The Organization as Weapon in White Collar Crime." *Michigan Law Review* 80(7):1403–26.

Franklin E. Zimring and Gordon Hawkins

Crime, Justice, and the Savings and Loan Crisis

ABSTRACT

The epidemic failure of savings and loan institutions during the 1980s was an important chapter in the financial and governmental history of the United States and an instructive context for discussing the costs of crime and for reconsidering longstanding controversies about causation in criminology. Key issues include the effect of deposit insurance on pressure for mobilization of the criminal law, the relationship between social harm from crime and levels of just punishment, the tendency for causal theories about the savings and loan failure to thrive without any empirical testing, the emphasis on regulatory rather than criminal justice failure explanations, the tendency for free market rhetoric to produce "second-best" regulatory environments that are more costly than tighter regulation, and widespread support for structural and environmental explanations of savings and loan crime that neoconservative critics attack as explanations of street crime.

The savings and loan (S&L) crisis of the 1980s and 1990s is one of the most significant chapters in the history of relations between government and financial institutions in the Western world. It will in time be studied from a variety of academic perspectives, including history, politics, economics, and the academic outposts of public administration. To date, however, the books and articles about the S&L crisis have been, in the main, nonscholarly. The early days of any historical event belong to journalists and activists, so the accumulating bookshelf

Franklin E. Zimring is William G. Simon Professor of Law, University of California, Berkeley. Gordon Hawkins is senior research associate, Earl Warren Legal Institute, University of California, Berkeley. Jan Vetter read and commented on an earlier draft. Gwyneth Hambley served ably as research assistant and phone coordinator.

on this crisis is both untheoretical and unconnected to the journals and jargon of the social and behavioral sciences. While some of the first generation of literature is of high quality (e.g., Mayer 1990; White 1991), published attempts in the social sciences to digest this chapter of American experience are not yet in evidence.

This essay reports our efforts to comprehend the S&L adventure as academic students of criminal law and criminal justice policy. In conducting a survey of the hearings and literature about the thrift crisis, we are interested both in what criminology can teach about the current crisis and in how data from the current crisis can inform legal and criminological theory.

In concentrating on our field of specialization, we do not mean to imply that the dramatic failure of American thrift institutions should be regarded as exclusively or even principally a criminological problem. We do, however, believe that the criminological perspective has special value in helping to comprehend both the S&L crisis and the governmental response to it. Contemporary discussion of that crisis reproduces themes that are frequently encountered in criminological debate. So the S&L crisis not only presents an opportunity to advance understanding by means of a criminological analysis but also provides a fresh setting in which to consider some issues that are recurrently discussed in criminological circles.

The essay proceeds in two sections. The first deals at length with two issues: first, the costs of the S&L crisis and how those costs can best be calculated; and second, the variety of competing explanations for the massive failure of thrift institutions in the late 1980s. Our discussion of these two issues shows how they parallel familiar debates about the costs of crime and the causes of criminal behavior in criminological literature.

Having dealt with those two issues at length in Section I, the second part of this essay gives somewhat less comprehensive attention to six theoretical issues generated by the longer discussions of cost and causation. In large part, the new ground that we break in Section II depends on the earlier elaboration of more familiar territory.

I. The Crisis as a Social and Governmental Problem

The two topics discussed in this section have great importance in the contemporary debate about the S&L crisis. There is large concern about the cost of the savings rescue, not only because public money is at risk, but also because cost is the only way that the magnitude of the problem can be measured. The S&L crisis is only a problem to the extent of its public cost, so calculating that cost is a central issue.

The search for causes involves not the calculation of magnitude but the fixing of responsibility; there is a felt need to assess blame or at least to tell the story of this man-made disaster so that it contains some account of why the loss was suffered. It is causation in the moral sense that seems to occupy observers in the thrift crisis just as causation as a moral account is a central theme in criminological debate.

A. The Issue of Cost

There seems to be universal agreement about at least one aspect of the current S&L industry crisis (also known as the S&L collapse, calamity, debacle, and scandal and by a thesaurus of other synonyms). That agreement relates to the centrality of the issue of cost to the public importance of the problem; it also relates to the likelihood that the cost of resolving the S&L failures will be very substantial, or, as one sober economist has put it, "horrendously large" (White 1991, p. 193).

When it comes to the question of the extent of the costs involved, however, unanimity gives way not so much to fundamental disagreement as to what seems much more like an auction with competing bidders. Indeed, the central importance of large numbers suggests that we are entering one of those fields, such as drug abuse, illegal gambling, and pornography, in which hyperbolism is pandemic and where, as we have noted elsewhere, "accounting commonly takes the form of dubious quantitative impressions and largely notional statistics" (Hawkins and Zimring 1988, p. 30).

In this instance, however, appearances are deceptive. It may be no great surprise that Ralph Nader, who sees "the S&L scandal" as the result of "an unprecedented frenzy of speculation and business criminality," speaks of "sums of money [that] boggle the mind." Nader is no stranger to hyperbole. But his reference to "this $500 billion bail out" (Nader 1990, pp. xiii and xv), although far in excess of the Federal Home Loan Bank Board's earlier estimate of $31 billion (U.S. Congress 1988, p. 3), actually reflects a relatively modest estimate of cost as compared with some other, by no means unreasonable, computations.

Thus, G. Christian Hill, San Francisco bureau chief of the *Wall Street Journal*, estimates the ultimate cost of the thrift rescue projected over forty years as what he refers to as "a grotesque total of more than $1 trillion" (Christian Hill 1990, p. 24). Nader's estimate is, in this case, far from what statisticians call an "outrider." During 1990 and 1991, estimates of the total cost of the S&L crisis varied from under $50 billion to $1.4 trillion, or by a factor of twenty-eight. And the existence of gross variations in cost estimates does not, in this case, merely represent indulgence in the adjectival use of zeros but reflects genuine differences not only in modes of computation but also in matters of substance.

Exploring the variations in the estimates of the costs generated by the S&L crisis is justified both because the issue is intrinsically important and because analyzing how people think about costs is a good way of determining their basic assumptions about the nature of the S&L crisis and also the appropriate role of government in response to it. The question of cost is also worthy of note because it is the only empirical question in the S&L crisis to become the subject of sustained public attention.

Discussions of the costs of the S&L crisis do not encounter two major difficulties that usually confound analysis of the costs of crime. The first problem typically encountered in discussions of the costs of crime is the difficulty with which such costs are diffusely spread over a variety of victims, including other citizens, insurers, governments, and social service providers. Both the quantum of costs in the aggregate and the harm suffered by individuals and institutions as a result of criminal offenses are difficult to sum up. In the S&L case, by virtue of the comprehensive insurance scheme, a single set of federal government institutions will absorb almost the entire cost of the episode; accurate centralized accounting of its economic impact should be the automatic result of that scheme.

A second problem with cost analysis of crime is that plausible monetary costs do not exist for fright, pain, or other major loss elements from crime. For the S&L crisis, however, not only will the aggregate cost of the failures be centrally tabulated, but it will also be accurately reflected in the monetary terms used in conventional cost accounting. Trying to determine the economic cost of events like rape or robbery must involve the translation of nonpecuniary harms such as physical and psychological injury into artificial dollar equivalents, or it will inevitably fail to give any economic account of the most harmful negative consequences of those activities. With very few exceptions, what is most significant about the negative consequences of the S&L failures is the moneys lost by the various enterprises that must be replaced by the government insurance scheme. Without doubt, institutional fail-

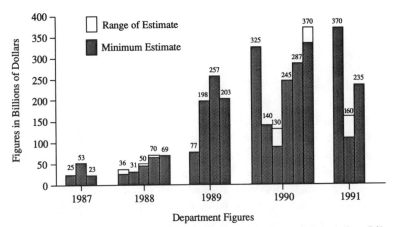

FIG. 1.—S&L bailout cost estimates. Sources: U.S. General Accounting Office (1989*a*, 1989*b*, 1991); Reischauer (1990); Barth (1991); U.S. Congressional Budget Office (1991); Wayne (1991); and various unpublished sources.

ures of this magnitude generated a large number of disappointed expectations and a considerable degree of emotional upset, but the heart of the matter was monetary and of a directly measurable nature.

So when compared with estimating the economic impact of most types of crime, analysis of the costs of the S&L crisis should be a relatively simple matter with a reasonable expectation of relatively precise answers. Yet our review of available estimates of the cost of the S&L failures reveals huge variations over short periods of time and discrepancies far in excess of 100 percent between cost estimates provided by responsible government officials, even when the estimates are based on the same data sets analyzed at the same time. While the discrepancies over time—with the total cost spiraling upward at a dizzying rate from 1987 onward—can be attributed to official Washington being reluctant to face the full magnitude of the problem until forced to by events, we show below that the cross-sectional differences in cost estimates among informed opinion reflect different views about what elements of governmental activity should be described as direct costs of the widespread S&L failures.

1. *Patterns over Time.* Figure 1 sets out cost estimates provided between 1987 and 1991 by different levels of government, either responsible federal administration officials or the U.S. General Accounting Office, as to the total dollar cost to the federal government of responding to the S&L failures. Where a single estimate was given, a bar corresponding to that estimate is placed in the figure. Where a

range estimate, for example, from $100 billion to $130 billion is provided, a dark bar is drawn to the minimum estimate and a lighter bar represents the distance from the minimum to the maximum cost estimate.

A preliminary point about the data in figure 1 is that most of the estimates of total cost—about three-quarters in the data—are single estimates rather than estimates of ranges. While there is a trend toward a range of estimate techniques being used in 1990 and 1991, there is still a pronounced pressure on observers to conflate all of their thinking into a single uniform measurement system. With the accumulating evidence that such loss estimates had been catastrophically erroneous all through the second half of the 1980s, it is remarkable that there still existed persons willing to make sharp point estimates; yet the pattern persisted.

A second feature of the pattern of official estimates over time is the very significant association between the passage of time and the escalation in cost estimates. Prior to 1987 none of the cost estimates that were officially presented exceeded $11 billion, and the official estimates that had been provided *prior* to early 1989 were all under $80 billion. By contrast, none of the eleven official cost estimates *after* early 1989 is under $80 billion. Between 1987 and 1990 the upward momentum was rather astonishing with the annual inflation rate in cost estimates averaging about 100 percent as it climbed from $33.6 billion to $250 billion over three years' time before leveling during the first half of 1991.

Steep rates of inflation over time mean that one year's Cassandra estimate, at least during the late 1980s, could easily come to be regarded by the very next year as Pollyanna optimism. One of the only methods of self-protection available in this atmosphere is repeating estimate procedures and updating the minimum cost. Thus, for senior administrators both in the Bush administration and in the U.S. Government Accounting Office the only effective defense against the estimate one's office made last year is to update the official figure and then to deny that its predecessor should have any continuing claim to public attention.

To some extent, rapid and steep escalation in bailout cost estimates can be attributed to underestimation of the number of institutions likely to fail. But more important than the increasing number of institutional failures was the increasing level of cost that various observers incorporated in their formulae. By 1991 there had been five individual

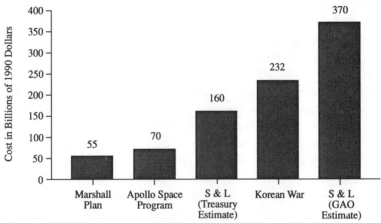

FIG. 2.—S&L bailout cost compared. Sources: Willis (1981, p. 369); U.S. Department of Commerce (1990, p. 336); U.S. National Aeronautics and Space Administration (1990, pp. 11–12); U.S. General Accounting Office (1991).

S&L failures where the bailout cost for a particular association exceeded the total cost of $1.6 billion for the bailout program predicted by the Federal Home Loan Bank Board in 1985.[1]

We would expect that the asymmetrical tendency to err on the low side in making bailout estimates would over time lead at least some observers to overestimate program costs so as not to appear to be subject to what may have looked like perennial shortfall. Yet in the contentious atmosphere of the S&L debates, no one has yet accused the Treasury or bank regulators of exaggerating when generating estimates that begin at the $130 billion level and surge relentlessly upward from there. So we have probably not yet seen a preemptively high bid in the guess-the-cost sweepstakes.

2. *Variations in Contemporary Estimates.*   Figure 2 illustrates both the financial scale of the S&L crisis and the variations in the size of estimated cost by comparing two estimates (as of mid-1991) of the S&L bailout with estimates of the cost of three other publicly funded programs: the Marshall Plan for European recovery, the Apollo space program, and U.S. expenditure for the prosecution of the Korean war—all estimates in 1990 dollars.

---

[1] The five S&L failures are Lincoln Savings and Loan, Irvine, California—$2.6 billion; University Federal Savings, Houston, Texas—$2.57 billion; Western Savings and Loan, Phoenix, Arizona—$1.73 billion; Centrust Federal Savings Bank, Miami, Florida—$1.7 billion; Empire of America, Buffalo, New York—$1.7 billion. Data were provided by Suzanne Brown, Resolution Trust Corporation.

The first lesson of figure 2 is that the economic impact of the S&L crisis is by any account substantial. The low-end estimate of public moneys to be expended exceeds American expenditure for the Marshall Plan by a large margin and represents more than one-half of the total public funds attributable to a multiyear American war effort in Korea. A second lesson of figure 2 relates to the variability in estimates; the high-end estimate in that figure is more than twice the size of the low end, and most of that difference does not stem from differences in the data concerning the current estimate of monetary loss but instead arises from the different principles and procedures used in estimating the total cost.

The most dramatic illustration of the impact of different procedures on estimates of total cost relates to the difference between Bush administration estimates of total program costs and congressional estimates of the cost of the same programs. The administration projected a total cost of about $160 billion for the program by estimating the amount the government will pay out to implement the recovery package over a small number of years in the near future. The U.S. Government Accounting Office estimate puts a $370 billion price tag on the same programs by measuring the cost in terms of total dollars to be paid back out of government sources to note and bond holders on account of the recovery program. So the administration estimate is in current dollars while the congressional total is an aggregate of government expenditures whenever incurred without an adjustment to discount to present value the obligation to pay a dollar at some future time.

Which of these two estimates is regarded as most appropriate depends to some extent on how an estimate is to be used. Since figure 2 speaks of the level of public expenditure directly attributable to a government program at the time resources are spent and restates historical experience so as to account for inflation, the more appropriate bailout cost estimate for comparative purposes is the lower estimate. A projection of the cost of the Korean War that included all interest payments on government indebtedness resulting from the War would produce a much higher figure. That much larger figure would be more properly compared with the larger S&L cost estimate.

However, in any discussion where the central issue is the extent and timing of federal government payments that are a consequence of S&L policy, the second estimate might be a more appropriate basis for analysis than the first even without the current value discounts that are usually important in economic analysis. If the question is how many federal dollars will be earmarked at what time and with what consequent opportunity costs for the federal budget, then the *future value* of *future dollars* spent may be more significant than their current discounted value.

There is a fine irony in the fact that lengthening the term in which the government will pay back obligations incurred in the S&L bailout increases in some estimates the aggregate cost, because the political and economic intention of the long-term payback provision is to reduce the visible economic pain associated with the program by minimizing the immediate budgetary and governmental consequences of the expenditure. A program of expenditure control that attempted to finance one-half of the S&L program by reducing levels of current governmental expenditure would bite with immediate and substantial impact. Seventy-five billion dollars next year in governmental expenditure cuts? From where and with what effects? Thus, the stretching out of repayment is a political necessity albeit one that by some measures more than doubles the cost of the enterprise.

A second conceptual issue encountered when attempting to calculate the cost of the S&L crisis is the question of how much of the total governmental cost of regulating, insuring, and reconstructing should be counted as a cost of the particular problems of the S&Ls in the 1980s. The usual technique here is to count the total cost of the regulatory mechanism as well as all the expenditures for reconstruction as part of the costs generated by the 1980s failures. But an analogy with the calculation of the cost of crime illustrates some potential difficulty with this.

Should we count all the sums spent on the police and courts and prisons as part of the costs of crime? This is a particular problem in criminal justice when scholars attempt to allocate the total cost of crime prevention and insurance to currently active offenders and the crimes they commit (see Zimring and Hawkins 1988, pp. 432–35). It is less of a problem with a limited jurisdiction regulatory regime such as the thrift industry during a period of catastrophic failure. Nevertheless, some part of the regulation and rehabilitation of that industry should be regarded as the cost of maintaining public confidence and business standards in the industry rather than a core cost of responding to thrift institution failure.

3. *The Contingent Significance of Cost.*   Comparing the projected cost of the S&L bailout with the usual estimates of the cost of crime both illustrates the scale of the current problem and highlights the absence

of a direct relationship between the extent of monetary cost and the palpable harm that citizens suffer and attribute to particular causes. A $200 billion round-number estimate for the S&L bailout amounts to a monetary cost of $750 per citizen, or $3,000 for a family of four. Those average figures represent a monetary loss greater than the direct cost of crime over a lifetime for all but a very small fraction of American individuals or families.

Yet the social response to the S&L crisis demonstrates a pattern of sustained attention and concern far lower than we would expect in relation to a problem that costs the average family $3,000 and much less than, for example, public fear of property crime. At the outset, we think that this shows that it is important to take into account how costs are distributed and the basis on which public payments to cope with losses are to be financed in predicting the public response to problems. We would argue that the combination of governmental insurance and long-term deficit funding produces the smallest and least palpable amount of immediate harm to individual citizens.

To begin with, the comprehensive insurance of S&Ls has meant that practically no private citizens have suffered out-of-pocket losses as a consequence of S&L failures. The comprehensive insurance scheme makes the S&L debacle the first major institutional failure in American history subject to 100 percent government reimbursement. In this respect, the S&L crisis is a laboratory experiment in the social impact of governmental insurance, under almost ideal circumstances, because most of the harm suffered is of insurable pecuniary form. The immediate aftermath of an S&L failing and government paying depositors is that none of the depositors suffers any loss. In these circumstances, S&L failures can for a period of time be a governmental problem without being a perceptible social problem, and one significant aspect of the current situation for the criminologist and student of criminal justice is as a case study of the effect of comprehensive insurance on the processes and pressures that are ordinarily immanent throughout the criminal justice system. We return to this topic in Section II.

But it is not just deposit insurance, what Martin Mayer (1990, p. 298) calls "the socialization of losses," that attenuates public perception of the harm attributable to the S&L crisis. For the decision essentially to deficit finance the government's 100 percent liability, and thus defer the cost of the bailout and avoid either immediate taxes or conspicuously forgone opportunities for other government services, also plays a significant role in modulating public awareness. Imagine the difference in social response if taxpayers were ordered to pay a surcharge that averaged $1,500 or $2,000 per family on federal income tax as an S&L bailout assessment. Clearly, the political salience of the issue would substantially increase. By contrast, "money paid ten years from now by today's voters' children seems to belong to a lower order of reality than money paid today by those voters themselves" (Thomas 1991b, p. 59). So it is deferral of loss in conjunction with socialization of loss that has deprived a $200 billion misadventure of immediate impact. In that sense, current government policy represents a considered, and probably correct, judgment that a $400 billion solution over the long run is less costly than a $200 billion commitment of current and near-term resources.

The S&L crisis provides an opportunity to study the characteristics and consequences of an almost painless public catastrophe. Does the diminished level of perceptible public harm reduce the pressure on the criminal justice system for prosecution and punishment? If so, might not some of the public outrage that goes into the calculation of just deserts in criminal cases be in part a social response to inadequate insurance? Conversely, perhaps the anesthetic effect of comprehensive deposit insurance leads to criminal justice authorities giving less priority to the S&L problem and its prosecution than a full account of the costs involved would demand. Evidently, contingencies other than the immediate effect of particular acts are an important ingredient of the social response to perceived problems. The student of criminal justice could not find, indeed has never had, a better example of the amelioration of immediate individual loss to serve as an object of study. The wider criminological relevance and significance of this point seem to us both obvious and important.

The performance of government as a cost absorber in the thrift crisis has to date been both impressive and equivocal. The federal government can centralize and defer the cost of making good on hundreds of billions of dollars of deposit insurance. Thus, this process has been almost painless in the sense of defined groups suffering palpable harm. The ultimate cost of this maneuver in individual and social terms is almost completely unknown. Even when more is known, we suspect the social cost of the deposit payouts of this era will be better measured in specific, forgone governmental opportunities than in strict dollar terms.

B. Ideology and Causation

The large and still growing body of books and articles dealing with the S&L crisis provides if nothing else a nice example of what Isaiah Berlin (1966, p. 9) has described as "the disordered mass of truth and falsehood that [goes] by the name of history." It also provides an interesting and varied array of examples of the use of what has been called "the most important explanatory notion in history . . . that of causation" (Scriven 1966, p. 238), more particularly of the influence of ideology in the choice of causal theory.

This sometimes takes the form of direct and explicit causal attribution as when federal deposit insurance is said to have been "the fundamental cause" (Barth and Brumbaugh 1990, p. 58) or "the underlying cause" (Schumer and Graham 1990, p. 69) of the S&Ls' problems, or when "the root cause" is identified as "structural flaws in the system" (Gorham 1989, p. xvii), or "a flawed political process" is nominated as "the most fundamental cause of all" (Christian Hill 1990, p. 22). Elsewhere, although the term "cause" may not itself be used, cognate expressions are, as when the S&L crisis is said to be "*the result of greed*" (Waldman 1990*b*, p. 4; emphasis added) or "*part of the legacy of deregulation*" (O'Connell 1988, p. xi; emphasis added), or when reference is made to "*the forces that led to* the downfall of the U.S. savings and loan industry" (Pilzer 1989, p. 58; emphasis added) or to "*the key component underlying* the thrift crisis" (Romer and Weingast 1990, p. 38; emphasis added).

1. *On Cause in Criminology.* Causation has been the subject of one of "the major theoretical controversies in criminology" (Short 1983, p. 558), and some aspects of that controversy are relevant to the subject matter of this essay. For the most part, controversy has related to the relative importance of one or another perspective, as, for example, when *personality* is said to be more significant than *social structure*. An even more fundamental disagreement took the form of a suggestion by Leslie Wilkins (1968, pp. 158–60) that "the concept of 'cause' be replaced" because " 'cause and effect' models . . . have revealed a startling lack of pay-off" in "criminological research." Wilkins's critique was elaborated somewhat by others (Burnham 1968; Carr-Hill 1968), but they added little of substance to his original statement.

For our purpose here, it is necessary to make only two points. The first is that, as H. L. A. Hart and Tony Honoré (1985, p. 11) have pointed out, "an inseparable feature of the historian's and the lawyer's and the plain man's use of causal notions" concerns "the particular context and purpose for which a particular causal inquiry is made and answered." In many cases the only "payoff" that is available, or can be reasonably expected, is that the causal explanation is coherent, in accordance with the available evidence, and satisfies the inquirer. Many causal explanations meet those criteria, which explains the omnipresence of causal notions in everyday language and thinking. Wilkins's (1968, p. 147) suggestion that "the concept of system" might provide a better "basis for models for use in the investigation of problems in the field of criminology," and presumably might provide more "payoff" than causal explanation, is simply an unsupported (and unlikely) assertion.

The second point is this. Wilkins argues that "there is a basic inconsistency in saying that criminal behavior is complex and then trying to organize that statement into a 'cause-effect' system which is essentially simple." He dismisses as a "*so-called* theory of crime causation" that which is known as the "theory of multiple causation." This "concept," he asserts, proves "to be futile if not absurd" (Wilkins 1968, p. 156; emphasis added). Wilkins had argued in an earlier publication that the theory of multiple causation is "no theory." At best it could be considered an antitheory that proposes that no theory can be formed regarding crime. Such an antitheory may be legitimately put forward as a kind of beatnik philosophy but not as a "scientific theory" (Wilkins 1965, p. 37). Yet it is really immaterial if the theory is not "scientific," in the sense that it is not a systematic formulation, supported by evidence, of apparent relationships or underlying principles of observed phenomena, or that it might better be referred to not as a "theory" but rather, in George Vold's (1958, pp. 99, 182) terms, as the "multiple factor orientation" or the "multiple factor approach."

For as Michael Scriven (1968, p. 80) pointed out in response to Wilkins's article, "The importance of cause doesn't mean one can assume a *single* cause for any phenomenon in any field, or that one can *easily* identify the causes or that their relation to the effect is *simple*" (emphasis in original). The truth is that "the concept of cause is fundamental to our conception of the world in much the same way as the concept of number" (Scriven 1966, p. 258). Moreover, although John Stuart Mill's analysis of causation may have been misleading in some respects, his doctrine of the plurality and complexity of causes accords with both common sense and ordinary usage (Mill 1886, pp. 214–18, 285–88; Hart and Honoré, 1985, pp. 20–21). And in criminological research "the general multi-causal model, which is basic to most research," is based on the presumption "that the phenomenon to be explained may have many causes [and] different instances of the phenomenon may be accounted for by different combinations of these many causal factors" (Miller 1983, p. 568).

The extensive literature on the causes of crime reveals, in addition to a vast miscellany of nominated causes or causal factors, what has been called a "dichotomization of theoretical approaches" (Finestone 1976, p. 45) in relation to causation. Some analysts emphasize the importance of personal or individual factors in the genesis of criminal behavior, and others maintain that the explanation of crime or delinquency is to be found in social, organizational, or structural conditions. At the same time, a review of the literature also reveals a remarkably close relationship between the political ideology of the observer and the tendency to subscribe to either the personal/individual or societal/institutional views of crime causation.

In an earlier essay on this topic, we gave some examples to illustrate this point. Thus, we noted that, whereas political liberals tend to emphasize the importance of such things as poverty, unemployment, lack of opportunity, and racism in producing criminal behavior, political conservatives by contrast emphasize the personal characteristics and qualities of the criminal. As an example of the liberal approach, we cited Ramsey Clark's *Crime in America:*

> Ramsey Clark provides an excellent example of the "liberal, root causes" approach. "If we are to deal meaningfully with crime," he says, we have to deal with what he refers to as both "the fountainheads of crime" and the "sources of crime." These comprise a vast miscellany that includes slums, racism, ignorance, congenital brain damage, prenatal neglect, sickness, disease, pollution, overcrowded housing, alcoholism, narcotics addiction, anxiety, fear, hopelessness, and injustice. Clark has also stated, "Today, change is the main cause of crime." Elsewhere he identifies "the automobile, the high-rise, television, and chemistry" as "causes of crime." In addition, he provides a list of the "elemental origins of crime," which are "heredity and environment, the interaction of individual and society, the totality of human nature and human experience." [Zimring and Hawkins 1979, p. 380]

Conservatives, by contrast, tend to speak in terms of selfishness, indiscipline, and lack of respect for the law. Thus,

Richard Nixon stated during his presidency that he totally disagreed with the view that "the criminal was not responsible for his crimes against society, but that society was responsible." "Society is guilty," he maintained, "only when we fail to bring the criminal to justice." In a similar vein, Ernest van den Haag argues that those idealists and reformers who believe that "bad social institutions . . . corrupt naturally good men" ignore "the possibility that naturally bad men corrupt good institutions. . . ." James Q. Wilson adds that "Wicked people exist. Nothing avails except to set them apart from innocent people. We have trifled with the wicked, [and] made sport of the innocent." [Zimring and Hawkins 1979, p. 372]

Having remarked on the conservatives' tendency to blame crime on individual wickedness, we then noted an apparent exception to the general pattern: the category of business or white-collar crime. In this connection, we said: " 'Conservatives' raise the question: 'Is white-collar crime really crime?' The implication is that such 'crime' is not criminal in nature. The 'white-collar criminal,' it is argued, may be a violator of conduct norms, but his behavior is really no more than venial; as such referring to him as criminal is mere name-calling, based on political prejudice. . . . For the 'conservative,' crime is something that, almost by definition, cannot be committed by one's friends and associates, and, if it is, cannot be real crime" (Zimring and Hawkins 1979, p. 373).
By contrast:

The "liberal" also adopts an approach to white-collar crime at variance with his attitude to other types of offenses. Indeed, the phrase "white-collar crime" is denounced as "a revealing example of dual-standard labeling by which actions are excused, mitigated or trivialized by reference not to the nature of the conduct but to the status of the actor." The "liberals" say that large-scale theft by deception or exploitation on the part of middle and upper-class persons goes unprosecuted. They emphasize that when it is prosecuted, generally more benign treatment is accorded white-collar offenders than traditional offenders. . . . The "liberal" . . . views the categorization of certain offenses as white-collar crime as a refusal to recognize that such offenses, and, thus, their perpetrators, are really criminal and that crime is a pervasive social phenomenon which is not a reflector of wealth, power or class. It is argued, therefore, that such a refusal indicates a systematic bias and helps to perpetuate the myth that crime is committed by a class of patently malevolent persons, significantly different from the rest of us. [Zimring and Hawkins 1979, pp. 376–77]

2. *The Thrift Crisis as White-Collar Crime.*   The S&L crisis has been described as "the biggest set of white-collar crimes ever uncovered" and "the white collar heist of the century" (Calavita and Pontell 1990, pp. 309, 328). Current debate about the causes of the crisis represents a continuation of the liberal versus conservative exchange over the nature and cause of white-collar crime; a continuation in which the transposition of approaches with the conservatives looking for structural causes and the liberals for bad people to blame is almost absolute. But the complexity of the S&L situation has in this case resulted in a range of causal nominations that can be conveniently considered under four headings: structural problems unrelated to significant human error, intentional thieving and wrongdoing, structural problems attributable to the culpable failure of responsible actors, and a variety of multifactorial nominations.

a. No-Fault Structural Accounts.   Both those who speak on behalf of S&L entrepreneurs and intrepid deregulators and some other more neutral commentators have put forward one of two forms of no-fault structural explanation of the massive thrift failures. The earliest form of no-fault account involved a species of geographic determinism in which the recession first in energy prices and then in commercial and residential real estate in Texas and other parts of the Southwest are treated as if they were the most important proximate causes of S&L failures. It is further assumed, in some of these accounts, albeit implicitly, that regional economic turndowns were not foreseeable events that should have generated contingency planning. "The Texas real estate bust," says Bert Ely (1991, p. 2), "caused most of the FSLIC's [Federal Savings and Loan Insurance Corporation] asset quality problems. A comparable bust occurred in other energy-producing states. S&L real estate lending in Texas (and elsewhere in the Southwest) exploded in 1983, two years after the Southwest energy boom peaked. Real estate lending should have been declining in the 1983–1986 period, not rising. This escalating lending fueled the building of unneeded real estate, which then suffered a price collapse that added far more to S&L losses than did crime."

In a similar vein, Lawrence J. White notes that,

> Fueled by favorable tax treatment and rosy expectations
> concerning oil prices, commercial real estate projects boomed—
> especially in the Southwest. Thrifts were major financiers of and
> investors in these projects. . . . Not only did the price of oil fail
> to rise to the heights that many had expected, but it fell to levels
> that were only half of those of the early 1980s. Again this could
> only mean a sharp fall in real estate values in the oilbelt. . . .
> Finally, the price index of real commercial properties in the
> Southwest sub-region—covering the states of Arkansas, Louisiana,
> Oklahoma and Texas—fell by almost a third. . . . Since many
> real estate projects of the early 1980s were based on assumptions
> of a *continuing rise* in real estate values, even a leveling of prices
> would have had serious consequences for their viability. A severe
> price decline meant devastation for these projects—and for their
> investors and lenders. Thrifts were prominent among these two
> groups. [1991, pp. 109–10; emphasis in original]

But while the fall in oil prices and the prices of residential and
commercial real estate in Texas and other states in the Southwest make
up a standard entrepreneurial explanation of thrift failures in 1986–87,
other accounts put less emphasis on regional factors and more on general recessionary pressures as the longest period of economic expansion
in postwar American history came to a close. The S&L crisis, says
Michael Robinson (1990, p. 292), "began with years of economic mis-
management in this country, bloated federal budgets, and finally the
ravages of inflation."

Paul Pilzer puts it as follows:

> The forces that led to the downfall of the U.S. savings and loan
> industry were set in motion in the 1960s by a national government
> that tried to fight a costly war in Vietnam without sacrificing
> peacetime prosperity at home. Combined with the impact of the
> 1973 Arab oil embargo, which ended forever the era of cheap
> energy, the result was an extraordinary inflationary thrust that
> spiraled upward almost without pause for more than fifteen years.
> But while the cost of living rose a spectacular 162 percent between
> 1965 and 1980, the rate of interest paid on consumer deposits by
> thrift institutions remained locked in by Depression-era regulations

[that] had a savage impact on both the thrift industry and the millions of trusting depositors. [1989, pp. 58, 60]

b. Intentional Wrongdoing.   At the other extreme are those incensed observers who blame the magnitude of the S&L crisis on the activities of thieves and scoundrels and see the S&L crisis as "a story of prodigious crimes and the hurt and tragedy that followed in their wake" (Maggin 1989, p. 1). Thus, Michael Waldman (1990*b*, p. 4) says that "the first thing to understand is that this crisis [the S&L debacle] was not merely the product of adverse economic conditions or an act of nature. Instead it was the result of greed on an epic scale—what Al Capone called 'the legitimate rackets.' Bank robbers use guns and physical force. The thrift robbers saw a new method—persuading the government to enact laws that actually *allowed* them to empty the till" (emphasis in original).

"Remember," says Nader (1990, p. xiii), "when our governmental leaders first let us in on the secret: did you notice that they called it the S&L 'crisis' and never the *crime* and looting of the savers' monies it was and is?" (emphasis in original). "A financial mafia of swindlers, mobsters, greedy S&L executives, and con men," say Stephen Pizzo and his associates (1989, p. 298), "capitalized on regulatory weaknesses created by deregulation and thoroughly fleeced the thrift industry. Savings and loans would not be in the mess they are today but for rampant fraud. Yet to this day diehard apologists . . . flatly refuse to admit that purposeful fraud was in fact chiefly to blame for the FSLIC's $200 to $300 billion debt . . . [an] orgy of avarice and fraud."

Other commentators writing in a similar vein emphasize the unprecedented scale of the criminal activity involved as compared with earlier historical examples. "One of the most shopworn cliches of the financial industry," says L. J. Davis (1990, pp. 50–51), "[is] that the best way to rob a bank is to own one. This maxim, like all maxims, is rooted in a basic truth about human nature: To wit, if criminals are given easy access to large sums of money, they will steal, and under such tempting circumstances even honest men may be corrupted. To forget this is to invite madness and ruin. In our time, such madness and ruin has visited in the form of the savings and loan scandal . . . *the most astounding financial scandal the nation has ever witnessed*—not simply a debacle but a series of debacles" (emphasis added).

"We have here . . . a decade of commercial lawlessness," writes Michael M. Thomas (1991*a*, p. 30), "*unmatched anywhere in our history.*

Nothing in the Gilded Era of Gould and Fisk, or in the 1920s of Insull and Ivar Krueger, or any of the celebrated 'bubbles' comes close in scale and breadth of effect. . . . A great many people conspired over at least two decades to bring down the nation's system of savings and loan institutions. . . . The mosaic of disaster was complex in the extreme, mixing simple thuggery with subtle feats of financial and legal prestidigitation. . . . It is an extremely difficult story to tell in a fashion that would provoke the kind of outrage it deserves" (emphasis added).

Again, Mayer says that

> the theft from the taxpayer by the community that fattened on the growth of the savings and loan (S&L) industry in the 1980s is *the worst public scandal in American history*. . . . The S&L outrage makes Teapot Dome and Credit Mobilier seem minor episodes. . . . Future sociologists, like today's journalists, will study the irruption of criminality into what had been conservative, even beneficent organizations. . . . They will tell of Texas cowboys, California sharpies, Beltway whores, and assorted mafiosi . . . and investment banks that permitted some of their partners and executives to conspire with criminals and even rewarded them for it, provided the income derived from the conspiracy was sufficiently great. [1990, pp. 1, 3; emphasis added]

Many commentators incidentally cite in support of their analyses the testimony of Frederick D. Wolf, assistant comptroller general of the U.S. General Accounting Office (GAO), who at the San Francisco Hearings of the House Banking Committee in February 1989, stated that the "GAO found that extensive, repeated and blatant violations of laws and regulations characterized the failed thrifts that we reviewed in each and every case. Virtually every one of the thrifts was operating in an unsafe and unsound manner. . . . Under the Bank Board's definitions alone, fraud or insider abuse existed at each and every one of the failed thrifts and allegations of criminal misconduct abounded" (Wolf 1989).

We assemble all these statements not only to illustrate the popularity of this type of ascription of blame but also to highlight the ideological significance of this portrayal of the S&L crisis as the result of intentional dishonesty. For this diagnosis of the nature of the crisis by critics of the general business community is characteristic of those who subscribe to the Nader paradigm of the American state and society.

c. Culpable Negligence.   Perhaps the largest group of observers and commentators on the S&L crisis to subscribe to a single-cause explanation emphasize the culpable stupidity of government and business leaders rather than larcenous hearts or impersonal economic forces. Thus, Ely writes that "early to mid-1983 would have been the ideal time for the federal government to have disposed of all then insolvent S&Ls. But it did not, and consequently this buried problem has continued to build." Ely ties the failure of the thrift institutions to the basic structure of the industry before the mid-1980s:

> The earliest source of FSLIC/Resolution Trust Corporation (RTC) losses, maturity mismatching (investing short-term passbook savings in long-term, fixed-rate home mortgages) finally caught up with the S&Ls in 1981. Although interest rates exploded in late 1979, the willingness of many people to keep deposits in S&L at below-market interest rates largely neutralized for almost two years the devastating effect that high interest rates had on the market value of the fixed-rate mortgages owned by S&Ls at that time. In the first half of 1981, S&L depositors on average were accepting yields almost 5 percent below market rates.
> By mid-1982, however, the willingness of depositors to subsidize S&Ls had substantially disappeared, which had the effect of making S&Ls deeply insolvent, based on the market value of their mortgages. At this peak, . . . almost every S&L in America was insolvent on a market-value basis; collectively, the industry was almost $100 billion underwater, an amount equal to 15 percent of the industry's deposits and other liabilities. [1991, pp. 1, 2]

But far more popular as a candidate for blame are the legislative changes that decontrolled interest rates paid by thrift institutions and also the financial risks they could take, while both continuing the pattern of depository insurance and substantially increasing the amount of coverage. "Probably the single most damaging provision in the law [the Garn-St. Germain Depository Institutions Act of 1982]," says Mayer (1990, pp. 97–98), "was the elimination of all regulation of the ratio between what an S&L could lend to a developer and the appraised value of the project for which the loan was made. . . . Garn-St. Germain was increasing greatly the proportion of their assets that S&Ls could have in commercial real estate—and at the same time eliminating all control over how much could be lent to build and carry commercial properties. And the Bank Board was permitting developers to buy S&Ls."

Another commentator on that legislation, James Ring Adams, puts it as follows:

> Garn-St. Germain unleashed a horde of habitual risk-takers without subjecting them to any risk. The Bank Board compounded the problem by relaxing capital requirements almost to nonexistence. With expanded deposit insurance and reductions in the amount of capital thrifts were required to keep on hand, the new owners had every incentive to be as reckless as possible. They would reap the benefits of a long-shot business deal but bear none of the cost. In the words of one regulator, "Heads, they win. Tails, FSLIC loses." Insurance professionals have a term for it, "moral hazard." The policy offers too much temptation to cheat. [1990, p. 22]

Many commentators emphasize the role of federal deposit insurance. Thus, James Barth and R. Dan Brumbaugh (1990, p. 58) refer to federal deposit insurance as "the fundamental cause of the savings and loan problem." Again, Charles Schumer and Brian Graham (1990, pp. 73, 79) say that "it was federal deposit insurance that made the thrift crisis possible. . . . The underlying cause of this massive crisis [is] the deposit insurance system."

The operating motive suggested here is not predatory greed but rather ideologically accented naïveté or stupidity. As Neil Eichler (1989, pp. viii–ix) puts it: "In the end it was not venality or evil intentions that produced losses approaching, if not exceeding, $100 billion most of which will fall on taxpayers; rather it was the power of an idea . . . deregulation. Ideological puritans in the Reagan administration went wild."

As for the president, "Reagan," says P. J. O'Rourke (1991, p. 206), "was the blind, deaf referee of the deregulatory wrestlemania match." "In the name of 'deregulation,'" say Norman Strunk and Fred Case (1988, pp. 2, 14), "almost overnight the [savings and loan] business was thrown into the jungle of open competition even though it was not equipped for it. . . . The single most important development that precipitated the wave of failures was 'deregulation' which first produced operating losses for most institutions and then attracted venturesome entrepreneurs to the business who led savings associations into unfamiliar business activities."

Nevertheless, many of those who subscribe to the idea that "the savings and loan failures of the 1980s are part of the legacy of deregulation" (O'Connell 1988, p. xi) see those failures as the result of culpable negligence, more than occasionally influenced by campaign contributions and other financial inducements. "The major blame for the debacle," says Barth (1991, p. 4), formerly chief economist of the Federal Home Loan Bank Board, "rests with the government—Congress, the administration, and the federal (and state) regulators and insurers of savings and loans."

Some commentators blame "the system." Thus, William Gorham (1989, p. xvii), president of the Urban Institute, says, "The root cause of the crisis is neither a few specific regulatory mistakes nor corruption by a group of unscrupulous people in the Savings and Loan industry. The problem is the result of structural flaws in the system. Because of these flaws, the industry and its regulators, which include the United States Congress, are faced with virtually irresistible incentives to ignore signals of pending insolvency, and to postpone the inevitable day of reckoning until 'someone else' takes over and becomes responsible."

Thomas Romer and Barry Weingast (1990, p. 38) also emphasize the political foundations of what they refer to as "the thrift debacle." "The key component underlying the thrift crisis," they assert, "[was that] massive gambling for resurrection was allowed to proceed because Congress intervened in the regulatory process. . . . First, Congress delayed and kept recapitalization funding at low levels thus ensuring that regulators could force only some insolvent savings and loans to close or reorganize. . . . Second, when regulators did propose to embark on a tougher policy, Congress intervened to prevent enforcement of existing rules and, through new legislation, relaxed many regulatory provisions."

Pilzer, too, stresses the political background of the crisis:

> Nor did Congress wish to have the thrift crisis laid bare and the enormous cost unveiled. Certainly the Democratic leadership could not be expected to see any profit in such an exercise. In the first place, Congress had always been the ultimate regulator of the thrift industry. It had set the rules for the Federal Home Loan Bank Board. It—or, rather, its Democratic majority—had allowed

the crisis to develop. . . . [But] the Democratic leadership's vulnerability on the thrift issue wasn't a weakness that could be exploited by the Republicans. After all, it had been the Reagan White House that had blocked Ed Gray's efforts to increase the size of the FHLBB's regulatory police force. There was also the troubling matter of Vice President George Bush's involvement. . . . The fact is that exposing the monstrous proportions the thrift crisis had reached by 1988 carried no political advantage for either party. [1989, pp. 208–9]

Moreover, Edwin Gray (1990, p. 138), who was chairman of the Federal Home Loan Bank Board from 1983 to 1987, has himself described the S&L crisis as "a story of unbridled power and influence corrupting the political process." And Joseph Grundfest (1990, p. 25), who was a commissioner of the Securities and Exchange Commission from 1985 to 1990, sees the crisis as the result of "political failure endemic to congressional decision making: under current budgeting procedures some constituencies can manipulate Congress to provide massive private benefits at substantial public cost."

Others have made more explicit charges. For example, Waldman (1990a, p. 47), director of Public Citizen's Congress Watch, has said that "voters are now coming to realize that Capitol Hill corruption will soon cost them thousands of dollars each. The present system of special interest financing of congressional campaigns, routine congressional intervention on behalf of wealthy contributors, and a capitol besieged by business lobbyists of every pinstripe, has led to this unprecedented bailout and a scandal of historic dimensions."

Again, "The S&L disaster couldn't have happened without a posse of thrift allies on Capitol Hill—lawmakers purchased by campaign contributions, personal gifts, entertainment, and speech fees. In the 1980s Congress was a thoroughly corrupted institution. . . . Financial industry political action committees as a whole gave current Senate [Banking] Committee members $3,836,598 between 1985 and 1990 and gave current House Banking Committee members $5,193,258" (Waldman 1990b, pp. 60, 63).

The same point is made in a somewhat breezier style by O'Rourke (1991, pp. 208, 210), the White House correspondent for *Rolling Stone:* "If we want somebody to blame who can stand the blaming, let's look to the jacklegs in Congress. Beginning in the late 1980s savings-and-loan lobbyists produced a bloody flux of political-action-committee funds and other influence effluvia, and members of the House and Senate stood by like toilets with lids up. . . . There is not room in this book for a complete list of elected offenders. There are 535 members of the House and Senate; as many as a dozen of them are blameless."

Finally, Adams offers an explanation:

> Congress was an easy mark. After a decade of campaign finance hypocrisy, its members needed the money more than ever. The growth of television advertising has made the multi-billion dollar campaign a common event. With the right technology, an incumbent could virtually guarantee his seat; the rate of re-election in the 1988 House campaign exceeded 98 percent. . . . Just on the face of it—the thrift industry ruined at a public cost of $300 billion—the result was an incredible scandal. Congress had been willfully irresponsible; in the face of urgent warnings, it had delayed the rescue of FSLIC and then had saddled it with the harmful CEBA, and all to protect the worst elements of the industry. It is hard to think of a grosser betrayal of the public interest. The one-hundredth Congress may well be remembered as the most corrupt since the days of the Credit Mobilier scandal in the late nineteenth century. And the 101st Congress is an accomplice after the fact. [1990, pp. 51–52]

d. Multiple Causation. In concentrating on single-cause explanations of the S&L problems, we do not mean to imply either that the multiplicity of failures can best be understood as the product of a single cause or that most observers who have published accounts of the matter have adopted single-cause explanations. The implosion of so many financial institutions is a phenomenon that can accommodate a variety of different causal factors interacting in the historical context of the 1970s and 1980s. Moreover, many observers have been sensitive to the way in which different kinds of problems associated with different levels of personal culpability have interacted. But, as we shall see, the attribution to multiple cause lacks a central moral focus. If lots of elements are responsible, then no one agency or personification is to blame.

"The recent savings and loan crisis," writes Patricia Werhane (1990, p. 125), "is attributed to *a number of factors*, including: deregulation of the thrifts and subsequent changes in the minimum capital requirements; the raising of Federal Savings and Loan Insurance Corporation guarantees to $100,000 for depositors; increased costs of funds in a fixed mortgage interest rate market; the growth in popularity of high-yield junk bonds and money market funds; and insufficient oversight of savings and loans by regulatory agencies" (emphasis added).

Christian Hill (1990, pp. 21–23) says that "there is common agreement that the biggest mistakes leading to the thrift crisis were the decisions by the Federal Home Loan Bank Board from 1980 to 1989." But he adds that "there are at least *three other primary causes* of the thrift debacle. . . . The first is the lack of current market information about the value of assets owned by the thrift industry. . . . But beyond that, it is deposit insurance that has led to the most pressing problem for depository institutions. . . . Finally there is common underestimation of another primary cause of the thrift debacle—the extent to which the mortgage market is moribund" (emphasis added).

"The savings and loan crisis. How did we get here?" wrote James Glassman in the *New Republic*. "Through *a combination* of deregulation, short-sighted home-district politics, changing cultural values, macro-economics, and the deposit-insurance system," he states (Glassman 1990, p. 16; emphasis added). Whereas Lawrence White (1991, p. 117) says that the "thrifts largely failed because of *an amalgam* of deliberately high-risk strategies, poor business judgments, foolish strategies, excessive optimism, and sloppy and careless underwriting, compounded by deteriorating real estate markets" (emphasis added).

Perhaps the most popular multicausal explanation of the S&L crisis is in terms of the interaction of lack of regulatory control and supervision and entrepreneurial larceny in a situation where "the enhanced opportunities, capabilities and incentives for risk taking . . . created an explosive mix" (White 1991, p. 109). For the uneven regulatory pattern of the post-1981 legislation made the operation of an S&L an ideal business opportunity for entrepreneurs. As Adams (1990, p. 22) puts it: "Garn-St Germain shifted the focus to rebuilding capital. Reasoning that thrifts couldn't profit on their traditional mortgages, the bill greatly expanded the types of investments they could make. A new breed of owner was invited in, aggressive risk-takers who presumably would help the thrifts earn their way out of their hole." And entrepreneurs willing to take astronomic risks with insured deposits moved in, straddling the frontier between optimism and felony.

But a review of these multicausal accounts reveals that they lack a moral center of gravity in their descriptions of what went wrong—a bedrock notion of whom or what to blame. And here the parallel with the general debate about white-collar crime is most striking, in that subscription to one pattern of emphasis seems to involve the exclusion of the other. Thus, some structural accounts of the S&L mess seem to be at pains to argue not merely that larcenous hearts are not a good explanation of the crisis but rather as if a search for evildoers would divert from the proper appreciation of systemic problems. Ely (1991, p. 2), whose explanation of the S&L failures we noted earlier, says categorically, "Claims that crooks stole a big chunk of the money that the S&L cleanup is going to cost are simply not true."

Critics like Nader and Waldman, by contrast, are anxious not to have attention diverted from what is referred to as "epic corruption" and "an unprecedented frenzy of business criminality" (Nader 1990, p. xiii). While they recognize the role played by government error in, for example, "failing to shut down insolvent thrifts," they reject as morally inappropriate accounts that place the emphasis on negligence or mistake. "We don't say there isn't a mugging just because the foot patrolman is off at the donut shop" (Waldman 1990b, p. 53). Waldman (1990a, p. 48) acknowledges "the S&L crackup was the product of many factors" and mentions "speculative excess, high interest rates, and falling land values . . . magnified by reckless deregulation." At the same time, he poses, as though it were the crucial issue, the question "Who robbed America?" (Waldman 1990b, p. 3). The emphasis must remain singly on individual moral accountability.

The reversal of positions that occurs in the liberal-versus-conservative debate in relation to white-collar crime can be thought of as a *moralistic inversion* in which the liberals shift from an emphasis on societal/institutional factors to an emphasis on moral blame and personal responsibility while crime control conservatives move in the opposite direction. In the S&L affair, we would expect this reversal to be most pronounced when the focus of attention is high-status businessmen rather than some of the more socially marginal figures associated with S&L acquisitions in the early 1980s.

The morally indignant political liberals are at particular pains to label those who would describe themselves as business leaders in morally freighted language; to speak of "thrift robbers" (Waldman 1990b, p. 4) or the "financial mafia" (Pizzo, Fricker, and Muolo 1989, p. 298) is to create in language a moral linkage of those responsible for thrift institution losses with street criminals and Cosa Nostra dons.

Industry analysts, by contrast, tend to regard talk of "thrift robbers" as something of a distraction from the structural causes of large thrift losses. They speak of institutional causes such as partial deregulation and subsidized deposit insurance in the same tones that liberals might use to describe inequality of economic opportunity as a cause of street crime, a set of institutional forces more important than individual wrongdoing and on a different plane.

On one issue, however, proponents of wildly different causal accounts are in near total agreement. Nobody seems to believe that empirical tests of various causal accounts should be an important element in public discourse about the S&L crisis.

3. *The Prospect for Causal Testing.* While the considerable literature on the S&L scandal is awash with causal theories, very few observers have stepped over the boundary that separates theoretical speculation from statistical evidence and empirical testing. Indeed with the one exception of the issue of cost the absence of factual dispute in the S&L discussion is striking. Later in this essay we argue that there is a reason for this lacuna: factual evidence is irrelevant and superfluous when the crucial test of a theory's validity is ideological.

But quite apart from any motives that anyone might have for neglecting empirical testing of propositions about the causes of the S&L failures, there is the question whether there is available evidence relating to those failures that might be used by any observer wishing to carry out such tests. While the data available for testing existing causal theories is limited, there is much more data available for this purpose than has so far been used.

Two kinds of historical evidence could be used to test theories regarding factors nominated as causal in relation to the S&L collapses. In the first place, one can search for historical antecedents of the widespread S&L failures from the 1980s onward and critically examine the argument that in this case temporal order provides evidence for causal order. Some of the historical antecedents that have been nominated in this context include deficit spending, the activities of the Arab oil cartel, hyperinflation in the 1970s, and deregulation.

Causal arguments from historical antecedents are notorious for their inadequacy. Post hoc, ergo propter hoc is one of the most elementary fallacies, and the arguments involving this fallacy to be found in the literature on the S&L failures are no stronger than the usual post hoc candidate. But it is not merely unsophisticated post hoc argumentation that provides an inadequate empirical reference for causal inference in this area. For multivariate statistical analyses that attempt to control by statistical means changes in policy and in economic conditions other

TABLE 1

S&L Resolutions, GAAP Insolvencies, and Estimated Resolution Costs

	Texas	United States Other than Texas
Percentage of failure rate in the 1980s	34 (108/318)	11 (418/3,675)
Percentage of operating institutions insolvent under generally accepted accounting principles (GAAP) (1988)	56 (114/204)	12 (320/2,745)
Percentage of total funds estimated for resolutions (1989)	53 (2,953/5,608)*	47 (2,655/5,608)*

SOURCES.—Barth, Bartholomew, and Bradley (1989); Barth (1991).
* Millions of dollars.

than the hypotheses that are being tested also seem to us a singularly weak method for analyzing the empirical evidence regarding the causes of the S&L failures. Statistical sophistication and complexity hold little promise of overcoming the problems of post hoc reasoning. Almost anything that happened in the United States over the 1970s and 1980s is a candidate for post hoc causal responsibility for the thrift crisis.

A second kind of historical analysis seems more promising than efforts at post hoc reasoning. Cross-sectional analysis provides potentially helpful tests of the determinants of S&L failures. Despite the generality of the crisis, only a minority of thrift institutions in the United States have in fact failed, and failure rates differ for different kinds of institutions, in different areas, and with different management histories (White 1991, pp. 108, 113–15). Straightforward analysis of these cross-sectional differences could provide significant evidence about the relative contributions of various causal factors to the current level of failure and loss.

Consider by way of example what we would call the "geographical determinist hypothesis" as an explanation of the S&L failures. Table 1 shows three measures of S&L failure, comparing Texas to the rest of the United States. First, it shows the rate at which federally chartered S&Ls failed throughout the 1980s to the point of requiring "resolution" by the relevant federal agencies. The second measure in table 1 shows the percentage of Texas and non-Texas institutions regarded as insolvent for bookkeeping purposes by federal regulatory agencies in 1988. The third measure of comparative difficulty is the estimated dollar cost in constant dollars for Texas and non-Texas thrift rescues.

The analysis on the impact of geography begins with data on the S&L "resolutions" by the federal government. Thirty-four percent of Texas thrifts in existence in 1980 had to be put through "resolution"—about three times the "resolution" rate for the rest of the United States. Yet the same data show a modest role for any geographical influence in two respects. First, a Texas location was hardly a sufficient condition for S&L failure. Two-thirds of Texas thrifts survived the decade without being put into "resolution." Second, only a small fraction of all S&L institutions that were put through "resolution" were located in Texas, about 20 percent of total resolutions (108 out of 526) during that ten-year period. A Texas location was far from being a necessary condition for S&L failure.

At the same time, each of these reservations needs to be further qualified by the rest of the data in table 1. When the percentage of all Texas thrifts considered to be in a state of bookkeeping insolvency in 1988 is added to the 33 percent that had already failed and been resolved, the aggregate percentage of thrifts in serious difficulties over the 1980–90 period was greater than 75 percent. A Texas location was not a sufficient condition for financial difficulty, but Texas thrifts were much more likely than not to encounter very serious problems.

Moreover, the small percentage of total thrift failures occurring in Texas understates the contribution to the S&L crisis of Texas institutions when measured by cost. For, as the bottom figures in table 1 reveal, as of 1989, more than one-half of the aggregate dollar losses attributable to particular resolutions came from Texas institutions. So Texas thrift failures when they occurred were big ticket items for the federal insurance schemes.

The simple cross tabulations in table 1 are far from telling the whole story. S&Ls can be further subdivided where data are available in order to determine whether capital and managerial conditions that might be associated with a Texas location, rather than the Texas location itself, are the significant predictors of failure or serious trouble. This kind of specific analysis should be the next step in the discussion and investigation of the causes of thrift institution failure.

None of the published discussion or analysis to the time of this writing contains any multivariate disaggregation of S&L failure rates. Indeed, it is difficult to determine, from the available literature, the actuarial odds of S&L failure by any accounting or legal measure.

With few exceptions, for example, Lawrence White's *The S&L Debacle* (1991), there is no citation of data on the relative chances of thrift institution failure in the already substantial volume of discussion of the causes of the S&L crisis. We speculate later in this article about why very few of those who purport to explain S&L failures seem to require empirical data.

II. Some Criminal Justice Perspectives

This section discusses six hypotheses about the thrift crisis of particular interest to academic students of American crime and criminal justice. We hope here to illustrate the value of social science perspectives to the comprehension of the policy issues raised by the S&L crisis.

A. Deposit Insurance and the Mobilization of the Criminal Law

As we have earlier noted, there is considerable disagreement among contemporary observers about the amount of criminal conduct associated with the S&L failures and about the degree to which criminality can be said to be a cause of the large number of failures. At one extreme are trade figures like Ely's estimate that criminal conduct is the explanation for no more than 3 percent of S&L insolvency (Ely 1991, p. 2). At the other extreme are a substantial number of commentators who appear to suggest that criminal fraud or its substantial equivalent played a major role in most S&L failures (Calavita and Pontell 1990; Mayer 1990; Nader 1990; Waldman 1990*b*; Thomas 1991*a*, 1991*b*).

A part of the difference between such polar estimates can be accounted for by terms of reference. We think that Ely has in mind criminal diversion of S&L assets where the primary intention was to misrepresent and no thought was given to the repayment of loans or the straightening out of accounts. By contrast, practices included in Nader's condemnation cover a far wider spectrum of conduct. So it seems likely that the explanation of this polar opposition regarding the degree to which the S&L failures can be blamed on criminal misconduct depends to a significant extent on where the observer draws the line in defining the management of failed loans and other potentially blameworthy S&L conduct as criminal.

The federal criminal code contains several fraud statutes that define as a felony any known falsehood in a loan application that turns out to be material to securing a loan and that (for jurisdictional purposes) involves the use of the mails, the telephone, or another instrument of interstate commerce (e.g., 18 U.S.C. 1001, 1014). Since most of the S&L failures involve hundreds of loans that turned sour, the degree to which those failures can be regarded as the product of criminal activity depends very much on the discretionary view of federal and state prosecutors, judges, and juries. Was the developer who applied for a loan a liar, or merely an optimist, or both? Did the S&L officer who made the loan on the basis of what turned out to be an inflated market estimate know that the market estimate was too high? Did the S&L officers and board that declared and distributed profits know that those profits were an artifact of inflated asset values?

In such circumstances, the degree of criminality involved in an S&L failure is very much in the eye of the prosecutorial beholder. Moreover, the amount of punishment that might be regarded as socially required in response to such behavior is contingent on a number of other social variables. One of the major variables influencing the social pressure to prosecute and punish in this context is deposit insurance. When such insurance schemes cover individual losses, they absorb pecuniary losses that would otherwise be suffered by individual depositors and thereby diminish the pressure on investigators and prosecutors to seek out and prosecute questionable S&L behaviors as criminal acts. This in turn makes it more likely that regulatory rather than criminal law approaches will be adopted in the restructuring of the thrift industry.

A textbook example of the relationship between insured losses and pressure to prosecute concerns Charles Keating and the now-famous business practices of his Lincoln Savings and Loan. Of all the activities involving that organization and its officers, many of which appear to be potential subjects of criminal investigation and prosecution, it is significant that the first substantial indictment to be generated by the failure of the Lincoln Savings and Loan was a thirty-count fraud charge centrally concerned with the sale of holding company bonds to southern California residents. The outrage provoked by these bond sales was largely due to the fact that when the assets of the Lincoln management were seized the bondholders found themselves in possession of corporate obligations unlikely to repay one cent on the dollar and not covered by deposit insurance because they were corporate securities rather than association deposits.

The billions of dollars of Lincoln deposits that probably will not be covered by the S&L's assets will, by contrast, nonetheless be cashed out by Federal Deposit Insurance. Those losses have to the date of this writing been the subject of no criminal prosecution. And whatever public chagrin and disapproval may be attached to the spectacle of hundreds of millions of dollars of insured deposits poured into a hotel complex with break-even room rentals of $600 a night, it is the palpable harm represented by the losses of individual investors that produces pressures for criminal prosecution.

A significant feature in the politics of criminal prosecution is that federal and local prosecutors pay more attention to crimes when identified individuals are the victims (Benson, Cullen, and Maakestad 1990). Comprehensive insurance schemes may substantially diminish effective pressure for criminal prosecution. When insurance schemes are not subsidized, there may be some countervailing pressure for criminal prosecution generated by those who administer insurance funds or who contribute to them in ways that are sensitive to variations in cost. But such funds not only spread risks, they also diminish the levels of palpable harm that influence the allocation of prosecutorial and punishment resources.

Publicly subsidized insurance schemes where the costs of harm or damage will be absorbed at some unspecified future date should serve as a particularly effective anesthetic for the kinds of harm that usually produce public pressures for criminal prosecution. So the S&L crisis presents an opportunity for studying the way in which the insurance of individual losses affects the priority that federal and state prosecutors assign to thrift cases vis-à-vis other public and private harms that compete for attention and resources. We can also predict that the level of punishment meted out to convicted S&L miscreants will be moderated because the widows and orphans who deposited money in their institutions have been rendered fiscally whole by federal deposit insurance, a prospect we discuss in the next section.

Whether the deemphasis on punishment that social insurance may produce should be considered a distortion of the proper priorities of prosecution and punishment depends on whether there is in any meaningful sense an optimal level of prosecution and punishment for such financial crimes and also on whether the way in which that optimal level should be defined relates primarily to the level of gross pecuniary loss or to the palpable individual harm incurred. To say that such questions have not yet been answered is to misrepresent our current level of information. For such questions can only be considered in an informed and objective fashion in the aftermath of studies of the impact of insurance schemes on the operation of the institutions of criminal justice.

B. Harm and Punishment

It is a popular axiom in modern discussions that punishment should be calibrated in proportion to the amount of harm resulting from a particular criminal act perpetrated by a particular criminal actor (van den Haag 1975; von Hirsch 1976; Singer 1979). For property crime this has been taken to justify direct linkage between the amount of money or the value of the property taken in the course of an offense and the quantum of punishment called for. This sort of justification can be found in, among other places, the guidelines issued by the U.S. Sentencing Commission that took effect in November 1987 (U.S. Sentencing Commission 1987).

The role of deposit insurance in the S&L episode shows, however, that contingencies other than the amount of money or property taken can have a powerful influence on the level of harm suffered by identifiable victims. Where the level of harm suffered depends on factors outside the offender's control, why should the social results be considered an important element in assessing the degree of blame applicable to the offender? Consider an example from the previous subsection. If Keating is convicted of fraud in relation to insured deposits, should the level of punishment be reduced because the individual losses usually associated with predatory property crime were avoided because of the federal deposit insurance scheme? If he is convicted of fraud in connection with the uninsured losses of corporate security holders, should the punishment be increased because of the greater harm to individuals? One way of considering the question is to view it in light of the common thief's complaint when punished for stealing uninsured property, which is to the effect that part of the punishment imposed on him is not due to his wrongdoing but rather to inadequate insurance.

One ingenious answer to this problem in the S&L case seems inadequate. It might be argued that the existence of deposit insurance does not affect the quantum of social harm but merely the site where the ultimate costs are borne, so that the theft of insured property is just as socially injurious as the theft of uninsured property. But one problem with this formulation is that if we took it seriously, there would be no basis for insurance. Loss spreading does in fact diminish the social disutility caused by theft. A second way of magnifying the harm caused by theft in the context of insurance is to create a moral link between the offender's behavior and the fate of the general insurance scheme. Thus, a prosecutor may attempt to tie the behavior of individual offenders to the insolvency of the insurance fund in the late 1980s and early 1990s.

But this stratagem runs afoul of strict standards of causation because no single S&L failure was either the necessary or the sufficient cause of the failure of the insurance scheme. No single failure would have exhausted the insurance fund by itself even if the losses attributed to it were added to the historically normal loss rates for the rest of the industry. So the social harm attributable to any single S&L failure would have been quite modest if so many other S&Ls had not also failed. In this sense, the social harm attributable to the aggregate of S&L failures is considerably greater than the sum of its parts. But is each offender morally chargeable with notice that so many other S&Ls would fail?

Thus, the institution of insurance may be relevant not only to the amount of pressure for prosecution and punishment that in fact occurs but also with respect to the degree of punishment that should as a matter of principle be imposed. We would hope that the experience with insurance loss that we are currently enjoying will be seen to provide an opportunity for sustained analysis of these matters.

C. The Independence of Causal Theory

We have already distinguished between causal theories about the S&L crisis and tests of such causal theories using empirical data. The literature on the S&L failures is flooded with causal theories and hypotheses, yet the possibility of testing those theories empirically is never mentioned. This is a pattern that demands an explanation. The same factors that allow and even encourage the development of such theories without any substantial resources being invested in testing them can be found also in the circumstances of criminological discourse over the past few decades.

The motive that most observers have for constructing causal explanations of the S&L crisis is to provide explanations that are consistent with the observers' worldviews. The task is one of making the relevant events comprehensible within the observers' own ideological frame of reference. For the most part, their theories seem to have been cooked up for home consumption rather than developed for competitive trials among agnostics in the free marketplace of ideas. As soon as an explanation has been found that is consistent with the observers' general views, the problem of explaining the S&L crisis is taken to have been solved. In such circumstances, any empirical testing of the explanation is regarded as superfluous, indeed potentially dangerous.

As long as such explanations are designed for consumption by persons who share the observers' perspective, an appropriate causal explanation will be accepted as more or less self-validating. It is only when dialogue and debate between those whose perspectives differ produces disagreement about causation that the need for empirical testing of any kind comes to be recognized. But as long as those who subscribe to different causal explanations talk *past* each other rather than *to* each other, there will be no recognition of any such need. That seems to be the position in relation to the explanation of S&L failures in the United States in 1993.

It also seems to be closely analogous to the conditions that characterize much criminological discourse on the subject of causation in recent decades, particularly where ideologues of the left and right are concerned. Those who are substantially committed to either "Marxist" or to neoconservative positions seem to be principally concerned to discover or formulate theoretical accounts that can be integrated with their own general views. Once an explanation of crime is found that is consistent with their respective positions it can function quite satisfactorily without being subjected to any empirical testing as long as its principal audience consists of persons already predisposed to accept it.

It is only when dialogue or debate between those holding conflicting views become more important than exchanges within the opposed ideological camps that the question of empirical testing is likely to receive attention as an important criminological concern and even then it is by no means certain that it will do so (Allen 1974, pp. 1–23).

D. The Relationship between Regulatory and
Criminal Justice Responsibility

The S&L story has presented an unprecedented opportunity to observe the interaction of civil law regulatory regimes and the federal criminal justice system. Increasingly, modern government action is an important influence in creating the environment in which individual conduct including criminal conduct takes place. But the discussion of the causes of the S&L failures is the first time we can recall when the failure of the regulatory system has been widely seen as a principal cause of large-scale criminal conduct.

The notion of public causes of crime and, in particular, of government action or inaction as an influence on individual behavior is by no means novel, but it is usually associated with attenuated theories regarding the relationship between poverty or unemployment and street crime or inadequate supervision as part of a climate that allows that criminal conduct to occur. In the case of the S&L failures, however, many observers go well beyond that and speak of regulatory changes as a proximate cause of a wave of financial recklessness quite frequently including criminal conduct. It is a common understanding of the early 1990s not only that criminal conduct was an important part of the S&L failures but that this was one crime wave that was made in Washington.

William Seidman, the Federal Deposit Insurance Corporation (FDIC) chairman who led the initial Bush bailout effort, for example, put it as follows: "I suppose bad members of the industry are at fault, but they are at fault because the government allowed them in. The government said here's the candy and you can have all you want. What they didn't realize is that if you combine a credit card on the United States with no limits, the chance to invest that money just about any way you wanted, and then call off supervision because you decide you have deregulated the industry, you create almost an entrapment—a fatal attraction or whatever they call it in the law" (O'Shea 1991, pp. 289–90).

In most contemporary discussion of those failures, the actions and the inaction of the regulatory authorities are regarded as both costly and blameworthy, while the relative inaction of the criminal justice system is regarded as unimportant and certainly not particularly blameworthy. There are three attributes of the regulatory scheme that governed thrift institutions that make it an eminently suitable candidate for blame when things went wrong: thrift regulation was specific to savings institutions, was preventive in design, and historically had been effective.

All other things being equal, a specific regulatory mission should generate more responsibility for behavior within the agency's jurisdiction than a more general mandate. The Federal Home Loan Bank Board had only the responsibility for certain specified institutions, while U.S. attorneys and the FBI are charged with enforcing an enormously thick federal criminal code covering the full spectrum of social and individual conduct in violation of the criminal law. When something goes wrong with thrift institutions, it is both natural and appropriate that the public should expect more from the body with the more specific enforcement responsibilities.

The second reason for expecting more from the bank regulators than the enforcers of the criminal law in this context is that the regulatory scheme was designed to *prevent* harm while criminal law enforcement notoriously can only arrive after the fact of particular harms. The preventive rationale of regulation inevitably creates expectations of prevention and a tendency, when prevention fails, to blame those who maintain and operate the preventive apparatus.

A third reason why thrift regulators have received the brunt of the blame for S&L failures is that thrift regulation had succeeded, at least in avoiding scandal, for almost four decades before the 1982 deregulation. Since the regulatory mechanism was presumably effective for all those years, any epidemic of losses would naturally be seen as a culpable failure on the part of the regulators.

So state and federal criminal law enforcement has so far been assigned little of the blame for the catastrophic losses in the S&L industry. There are several aspects of this relatively low profile that are worthy of note. First, with the growth of regulatory government, the number and variety of circumstances in which other arms of government seem more importantly connected to specific areas of behavior than the criminal law have also grown and now include almost all forms of economic regulation. Sale of publicly owned securities, fraud in labeling and advertising, pollution of air and water, and standards of conduct in regulated industries are four of the main instances where specific civil regulatory authority is generally regarded as more important than criminal law enforcement.

Second, this displacement of primary responsibility can take place independently of whether criminal conduct is a recurrent and significant element in the regulatory problem. All three of the attributes we nominate as reasons for looking first to regulatory responsibility can occur even when most of the losses regulatory failure produces involved criminal conduct. The allocation of primary responsibility may then depend not on how the behavior may be characterized but rather on perceptions about how it can best be controlled.

Finally, one consequence of the relatively low profile of criminal justice agencies and processes in the S&L crisis is that it has encouraged caution on the part of criminal law enforcers. The surest way to attract attention and thus be seen as more responsible for outcomes in this crisis is to make loud noises. As long as inaction is unlikely to be perceived by the public as the cause of any great loss, the risks associated with any conspicuous activity are likely to suggest to more than one prosecutor that discretion may be the better part of valor.

E. Deregulation and the Theory of Second Best

The story of thrift institutions in the 1980s amounted to a large-scale demonstration project testing what economists call "the fallacy of second best" (Meade 1955, pp. 102–18; Lipsey and Lancaster 1956–57). The economic fallacy is to conclude that, even when conditions contain one distortion from a perfect market, the goal of policy should still be to make all other circumstances as close to free market conditions as possible. The lesson was that policy analysts could not assume that just because a perfect market would be the best outcome, an environment with only one distortion from a perfect market would be second best. Postwar economists demonstrated that under certain conditions "two small distortions" from market conditions "are preferable to one large one" (Stiglitz 1986, p. 389).

The distortion from market conditions inherent in the structure of S&Ls was the availability of deposit insurance sold at rates that do not reflect risks or costs. As long as this distortion was a characteristic of the S&L industry, other steps toward free market conditions such as interest rate deregulation, eased capital requirements, or the end of restrictions on S&L investments may not improve the efficiency of the system and could well make matters worse.

Nobody seriously suggested moving away from deposit insurance in the 1982 deregulation—indeed, deposit insurance coverage was substantially expanded from a maximum of $40,000 to $100,000 per deposit. Yet all the other restriction removals were justified in classic fallacy of second-best terms.

This is perfectly exemplified in the 1984 Report of the Task Group on Regulation of Financial Services that was chaired by Vice-President Bush (Bush 1984). Although, in a prefatory letter to the president, the vice-president says that "our goal was to develop practical proposals to *strengthen the effectiveness of federal regulation*" (emphasis added), that is the only reference to strengthening federal regulation in the entire document. The whole tenor of the report is inimical to, indeed represents an explicit repudiation of, the notion of federal regulation (Pilzer 1989, p. 208; Pizzo, Fricker, and Muolo 1989, p. 250).

It is no exaggeration to say that the dominant, recurring, and unifying theme of the report, so far from being the need "to strengthen the effectiveness of federal regulation," is by contrast what is referred to as the "need for regulatory relief" and for the removal of "excessive regulatory controls," as well as the need for "the removal of unnecessary barriers to competition" and the "reduction of unnecessary regulatory costs" (Bush 1984, pp. 27, 28, 41).

In the report's summary of recommendations, the emphasis throughout is on the achievement of "a deregulated environment" by such means as reducing "unnecessarily burdensome restrictions" and "eliminating redundant federal oversight." Thus, it is said that "the Task Group recommendations would eliminate or narrow the application of various regulatory controls to reduce unnecessarily burdensome regulatory controls." Again, "The Task Group recommendations would substantially reduce . . . the overall regulatory burden on regulated institutions and their customers" (Bush 1984, pp. 63–65).

Moreover, the rationale underlying the recommendations is clearly stated in Section I of the report: "In the five decades since the 1930s federal government policy has been largely interventionist, imposing restrictions on financial markets. . . . Federal controls on interest rates and legislative creation of various areas of restricted competition helped to stabilize the chaotic marketplace conditions that followed the stock market crash of 1929 and the wave of bank failures that occurred over the succeeding few years." It is suggested, however, that viewed in retrospect "these actions were more restrictive of competition than necessary" and that an unfortunate aftereffect is that, well over half a century later, "bank and thrift institutions remain some of the most extensively regulated businesses in America. Extensive controls remain."

By contrast, a future is envisaged in which "most federal restrictions on pricing by depository institutions will end," as will other "outdated or unnecessary regulatory controls." "Unnecessary restrictions on financial competition" will be eliminated, and "unrestrained entry into financial services markets will produce efficient markets, free of the distortions and inefficiencies that are usually created by government attempts to organize market activity." Indeed, "Congress is considering Administration-sponsored legislation to reduce the current restrictions" (Bush 1984, pp. 23–27).

As a result, of course, the other deregulations of the 1980s greatly magnified the level of public resources absorbed by the S&L failures, a case of second best with a vengeance.

The interesting question is why such an expensive object lesson of a rather uncontroversial economic theorem was required during the 1980s. The most plausible explanation would stress the important distinction between the free market as an economic system and free market terms and metaphors as a rhetorical system. In the political arena of the 1980s and 1990s, terms like "competition," "market," "regulation," and "incentives" were part of a rhetorical system not grounded in economic theory. They were among a set of symbols to be turned to advantage by contending interest groups.

In this context, no industry group ever regards perfect competition as a best-case political outcome. Government subsidies such as underpriced deposit insurance and barriers to the free entry of potential competitors are high on the wish list of every industry lobby. The "noncompetitive regulations" under attack in the early 1980s were those that limited the ability of thrift institutions and their managements to attract funds, take risks, and have unrestricted dispositional power over their deposits. So the economists' notion of efficiency was not seen as an important value in the debate on deregulation, and technical economists were not regarded as a significant constituency to be consulted in the deregulation process.

Further, if it is only the metaphorical and symbolic significance of terms like "competition" and "market" that is of paramount importance, then it is to be expected that close but imperfect approximation of markets would be enormously appealing. And this seems just as true of efforts like the Bush Task Group after the fact of deregulation as it was in the administration and congressional activities of deregulation in 1982. So the politics of deregulation with respect to thrift institutions were on a collision course with informed economic analysis from the start. As is usual in the United States when rhetoric and substance pull in opposite directions, a rhetorical outcome was preferred.

When deregulation of financial institutions functions as a rhetorical rather than an economic exercise, close parallels can be observed between rhetoric on deregulation and the chronically theatrical debates about crime policy. Just as the symbolic politics of crime dominates discussion of legislation and judicial opinions, the symbolic politics of deregulation preempted the field and were manipulated by industry groups. For a not insignificant period in the 1980s, some economic policy in the United States was too important to permit the participation of economists in its analysis and formulation.

F. The Triumph of Structural Explanation

Earlier, we referred to competition between structural and individual theories of crime causation. When asked to list the causes of, for example, automobile theft, a person favoring structural explanations would prefer accounts featuring the widespread ownership of automobiles, inequality of incomes, inadequate security devices, and the like, whereas those who regard crime as caused primarily by individual character defects would stress such things as moral deficiencies, lack of parental discipline, and possibly other familial conditions that might encourage delinquent character development. In debates about most types of crime it is commonly liberals who emphasize structural factors and conservatives who stress individual moral weakness. This pattern is frequently reversed in the case of white-collar crime, with liberals putting the emphasis on personal immorality as the proximate cause of white-collar offenses (see Zimring and Hawkins 1979).

Some of this type of moral inversion on the part of liberals is a feature of the S&L crisis. But a much more significant reaction to the events of the past few years has been the universal acceptance by all who have seriously studied the issue that the structure of incentives produced by the 1982 deregulation was the most important explanation of the behavior that resulted in epic financial losses. Just as Richard Nixon ruefully observed in the early 1970s that "we are all Keynesians now" (Passell 1991), it can be said in the wake of the S&L crisis that we are all, or nearly all, structuralists. Indeed, nothing so powerfully confirms the importance of the structural elements in the thrift story as the reality that ignoring such factors would cause observers to be classified for that reason as part of a lunatic fringe.

The popularity of structural explanations for thrift failures stems in part from the pervasive importance of regulation in the history of the industry and the abrupt shift in policies that so immediately preceded the epidemic of failures. What remains to be noted is the hostility of some observers to accounts that stress criminal wrongdoing.

There is, of course, no inconsistency in holding to structural explanations of behavior and labeling that behavior as criminal. No matter the social forces and lapses in law enforcement that may influence the rate of purse snatching, the act itself is properly labeled and condemned as a crime. Yet many of the industry analysts minimize the role of crime in the dimensions of the S&L collapse. Thus, White says that any treatment of the S&L debacle that focuses largely or exclusively on the fraudulent and criminal activities is misguided and misleading. It perpetuates the incorrect notion, implicitly held by many, that virtually all the thrift insolvencies were caused by "crooks" whose ill-gotten gains are deposited in Swiss bank accounts (and if we could somehow find those bank accounts, we could recover all the moneys that are necessary to clean up the insolvencies). It also diverts attention from an understanding of how and why government policies went awry and distracts policy makers from the difficult but necessary policy reforms . . . that are relevant for all of bank and thrift regulation. [1991, p. 117]

At one level, this analysis misses the obvious point that behavior can be both structurally caused and morally blameworthy. At a deeper level, however, there *is* a competition for moral attention taking place in the S&L crisis in which regulation and condemnation are competing paradigms for public policy. To address the problem as if bad men and Swiss bank accounts were the heart of the matter will divert our attention and resources from changes in society and government that can better protect us from loss.

This is, of course, the very point the liberal criminologists have been making in critiques of the politics of law and order for two decades. There is novelty, if not irony, in the prospect that massive failure of financial institutions may be the vehicle that restores the respectability of this perspective.

REFERENCES

Adams, James Ring. 1990. *The Big Fix: Inside the S&L Scandal.* New York: Wiley.
Allen, Francis A. 1974. *The Crimes of Politics: Political Dimensions of Criminal Justice.* Cambridge, Mass.: Harvard University Press.
Barth, James R. 1991. *The Great Savings and Loan Debacle.* Washington, D.C.: American Enterprise Institute Press.
Barth, James R., Philip F. Bartholomew, and Michael G. Bradley. 1989. *The Determinants of Thrift Resolution Costs.* Research Paper no. 89-03. Washington, D.C.: Department of the Treasury, Office of Thrift Supervision.
Barth, James R., and R. Dan Brumbaugh, Jr. 1990. "The Rough Road from

FIRREA to Deposit Insurance Reform." *Stanford Law and Policy Review* 2(1):58–67.

Benson, Michael L., Francis T. Cullen, and William J. Maakestad. 1990. "Local Prosecutors and Corporate Crimes." *Crime and Delinquency* 36:356–72.

Berlin, Sir Isaiah. 1966. "The Concept of Scientific History." In *Philosophical Analysis and History*, edited by William H. Dray. New York: Harper & Row.

Burnham, R. W. 1968. "Further Thoughts on the Concept of Cause—a Philosophical Approach." *Issues in Criminology* 3(2):173–82.

Bush, George. 1984. *Report of the Bush Task Group on Regulation of Financial Services*. Washington, D.C.: U.S. Government Printing Office.

Calavita, Kitty, and Henry N. Pontell. 1990. "Heads I Win, Tails You Lose: Deregulation, Crime, and Crisis in the Savings and Loan Industry." *Crime and Delinquency* 36:309–41.

Carr-Hill, Roy. 1968. "The Concept of Cause in Criminology—a Comment." *Issues in Criminology* 3(2):167–71.

Christian Hill, G. 1990. "A Never Ending Story: An Introduction to the S&L Symposium." *Stanford Law and Policy Review* 2(1):21–24.

Davis, L. J. 1990. "Chronicle of a Debacle Foretold: How Deregulation Begat the S&L." *Harpers Magazine* (September), pp. 50–66.

Eichler, Neil. 1989. *The Thrift Debacle*. Berkeley and Los Angeles: University of California Press.

Ely, Bert. 1991. "FSLIC's Losses—When and How They Accumulated." Mimeographed. Alexandria, Va.: Ely & Co.

Finestone, Harold. 1976. "The Delinquent and Society: The Shaw and McKay Tradition." In *Delinquency, Crime and Society*, edited by James F. Short. Chicago: University of Chicago Press.

Glassman, James K. 1990. "The Great Bank Robbery: Deconstructing the S&L Crisis." *New Republic* (October 8), pp. 16–21.

Gorham, William. 1989. "Foreword" to *The S&L Insurance Mess: How Did It Happen?* edited by Edward J. Kane. Washington, D.C.: Urban Institute Press.

Gray, Edwin J. 1990. "Warnings Ignored: The Politics of the Crisis." *Stanford Law and Policy Review* 2(1):138–46.

Grundfest, Joseph A. 1990. "Lobbying into Limbo: The Political Ecology of the Savings and Loan Crisis." *Stanford Law and Policy Review* 2(1):25–36.

Hart, H. L. A., and Tony Honoré. 1985. *Causation in the Law*. 2d ed. Oxford: Clarendon.

Hawkins, Gordon, and Franklin E. Zimring. 1988. *Pornography in a Free Society*. Cambridge: Cambridge University Press.

Lipsey, R. G., and Kelvin Lancaster. 1956–57. "The General Theory of Second Best." *Review of Economic Studies* 24:11–32.

Maggin, Donald L. 1989. *Bankers, Builders, Knaves, and Thieves: The $300 Million Scam at ESM*. Chicago: Contemporary Books.

Mayer, Martin. 1990. *The Greatest-ever Bank Robbery: The Collapse of the Savings and Loan Industry*. New York: Scribner's.

Meade, James E. 1955. *Trade and Welfare*. Oxford: Oxford University Press.

Mill, J. S. 1886. *A System of Logic Ratiocinative and Inductive*. 8th ed. London: Longmans.

Miller, Alden D. 1983. "Criminology (3): Research Methods." In *Encyclopedia of Crime and Justice*, edited by Sanford H. Kadish. New York: Free Press.

Nader, Ralph. 1990. "Introduction" to *Who Killed America? A Citizen's Guide to the S&L Scandal*, edited by Michael Waldman. New York: Random House.

O'Connell, William B. 1988. "Preface" to *Where Deregulation Went Wrong: A Look at the Causes behind Savings and Loan Failures in the 1980s*, by Norman Strunk and Fred Case. Washington, D.C.: U.S. League of Savings Institutions.

O'Rourke, P. J. 1991. *Parliament of Whores*. New York: Atlantic Monthly Press.

O'Shea, James. 1991. *The Daisy Chain: How Borrowed Billions Sank a Texas S&L*. New York: Pocket Books.

Passell, Peter. 1991. "Does Government Have the Stuff to End a Recession?" *New York Times*, national ed. (February 11), p. 17.

Pilzer, Paul Zane, with Robert Deitz. 1989. *Other People's Money: The Inside Story of the S&L Mess*. New York: Simon & Schuster.

Pizzo, Stephen, Mary Fricker, and Paul Muolo. 1989. *Inside Job: The Looting of America's Savings and Loans*. New York: McGraw-Hill.

Reischauer, Robert D. 1990. Letter from Robert D. Reischauer, director, U.S. Congressional Budget Office, to Henry B. Gonzalez, chairman, Committee on Banking, Finance, and Urban Affairs, U.S. House of Representatives, June 13.

Robinson, Michael A. 1990. *Overdrawn: The Bailout of American Savings*. New York: Dutton.

Romer, Thomas, and Barry R. Weingast. 1990. "Congress: The Genesis of the Thrift Crisis." *Stanford Law and Policy Review* 2(1):37–46.

Schumer, Charles E., and J. Brian Graham. 1990. "The Unfinished Business of FIRREA." *Stanford Law and Policy Review* 2(1):68–81.

Scriven, Michael. 1966. "Causes, Connections, and Conditions in History." In *Philosophical Analysis and History*, edited by William H. Dray. New York: Harper & Row.

———. 1968. "In Defense of All Causes." *Issues in Criminology* 4(1):79–81.

Short, James F. 1983. "Criminology (2). Modern Controversies." In *Encyclopedia of Crime and Justice*, 2:556–66, edited by Sanford H. Kadish. New York: Free Press.

Singer, Richard. 1979. *Just Deserts: Sentencing Based on Equality and Desert*. Cambridge, Mass.: Ballinger.

Stiglitz, Joseph E. 1986. *Economics of the Public Sector*. New York: W. W. North.

Strunk, Norman, and Fred Case. 1988. *Where Deregulation Went Wrong: A Look at the Causes behind Savings and Loan Failures in the 1980s*. Washington, D.C.: U.S. League of Savings Institutions.

Thomas, Michael M. 1991a. "The Greatest American Shambles." *New York Review of Books* 37(3):30–35.

————. 1991*b*. "The Greatest American Shambles: An Exchange." *New York Review of Books* 38(11):59–60.

U.S. Congress, House Committee on Government Operations. 1988. *Combating Fraud, Abuse and Misconduct in the Nation's Financial Institutions: Current Federal Efforts Are Inadequate.* Report no. 100-1088. Washington, D.C.: U.S. Government Printing Office.

U.S. Congressional Budget Office. 1991. Telephone interview with staff of U.S. Congressional Budget Office, August 15.

U.S. Department of Commerce. 1990. *Statistical Abstract of the United States, 1990: The National Data Book.* Washington, D.C.: U.S. Government Printing Office.

U.S. General Accounting Office. 1989*a*. *Troubled Thrifts. Bank Board Use of Enforcement Actions.* Briefing report to the Honorable Henry B. Gonzales, chairman, Committee on Banking, Finance, and Urban Affairs, House of Representatives. GAO/GGD-89-68BR.

————. 1989*b*. *Thrift Failures: Cost Failures Resulted from Regulatory Violations and Unsafe Practices.* Report to the Congress. GAO/AFMD-89-62.

————. 1991. Telephone interview with staff of U.S. General Accounting Office, August 23.

U.S. National Aeronautics and Space Administration. 1988. *NASA Historical Data Book,* vol. 3, edited by Linda Neuman Ezell. Washington, D.C.: U.S. Government Printing Office.

————. 1990. *Report of the Advisory Committee on the Future of the U.S. Space Program.* Washington, D.C.: U.S. Government Printing Office.

U.S. Sentencing Commission. 1987. *Supplementary Report on the Initial Sentencing Guidelines and Policy Statements.* Washington, D.C.: U.S. Sentencing Commission.

van den Haag, Ernest. 1975. *Punishing Criminals.* New York: Basic.

Vold, George B. 1958. *Theoretical Criminology.* New York: Oxford University Press.

von Hirsch, Andrew. 1976. *Doing Justice: The Choice of Punishments.* New York: Hill & Wang.

Waldman, Michael. 1990*a*. "The S&L Collapse: The Cost of a Congress for Sale." *Stanford Law and Policy Review* 2(1):47–57.

————. 1990*b*. *Who Killed America? A Citizen's Guide to the S&L Scandal.* New York: Random House.

Wayne, Leslie. 1991. "Seidman Asks for Hiring of a 'Strong' Bailout Chief." *New York Times,* national ed. (June 22), p. 33.

Werhane, Patricia H. 1990. "Introducing Morality to Thrift Decision Making." *Stanford Law and Policy Review* 2(1):125–31.

White, Lawrence J. 1991. *The S&L Debacle: Public Policy Lessons for Bank and Thrift Regulation.* New York: Oxford University Press.

Wilkins, Leslie T. 1965. *Social Deviance: Social Policy, Action, and Research.* Englewood Cliffs, N.J.: Prentice-Hall.

————. 1968. "The Concept of Cause in Criminology." *Issues in Criminology* 3(2):147–65.

Willis, F. Roy. 1981. "Marshall Plan." In *The Encyclopedia Americana,* vol. 18. Danbury, Conn.: Grolier Inc.

Wolf, Frederick D. 1989. Testimony of Frederick D. Wolf, assistant comptroller general, U.S. General Accounting Office, San Francisco Hearings of the House Banking Committee, February 1989.

Zimring, Franklin E., and Gordon Hawkins. 1979. "Ideology and Euphoria in Crime Control." *University of Toledo Law Review* 10:370–88.

———. 1988. "The New Mathematics of Imprisonment." *Crime and Delinquency* 34:425–36.

Author Index

Subject Index